Clinical Applications Cancer Genetic Testing

This text provides a clear and concise guide to the evolving role of genetic testing in oncology. Bridging research and clinical practice, it offers essential insights into genetic diagnostics, risk assessment, and personalized treatment. Designed for healthcare professionals, researchers, and students, this book simplifies complex concepts, making cutting-edge advancements in cancer genetics more accessible and applicable to patient care.

Dr. Parul Sharma is dedicated to advancing the field of cancer genetics, driven by a commitment to bridging research and clinical practice. Through this text Dr. Sharma aims to make genetic insights more impactful in oncology. Her contributions to research have been recognized with the Young Researcher Award, the Research Luminary Award, and the Young Scientist Award, reflecting her passion for meaningful scientific progress. For her, every breakthrough in this field brings us closer to a future where cancer is no longer a life-defining diagnosis.

Clinical Applications of Cancer Genetic Testing

Edited by
Parul Sharma, PhD
Assistant Professor, Chandigarh University,
Punjab, India

CRC Press
Taylor & Francis Group
Boca Raton London New York

CRC Press is an imprint of the
Taylor & Francis Group, an **informa** business

Designed cover image: Shutterstock

First edition published 2026
by CRC Press
2385 NW Executive Center Drive, Suite 320, Boca Raton FL 33431

and by CRC Press
4 Park Square, Milton Park, Abingdon, Oxon, OX14 4RN

CRC Press is an imprint of Taylor & Francis Group, LLC

ISBN: 978-1-032-89312-9 (hbk)
ISBN: 978-1-032-89303-7 (pbk)
ISBN: 978-1-003-54216-2 (ebk)

DOI: 10.1201/9781003542162

Typeset in Palatino
by Deanta Global Publishing Services, Chennai, India

Contents

Preface vi

Acknowledgment vii

Contributors viii

1 Introduction to Cancer Genetic Testing 1
  Preeti Rajesh, Harsimran Kaur, and Changanamkandath Rajesh

2 Molecular Basis of Cancer: Genetic Alterations and Tumor Development 23
  Samkeliso Takaidza, Nnana M. Molefe, and Patience Chihomvu

3 Fundamentals of Cancer Genetics 45
  Lata Kumari, Dipansh Katoch, Gangandeep Singh, Arshiya Sood, and Neelam Thakur

4 Inherited Cancer Syndromes: Recognition and Management. 67
  Muskan Verma and Parul Sharma

5 Molecular Diagnostic Tools in Cancer Detection 85
  Aastha Dagar, Ashutosh Kumar Tiwari, Vivek Uttam, Manasranjan Parida, Kanupriya Medhi, Sia Daffara, Sanjana Bana, Sagarika Mukherjee, Raman Tikoria, and Aklank Jain

6 Cytogenetic Diagnostic Testing in Cancer 112
  Sweety Mehra, Priyanka Bhardwaj, Madhu Sharma, Muskan Budhwar, Anupriya Rana, and Mani Chopra

7 Genomic Profiling: A Paradigm Shift in Precision Oncology 124
  Arshiya Sood, Gangandeep Singh, Dipansh Katoch, Lata Kumari, and Neelam Thakur

8 Pharmacogenomics and Personalized Cancer Treatment 138
  Rituparna Choudhury, Chandan Kumar Bahadi, and Kumar Nikhil

9 Genetic Counseling in Oncology 156
  Depanshi Pandit, Ambica Koul, Sneha S. Kagale, and Ravindranath B.S

10 Ethical, Legal, and Social Implications of Cancer Genetic Testing. 191
  Anmol Bhatia and Parul Sharma

11 Implementing Cancer Genetic Testing in Clinical Practice 215
  Changanamkandath Rajesh, Harsimran Kaur, and Preeti Rajesh

Index 227

Preface

Cancer genetics has emerged as a crucial field in understanding the molecular mechanisms underlying cancer development and progression. Advances in clinical testing have transformed the landscape of cancer diagnosis, prognosis, and treatment, allowing for more precise and personalized therapeutic strategies. This book, *Clinical Applications of Cancer Genetic Testing*, aims to provide a comprehensive overview of the methodologies, technologies, and clinical applications of genetic testing in oncology.

This volume brings together insights from leading experts in the field, covering topics such as genetic predisposition, tumor profiling, next-generation sequencing, and ethical considerations in genetic counseling. The chapters are designed to serve as a valuable resource for researchers, clinicians, genetic counselors, and students, offering both foundational knowledge and recent advancements in cancer genetic testing.

I hope this book will serve as a useful guide in bridging the gap between research and clinical practice, ultimately contributing to improved patient care and outcomes in oncology.

Parul Sharma

Acknowledgment

The completion of this book would not have been possible without the valuable contributions of numerous individuals. I extend my deepest gratitude to all the authors who shared their expertise and insights, ensuring the highest quality of content. Their dedication and meticulous work have been instrumental in shaping this book.

Special appreciation goes to the editorial and publishing team, whose guidance and commitment have been essential in bringing this work to fruition.

I am also deeply grateful to my family for their unwavering support and encouragement throughout this journey. Their motivation and positivity have been invaluable in bringing this book to completion.

It is my sincere hope that this book will serve as a valuable resource for the scientific and medical community, fostering further advancements in the field of cancer genetics.

Dr. Parul Sharma

Contributors

Chandan Kumar Bahadi
School of Biotechnology
Kalinga Institute of Industrial Technology
(KIIT) Deemed-to-be-University
Bhubaneswar, Odisha, India

Sanjana Bana
Non-coding RNA and Cancer Biology Lab
Department of Zoology, Central University of
Punjab
Ghudda, Bhatinda, India

Anmol Bhatia
Department of Biotechnology, Thapar Institute
of Engineering and Technology
Patiala, Punjab, India

Priyanka Bhardwaj
Cell and Molecular Biology lab, Department of
Zoology
Panjab University, Chandigarh, India

Muskan Budhwar
Cell and Molecular Biology lab, Department of
Zoology
Panjab University, Chandigarh, India

Ravindranath B.S
Department of Biotechnology
Manipal Institute of Technology
Karnataka, India

Patience Chihomvu
Vaal University of Technology
Department of Natural Sciences
Vanderbijlpark, Gauteng, South Africa

Mani Chopra
Cell and Molecular Biology lab, Department of
Zoology
Panjab University, Chandigarh, India

Rituparna Choudhury
School of Biotechnology
Kalinga Institute of Industrial Technology
(KIIT) Deemed-to-be-University
Bhubaneswar, Odisha, India

Sia Daffara
Non-coding RNA and Cancer Biology Lab
Department of Zoology, Central University of
Punjab
Ghudda, Bhatinda, India

Aastha Dagar
Non-coding RNA and Cancer Biology Lab
Department of Zoology, Central University of
Punjab
Ghudda, Bhatinda, India

Aklank Jain
Non-coding RNA and Cancer Biology Lab
Department of Zoology, Central University of
Punjab
Ghudda, Bhatinda, India

Sneha S. Kagale
Department of Biotechnology Engineering
Kolhapur Institute of Technology's College of
Engineering
Gokul-Shiragaon, Maharashtra, India

Dipansh Katoch
Department of Zoology, Sardar Patel University
Paddal Kartarpur, Mandi, Himachal Pradesh,
India

Harsimran Kaur
Department of Biotechnology, University
Institute of Biotechnology
Chandigarh University, Mohali, Punjab, India

Ambica Koul
Government Medical College
Baramulla, Kashmir, Jammu and Kashmir,
India

Lata Kumari
Department of Zoology, Sardar Patel University
Paddal Kartarpur, Mandi, Himachal Pradesh,
India

Kanupriya Medhi
Non-coding RNA and Cancer Biology Lab
Department of Zoology, Central University of
Punjab
Ghudda, Bhatinda, India

Sweety Mehra
Neonatology Lab, Department of Pediatrics,
PGIMER
Chandigarh, India

Nnana M. Molefe
Vaal University of Technology
Department of Natural Sciences
Vanderbijlpark, Gauteng, South Africa

Sagarika Mukherjee
Non-coding RNA and Cancer Biology Lab
Department of Zoology, Central University of
    Punjab
Ghudda, Bhatinda, India

Kumar Nikhil
School of Biotechnology
Kalinga Institute of Industrial Technology
    (KIIT) Deemed-to-be-University
Bhubaneswar, Odisha, India

Depanshi Pandit
Department of Biotechnology
Manipal Institute of Technology
Karnataka, India

Manasranjan Parida
Non-coding RNA and Cancer Biology Lab
Department of Zoology, Central University of
    Punjab
Ghudda, Bhatinda, India

Changanamkandath Rajesh
Department of Biotechnology, Brainware
    University
Barasat, Kolkata, West Bengal, India

Preeti Rajesh
Department of Biotechnology, Brainware
    University
Barasat, Kolkata, West Bengal, India

Anupriya Rana
Cell and Molecular Biology lab, Department of
    Zoology
Panjab University, Chandigarh, India

Madhu Sharma
Cell and Molecular Biology lab, Department of
    Zoology
Panjab University, Chandigarh, India

Gangandeep Singh
Department of Zoology, Sardar Patel University
Paddal Kartarpur, Mandi, Himachal Pradesh,
    India

Arshiya Sood
Department of Zoology, Sardar Patel University
Paddal Kartarpur, Mandi, Himachal Pradesh,
    India

Samkeliso Takaidza
Vaal University of Technology
Department of Natural Sciences
Vanderbijlpark, Gauteng, South Africa

Neelam Thakur
Department of Zoology, Sardar Patel University
Paddal Kartarpur, Mandi, Himachal Pradesh,
    India

Raman Tikoria
Non-coding RNA and Cancer Biology Lab
Department of Zoology, Central University of
    Punjab,
Ghudda, Bhatinda, India

Ashutosh Kumar Tiwari
Non-coding RNA and Cancer Biology Lab
Department of Zoology, Central University of
    Punjab
Ghudda, Bhatinda, India

Vivek Uttam
Non-coding RNA and Cancer Biology Lab
Department of Zoology, Central University of
    Punjab
Ghudda, Bhatinda, India

Muskan Verma
La Trobe University
Melbourne, Victoria, Australia

1

Introduction to Cancer Genetic Testing

Preeti Rajesh, Harsimran Kaur, and Changanamkandath Rajesh

1.1 INTRODUCTION—GENETIC TESTING IN CANCER

Cancer is fundamentally a genetic disease. It can arise from both inherited and somatically acquired mutations at different genetic loci. Cancer cells exhibit significant variation in the types and frequencies of genetic alterations. While some of these genetic changes act as "drivers" that promote neoplastic growth, others serve as "passengers" without contributing to tumorigenesis. Although most of the genetic mutations that are identified in tumors are acquired through somatic events, some cancers arise due to germline pathogenic variants in genes whose function is critical to the integrity of key cellular processes, including DNA repair and tumor suppression. Germline variants are inherited and exist in all nucleated cells throughout the organism. Cells with one nonfunctional allele have the propensity to lose the second allele, leading to an increased risk of cancer development in individuals with inherited genetic alterations, often manifesting at younger ages (Pon & Marra, 2015).

Clinical cancer genetics is becoming an integral part of the care of cancer patients. Over the past few decades, the field has witnessed exponential growth, reflected in the increasing number of publications indexed in PubMed on genetic testing and cancer. This surge underscores the continuous advancements in understanding cancer genetics, the identification of hereditary cancer syndromes, and the development of personalized interventions. From the early focus on high-penetrance genes such as BRCA1/2 to the broader exploration of multigene panels, genetic testing has become indispensable in oncology practice and research. A combination of the search terms "genetic testing" AND "cancer" shows 15,673 results from 1946 to 2024, highlighting the exponentially growing scientific interest in this issue (Figure 1.1).

Over the last two decades, genetic testing has become increasingly essential in oncology, offering significant insights into cancer susceptibility, risk assessment, diagnosis, prognosis, and therapeutic strategies (Figure 1.2).

By examining an individual's genetic makeup, such testing can identify mutations or modifications that might elevate the likelihood of developing specific types of cancer or affect the progression of the illness. Hereditary genetic testing in oncology is equally applicable to both males and females. Genetic testing plays an instrumental role in the identification of genetic changes associated with the development of many cancer types including breast, ovarian, endometrial, colon, pancreatic, and prostate cancers (Crawford & Warren, 2023; Kurian et al., 2023). The correlations

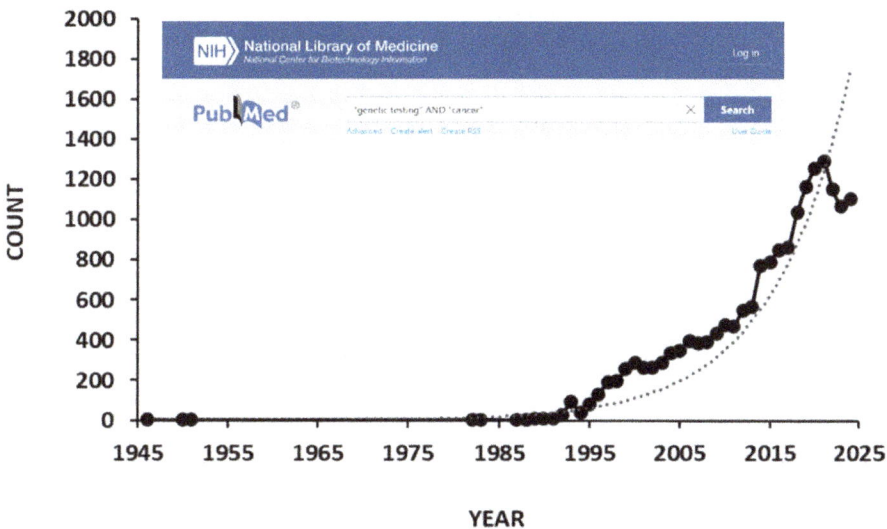

Figure 1.1 Bibliometric analysis of the PubMed database.

DOI: 10.1201/9781003542162-1

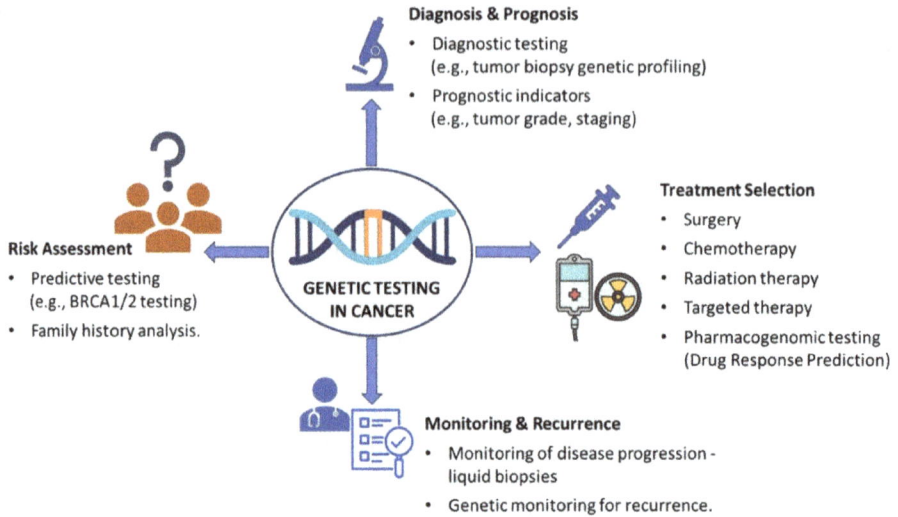

Figure 1.2 A flowchart illustrating the multifaceted role of genetic testing in cancer.

between histopathologic tumor features and the prevalence of germline cancer risk variants are emerging, which can guide cancer treatment and follow-up care. Although in many cancer types the incidence of targeted gene abnormalities is low, genetic testing may aid in identifying potential therapeutic agents and guide personalized approaches for treatment. Multigene panels are largely utilized in clinical settings for the identification of somatic and germline mutations in GI cancers. In gastrointestinal cancers and genitourinary malignancies, genetic testing provides great benefit in offering clinical decision support, cancer screening, surgical interventions, monitoring disease status, and enhancing patient survival outcomes (Adashek et al., 2020; Matsuoka & Yashiro, 2024). The first targeted therapy for urothelial carcinomas, erdafitinib, was approved by the FDA for the treatment of tumors harboring FGFR2 and FGFR3 alterations (Loriot et al., 2019).

Advances in next-generation sequencing technologies are enabling rapid and cost-effective analysis of multiple genes or even the entire cancer genomes. For breast, ovarian, and prostate cancers, next-generation sequencing is being widely used in clinical practice for multigene panel analysis, providing prognostic and predictive information that guides therapy decisions (Ece Solmaz et al., 2021; Tsaousis et al., 2019). Interestingly, the rapid advancement of genomic profiling technologies has led to new challenges. The detection of genetic variants of uncertain significance and the lack of clear clinical guidelines for their interpretation pose difficulties for healthcare providers (Catana et al., 2019; Marcom, 2017). Additionally, the recognition of germline variants in somatic tumor testing results (occurring in up to 12% of cases) requires oncologists to develop new skills in genetics interpretation and counseling (DeLeonardis et al., 2019). The molecular data generated from tumor profiling with next-generation sequencing (NGS) has become the main catalyst for precision oncology, opening opportunities for individualized, patient-tailored cancer care. It ishowever, challenging to interpret complex genetic data and translate it into actionable clinical decisions. Molecularly focused interdisciplinary meetings—molecular tumor boards (MTBs)—have been established internationally to meet this challenge. These MTBs facilitate the integration of genomics information into clinical practice and provide molecularly driven treatment recommendations (Boos & Wicki, 2024). The rapidly progressing technology is generating expansive opportunities to characterize the molecular attributes of cancer. With this progress, there is a growing need to integrate the principles of precision oncology into physicians' training, generate a multidisciplinary approach including (molecular) pathologists, molecular biologists, scientists, bioinformaticians, and technical staff, and develop new clinical models to communicate and utilize genetic information in cancer care effectively (Casolino et al., 2024).

1.2 UNDERSTANDING THE GENETIC BASIS OF CANCER

The advancements in the field of genetics drove the investigations into the origins of cancer and allowed the understanding of the molecular mechanisms underlying cancer development and progression. The oldest known scientifically documented case of disseminated cancer involves a

Scythian king (approx. 40–50 years old), who lived in the steppes of Southern Siberia roughly 2700 years ago. Advanced microscopic and proteomic methodologies have substantiated the cancerous nature of his disseminated skeletal lesions, confirming their prostatic origin. Alfred Armand Louis Marie Velpeau (1795–1867) scrutinized 400 malignant and 100 benign tumors through a microscope, expressing the genetic underpinnings of cancer (Faguet, 2015). He stated,

> The so-called cancer cell is merely a secondary product rather than the essential element in the disease. Beneath it, there must exist some more intimate element which science would need in order to define the nature of cancer.
>
> *(Velpeau, 1854)*

The exploration of the genetic foundations of cancer began to emerge even before the principles of inheritance articulated by Mendel gained widespread acceptance. In the early 1900s, Peyton Rous demonstrated the ability to transfer tumors to healthy birds using cell-free extracts from diseased animals, suggesting that agents smaller than cells were implicated in tumor formation (Martin, 2004). Around the same period, before Morgan's research on chromosomes as the carriers of genetic information, Theodor Boveri theorized that cancer could stem from improper combinations of chromosomes (Weinberg, 2008). Additionally, experiments with chemical carcinogens indicated that modifications in DNA sequences could lead to cellular transformation. These findings collectively anchored the understanding of cancer within the genetic domain (Bouck & Di Mayorca, 1976; Cooper et al., 1980). Almost half a century after the discovery of Rous Sarcoma Virus (RSV), the underlying principles of oncogenicity were explored. In 1970, Duesberg and Vogt reported the identification of the first oncogene *src* (Duesberg & Vogt, 1970). The biochemical identification of the cancer gene provided the key evidence for a physical basis of the cancer gene hypothesis establishing the molecular foundation of human carcinogenesis bringing the basis of cancer firmly within the realm of genetics (Bister, 2015).

1.2.1 Mutation Spectrum of Cancer

It is now established that cancer is the result of various mutations that affect specific genes, which are categorized as proto-oncogenes and tumor suppressor genes. As a genetic condition, cancer displays considerable diversity in the number and types of genetic changes observed in tumors. Nevertheless, it is essential to recognize that not every mutation within cancer genomes contributes to the onset or advancement of malignancy, as mutational processes can also impact cellular functions unrelated to cancer development. A pivotal step in comprehending tumor biology and formulating targeted therapies involves the identification of mutations that are instrumental in cancer progression. Those mutations that enhance growth potential and thus facilitate cancer development are classified as driver mutations, whereas those that do not influence this process are termed passenger mutations (De & Ganesan, 2017; Kontomanolis et al., 2020). The genetic changes in the cancer genome can manifest in the form of point mutations, amplifications, deletions, translocations, complex rearrangements, ploidy changes, or a combination of those. These genetics changes in the DNA of a malignant cells form a unique cancer molecular blueprint (Figure 1.3).

In the normal cell, the proto-oncogenes may function as growth factors, transducers of cellular signals, or nuclear transcription factors and regulate key biological processes. The mutational activation brings about their change into oncogenes, which go on to drive cell multiplication and assume a pivotal role in the pathogenesis of cancer as driver genes. However, tumor suppressor genes are driver genes that accumulate inactivating mutations. Oncogenes are typically influenced by focal amplifications or missense mutations occurring at a limited set of codons, while tumor suppressors are more frequently impacted by focal deletions or various types of mutations, including nonsense, frameshift, and splice-site mutations, which are distributed throughout the gene (Kern & Winter, 2006). Sometimes there are exceptions, such as the occurrence of missense mutations in the tumor suppressor p53, truncations that result in gain-of-function activities, and splice-site mutations that enhance the production of oncogenic isoforms (Kern & Winter, 2006; Ruark et al., 2013; Venables et al., 2009). The predominant type of activating or inactivating mutation varies among different driver genes. For example, the MYC oncogene is primarily associated with non-Hodgkin lymphoma through gene rearrangements, whereas the BRAF oncogene is most often affected by the V600E mutation (Ott et al., 2013; Pakneshan et al., 2013). The identification of driver genes may be contingent upon analyzing the specific mutations that predominantly influence

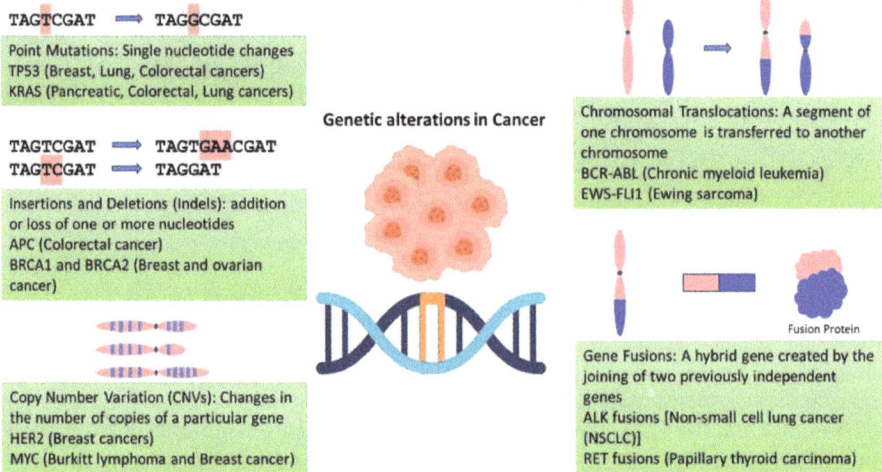

TAGTCGAT ⟹ TAGGCGAT

Point Mutations: Single nucleotide changes
TP53 (Breast, Lung, Colorectal cancers)
KRAS (Pancreatic, Colorectal, Lung cancers)

TAGTCGAT ⟹ TAGTGAACGAT
TAGTCGAT ⟹ TAGGAT

Insertions and Deletions (Indels): addition
or loss of one or more nucleotides
APC (Colorectal cancer)
BRCA1 and BRCA2 (Breast and ovarian
cancer)

Copy Number Variation (CNVs): Changes in
the number of copies of a particular gene
HER2 (Breast cancers)
MYC (Burkitt lymphoma and Breast cancer)

Genetic alterations in Cancer

Chromosomal Translocations: A segment of
one chromosome is transferred to another
chromosome
BCR-ABL (Chronic myeloid leukemia)
EWS-FLI1 (Ewing sarcoma)

Fusion Protein

Gene Fusions: A hybrid gene created by the
joining of two previously independent
genes
ALK fusions [Non-small cell lung cancer
(NSCLC)]
RET fusions (Papillary thyroid carcinoma)

Figure 1.3 Genetic alterations in cancer. The figure summarizes the different types of genetic alterations present in cancer, including point mutations, insertions and deletions, copy number variations, chromosomal translocations, and gene fusions, along with their examples.

them. The genetic mechanisms underlying cancer involve a myriad of molecular changes that are integral to numerous essential cellular activities and are remarkably intricate and complex. Various molecular components that regulate proliferation, apoptosis, differentiation, angiogenesis, cellular motility, and immune responses can be targeted in specific cancers that exhibit distinct mutational signatures. The array of genetic alterations observed is commonly referred to as "cancer genome landscapes" (Vogelstein et al., 2013). As a result, cancer is increasingly recognized not as a singular disease but as a diverse group of diseases characterized by unique genetic profiles. Our understanding of cancer genomics is currently expanding at an unprecedented rate, with the aim of elucidating its biological mechanisms, enhancing diagnostic and prognostic methodologies, and formulating novel therapeutic approaches tailored to the individual needs of patients.

Another critical aspect of the genetic etiology of cancer is the categorization of the variants into germline and somatic mutations. While most of the genetic mutations detected in the tumors are classified as acquired (somatic) events, some cancers can be traced back to germline (constitutional) pathogenic variants in genes critical for the proper functioning of key cellular mechanisms, including DNA repair (Stoffel & Carethers, 2020). The germline variants are heritable alterations arising in the germ cells and present in every nucleated cell in the body. The somatic mutations, however, are localized changes affecting only a portion of cells and are acquired during an individual's lifetime due to environmental or lifestyle factors (Figure 1.4). The distinction between germline and somatic mutations is essential during genetic testing, as it plays a significant role in identifying hereditary cancer risks and informing treatment approaches. It is possible to misclassify germline variants as somatic mutations in tumor-only genomic testing.

1.2.2 Clinical Significance of Germline and Somatic Mutations

Genetic testing is progressively becoming an indispensable component of cancer management for better clinical outcomes and patient care. Germline mutations in multiple genes are associated with a significant risk of cancer development, and testing for these mutations can help in patient screening and appropriate risk reduction interventions. While actionable somatic mutations are increasingly implicated and tested in targeted therapy for considerable therapeutic benefit, both germline and somatic mutations can contribute to interindividual differences in anti-cancer drug response. These mutations can not only lead to drug resistance but also to adverse drug effects. The mutation landscape of cancer can comprise a complex combination of germline variants from the patient and somatic mutations in tumor cells (Kaehler & Cascorbi, 2019).

Ten percent of all cancers have a hereditary component, with mutations increasing the risk of cancer development (Garber & Offit, 2005). In 1969, a multicancer predisposition syndrome known as Li-Fraumeni syndrome (LFS) was reported (Li & Fraumeni, 1969). LFS has an autosomal dominant pattern of inheritance and is associated with a high risk for a broad spectrum of

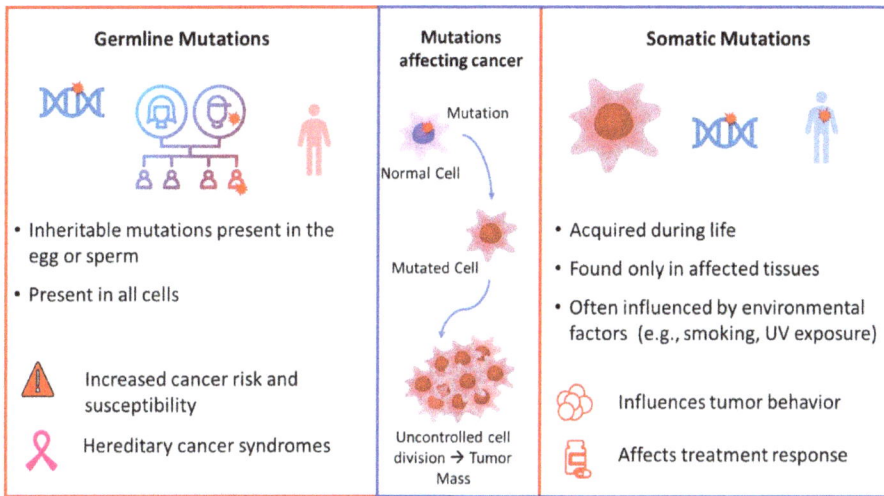

Figure 1.4 Germline and somatic mutations in cancer. Each person receives one allele of a gene pair from the mother and another from the father. A germline mutation is a genetic alteration in the germ cells, i.e., eggs or sperm, and is passed down to the child. Having an inherited germline mutation of oncogenes, tumor suppressor genes, or genes that play a role in DNA repair may predispose an individual to an increased risk of cancer during their lifetime. Conversely, a somatic mutation is called an acquired mutation and occurs within somatic, not germ cells, and is not passed on to offspring. These mutations are often caused by environmental stimuli; for example, tobacco smoking or exposure to substances that may be known carcinogens.

cancers, including breast cancer, central nervous system tumors, osteosarcomas, colorectal cancer, stomach cancer, lung cancer, melanoma, pancreatic cancer, and prostate cancer. After undergoing treatment, cancer survivors are further at increased risk for developing additional primary cancers and treatment-related secondary cancers. The clinical diagnosis of LFS requires genetic testing of mutations distributed across the *TP53* gene (Guha & Malkin, 2017; Schneider et al., 1999). Many cancers including breast, ovarian, pancreatic, prostate, colorectal, renal, gastric, and neuro-endocrine tumors, have a strong genetic component and are associated with multiple hereditary cancer syndromes (Garutti et al., 2023). Identification of a genetic mutation predisposing a patient to cancer can have significant clinical implications such as:

a) The gene variants could predict the efficacy of cancer treatment; for example, *BRCA1/2* for PARP inhibitors. In fact, as per the guidelines developed by the American Society of Clinical Oncology (ASCO), BRCA1/2 germline mutation testing should be offered to all newly diagnosed patients with breast cancer ≤65 years and select patients >65 years based on personal history, family history, ancestry, or eligibility for poly (ADP-ribose) polymerase (PARP) inhibitor therapy (Bedrosian et al., 2024).

b) Identification of germline mutations can guide a tailored preventive program entailing organ-specific surveillance and prophylactic surgeries. For example, guidelines exist for colonoscopy surveillance for patients with Lynch Syndrome and urologic screening for patients with *MSH2* variants. Also, bilateral risk-reducing mastectomy (BRRM) may be considered for women with high-risk pathogenic/likely pathogenic germline genetic mutations in genes including *BRCA1*, *BRCA2*, *CDH1*, *PALB2*, *PTEN*, and *TP53* (Peltomäki et al., 2023; Rooney et al., 2023).

c) Cascade genetic testing facilitates the assessment of familial risk and allows for testing the same gene variant identified in the patient in family members, thus providing relatives with the opportunity for early detection and prevention of cancer (Frey et al., 2022; Schmidlen et al., 2022).

Somatic mutation testing, on the other hand, via sequencing of tumor samples has become part of the standard cancer management protocol for non-small cell lung cancer (NSCLC), colorectal cancer, melanoma, and many other solid tumors. Such testing aims to detect genetic biomarkers that can predict response to targeted therapies. For instance, driver point mutations within the

ERCC2 gene are contributing factors in approximately 10% of bladder cancers (BLCAs) and serve as a promising biomarker for predicting responses to cisplatin treatment (Barbour et al., 2024). Additionally, activating somatic mutations in the *EGFR* gene, including *EGFR* exon 19 deletions or L858R in patients diagnosed with non-small-cell lung cancer, are associated with favorable clinical outcomes when treated with tyrosine kinase inhibitors including gefitinib, efitinib, erlotinib, and afatinib (Jorge et al., 2014; Lynch et al., 2004). Also, coexisting *KRAS* mutations with *BRAF* or *RBM10* mutations lead to the ineffectiveness of bevacizumab which is a standard regimen for patients with *BRAF*-mutant CRC (Guo et al., 2023). In addition to targeted therapy, molecular characterization through somatic cancer gene panels can provide prognostic and/or diagnostic information. Such information is also instrumental in the diagnosis of synchronous tumors and aids in the surgical decision (Al-Shinnag et al., 2024). In the case of metastatic colorectal cancer single-gene somatic mutations in genes *BRAF* and *RBM10* are associated with shorter progression-free survival and a high risk of secondary metastasis or recurrence (Guo et al., 2023). In the case of endometrial cancer, the evaluation of somatic mutations can be done in cervicovaginal samples. This assessment of molecular markers acts as a diagnostic tool and provides a clinically applicable molecular-based classification. The identification of a pathogenic mutation within the exonuclease domain of the *POLE* gene facilitates the diagnosis of *POLE*-mutated endometrial carcinoma (EC). Notably, patients exhibiting mutations in *POLE* demonstrate a favorable prognosis, while those harboring *TP53* mutations face significantly poorer clinical outcomes (Oaknin et al., 2022; Pelegrina et al., 2023). Another important aspect of tumor testing to assess somatic genetic changes is to identify therapy-induced mutations that can lead to chemoresistance. Resistance to therapy can emerge at the initiation of treatment or arise during treatment because of somatic mutations after an initial favorable clinical outcome. Development of the *ALK* TKI therapy significantly altered the management of advanced *ALK*-positive non-small cell lung cancer. Despite initial promise, these drugs could not ensure progression-free survival due to the development of drug resistance. The cancer can acquire resistance to therapy through both on-target (*ALK* mutations) or off-target (*MET, EGFR*) mutations (Batist et al., 2011; Poei et al., 2024). Understanding the somatic mutational signature of cancer through tumor sequencing can also help prevent some drug-resistance mutations by adjusting treatment regimens. For example, in the case of cancers with mutations in the mismatch repair pathway genes, avoiding temozolomide treatment may prevent the development of additional driver mutations (Brady et al., 2022).

1.3 CANCER GENETIC TESTING

Oncology genetic testing involves the assessment of an individual's genetic profile for specific mutations or comprehensive mutational signatures associated with the development and progression of cancer. As discussed in the previous section it offers critical insights into an individual's cancer risk, aids in diagnosis, informs prognosis, and enhances the effectiveness of treatment strategies. We can broadly categorize cancer genetic testing by the genetic source and clinical application. Clinical application-based testing such as predictive, prognostic, and pharmacogenomic testing is often used to guide treatment decisions, characterize disease outcomes, and tailor drug therapies. Genetic source-based testing addresses whether mutations are inherited (germline) or acquired (somatic) and represents a widely discussed framework in genetics research and cancer genomics. It is essential to distinguish between the somatic and germline mutations associated with cancer to understand its genetic basis, perform risk assessment, and personalized therapy.

1.3.1 Source-Based Genetic Testing in Oncology

In the established paradigm of source-based cancer genetic testing, two primary modes are recognized: somatic and germline testing. Somatic testing (or tumor testing) is typically performed on tumor tissue: cancer-containing biopsies, surgical material, or, in some cases, circulating tumor cells or circulating tumor DNA (ctDNA) in the blood. Testing of tumor tissue from primary or metastatic sites or blood may help provide personalized care and focus on guiding treatment decisions. This type of testing yields critical insights into targeted therapies and identifies the tissue origin of the tumor, thereby aiding in the selection of suitable treatments and providing prognostic information regarding the likelihood of recurrence. Findings in archival primary tissue obtained years earlier may differ from those in a metastatic site, and repeat testing of tumor DNA may be appropriate during the disease because somatic mutations observed in tumor tissue may change over time due to genetic instability and selective pressure from therapy. This is particularly important in the context of targeted therapies, where the genetic properties of metastases, rather than primary tumors, may be more relevant for treatment decisions (Cheng et al., 2019; Vermaat et al., 2012).

Germline genetic testing helps identify inherited pathogenic variants (mutations) in genes associated with cancer risk. Testing can be performed on lymphocyte DNA from blood or a combination of lymphocyte and buccal cells from saliva because germline DNA is nearly identical in all nucleated cells of an individual. Germline testing can also be performed on cultured fibroblasts in case of individuals with a hematological malignancy, to assess for an underlying hereditary cancer predisposition syndrome. This testing serves to elucidate the reasons behind the patient's current cancer diagnosis, assist in identifying potential targeted therapies, and assess the risk of developing additional malignancies. Consequently, patients may opt for enhanced surveillance or preventive surgical interventions to mitigate their risks, while also determining whether family members may be susceptible to hereditary cancer (Cheng et al., 2019).

The genomic testing of tumors can be approached in two distinct ways. The tumor-only approach sequences of tumor tissue only, wherein the tumor sequence analysis includes somatic and germline alterations. The parallel approach involves the sequencing of the tumor and matched normal tissue with the subsequent subtraction of germline alterations from somatic alterations, resulting in the identification of somatic mutations only on tumor assessment. Notably, although germline sequencing occurs in both the tumor-only and the tumor-normal matched approach, in the former, the germline assessment is an indirect result of the tumor sequencing and in the tumor-normal analysis, the germline is directly interrogated. The parallel tumor-normal matched approach allows for direct differentiation of somatic versus germline findings and the potential for the return of germline-specific genetic test results to the patient (Liu & Stadler, 2021). The growing implementation of parallel testing has uncovered a significant number of germline mutations in patients who would not have qualified for testing under traditional clinical criteria. This finding has substantial implications for the screening and subsequent testing of at-risk family members, as well as for advancements in gene discovery. Furthermore, it underscores the critical role of germline testing in informing therapeutic strategies. With the rising recommendations for universal genetic testing across various cancer types and an increase in therapies with germline indications, a gradual shift towards the adoption of parallel tumor-normal genetic testing for all cancer patients appears imminent.

1.3.2 Clinical Application-Based Genetic Testing in Oncology
1.3.2.1 Predictive Testing

Genetic testing for predictive biomarkers measures the likelihood of response or lack of response to a particular therapy (Table 1.1). It allows to distinguish patients who are most likely to respond to anti-cancer therapy enhancing therapeutic efficiency, decreasing treatment costs, and avoiding adverse events. Thus, these predictive biomarkers can guide and optimize therapy decisions for specific chemotherapeutics (Nalejska et al., 2014; Verdaguer et al., 2017). The scope of genetic testing techniques includes single-gene testing, targeted multigene panels, and mutational signatures. Single-gene testing is often conducted when a specific targeted therapy is being considered for a known mutation. For example, *BRAF V600E* mutation in melanoma to guide vemurafenib or dabrafenib therapy, *EGFR* mutation testing in non-small cell lung cancer (NSCLC) before prescribing tyrosine kinase inhibitors (TKIs) like Osimertinib or *BRCA1/BRCA2* mutations in ovarian cancer to determine eligibility for PARP inhibitors like Olaparib (L. Cheng et al., 2018; Ragupathi et al., 2023; Santarpia et al., 2017).

1.3.2.2 Prognostic Testing

Genetic testing for prognostic biomarkers can predict the likely course of cancer, its aggressiveness, and patient outcomes through guided therapy. Cancer patients can be stratified based on prognostic testing enabling the selection of efficacious treatment strategies and more effective treatments for individual cancer patients with minimal side effects. The prognostic genetic testing approach can range from single-gene testing to advanced mutational analysis. Specific mutations can be tested in patients using Sanger sequencing for prognostic assessment (Table 1.2). For example, somatic activating mutations in 12 and 13 codons of *KRAS* can be detected in different cancer types and are most frequently associated with poor survival prognosis (Guan et al., 2013). The advances in genomic technologies have shifted the paradigm to multigene panels and even comprehensive genomic profiling (CGP) using next-generation sequencing by simultaneously detecting genetic alterations in hundreds of genes and multiple molecular biomarkers. CGP

Table 1.1: Examples of Predictive Genetic Tests in Personalized Oncology

Biomarker/ Gene Mutation	Associated Cancer(s)	Predictive for Therapy	Targeted Therapy	Testing Methods	References
EGFR	NSCLC	EGFR mutations predict response to TKIs	Osimertinib, Erlotinib, Gefitinib	qPCR, NGS, Sanger Sequencing	(Mok et al., 2009)
ALK	NSCLC, ALCL	ALK rearrangements predict TKI response	Crizotinib, Alectinib, Lorlatinib	FISH, IHC, NGS	(Shaw et al., 2013)
ROS1	NSCLC	ROS1 fusions predict response to TKIs	Crizotinib, Entrectinib	FISH, NGS	(Shaw et al., 2014)
BRAF V600E	Melanoma, CRC, NSCLC, Thyroid	BRAF mutations predict response to inhibitors	Vemurafenib, Dabrafenib	qPCR, NGS	(Chapman et al., 2011)
KRAS (G12C, others)	CRC, Lung, Pancreatic	KRAS G12C mutations predict inhibitor response	Sotorasib, Adagrasib	NGS, qPCR	(Canon et al., 2019)
NRAS	Melanoma, CRC	Resistance to anti-EGFR therapy	Avoid Cetuximab, Panitumumab	NGS, qPCR	(Douillard et al., 2013)
HER2 (ERBB2)	Breast, Gastric, CRC, Lung	HER2 amplification predicts response	Trastuzumab, Pertuzumab, Tucatinib	IHC, FISH, NGS	(Slamon et al., 2001)
BRCA1/BRCA2	Breast, Ovarian, Prostate, Pancreatic	DNA repair deficiency predicts PARP inhibitor response	Olaparib, Rucaparib	NGS, MLPA, qPCR	(Robson et al., 2017)
PD-L1 Expression	Lung, Melanoma, Bladder, Gastric	High PD-L1 predicts immunotherapy response	Pembrolizumab, Nivolumab, Atezolizumab	IHC	(Reck et al., 2016)
MET Exon 14 Skipping	NSCLC	MET alterations predict response	Capmatinib, Tepotinib	NGS, PCR	(Paik et al., 2020)
RET Fusions	Thyroid, NSCLC	RET fusions predict response	Selpercatinib, Pralsetinib	NGS, FISH	(Subbiah et al., 2021)
NTRK Fusions	Various (Pediatric & Adult)	NTRK fusions predict response	Larotrectinib, Entrectinib	NGS, FISH	(Drilon et al., 2018)
IDH1/IDH2 Mutations	Glioma, AML	IDH mutations predict response to inhibitors	Ivosidenib, Enasidenib	NGS, qPCR	(Stein et al., 2021)
FGFR Alterations	Bladder, Cholangiocarcinoma	FGFR mutations predict response	Erdafitinib, Pemigatinib	NGS, FISH	(Loriot et al., 2019)
PIK3CA	Breast Cancer	Predicts response to PI3K inhibitors	Alpelisib	NGS, PCR	(André et al., 2019)
CDK4l6 Amplification	Breast Cancer	CDK4/6 amplification predicts CDK4/6 inhibitor response	Palbociclib, Ribociclib	NGS	(Turner et al., 2015)

Table 1.2: Genetic Testing of Molecular Biomarkers in Cancer Prognosis

Biomarker	Cancer Type	Specific Mutation/Alteration	Prognostic Significance	Testing Method	Reference
TP53	Breast, lung, colorectal cancer	Missense mutations (e.g., R175H, R248Q, R273H)	Poor prognosis, therapy resistance	NGS, IHC, PCR, Sanger sequencing	(Chen et al., 2022; Chiang et al., 2021)
KRAS	Colorectal, lung, pancreatic cancer	G12D, G12V, G13D mutations	Poor response to EGFR inhibitors, aggressive tumors	qPCR, ddPCR, NGS	(Valtorta et al., 2013)
BRCA1/BRCA2	Breast, ovarian cancer	BRCA1 (185delAG, 5382insC), BRCA2 (6174delT)	High recurrence risk, predicts PARP inhibitor response	NGS, MLPA, Sanger sequencing	(Lin et al., 2019)
HER2 (ERBB2)	Breast, gastric cancer	HER2 amplification	Poor prognosis but predicts trastuzumab response	IHC, FISH, CISH, NGS	(Gomez-Martin et al., 2013; Lee et al., 2014)
BRAF	Melanoma, colorectal cancer	V600E mutation	Poor prognosis, aggressive tumor growth	qPCR, NGS, IHC	(Samowitz et al., 2005)
EGFR	Lung cancer	L858R, exon 19 deletions	Sensitivity to TKIs but poor prognosis if untreated	qPCR, NGS, FISH, IHC	(Huang et al., 2022)
ALK	Lung cancer	EML4-ALK fusion	Predicts response to ALK inhibitors	FISH, IHC, NGS	(Bayliss et al., 2016)
PTEN	Prostate, endometrial, glioblastoma	Deletions, frameshift mutations	Loss linked to poor prognosis, therapy resistance	IHC, FISH, NGS	(Bazzichetto et al., 2019)
MYC	Lymphoma, breast, colorectal cancer	MYC amplification, translocations	Tumor aggressiveness, poor survival	FISH, NGS, IHC	(Petrich et al., 2014)
CTNNB1 (Beta-catenin)	Colorectal, liver cancer	S45F, T41A mutations	Worse prognosis, enhanced Wnt signaling	NGS, IHC, Sanger sequencing	(Gajos-Michniewicz & Czyz, 2024)

can identify mutational signatures and tumor mutational burden (TMB) with reduced specimen requirements and shorter turnaround times (Tjota et al., 2024). The multiple mutational processes generate a characteristic signature of somatic mutations in each cancer genome caused by specific etiologies or exposures. Genome sequencing can decipher these mutational signatures to yield therapeutic and prognostic insights (Brady et al., 2022). The association between TMB (No. of Som Mut/Mb) and the survival of patients with melanoma, lung, colon cancer, and breast cancer has been investigated (Ke et al., 2022). A prospective randomized clinical trial found that a TMB threshold of ≥10 mutations per Mb was indicative of good prognosis and longer progression-free survival in patients with non-small cell lung cancer (Klempner et al., 2020).

1.3.2.3 Pharmacogenomic Testing

Genetic testing in the context of cancer pharmacogenomics evaluates an individual's genetic variations to predict their response to specific drugs. Genetic alterations can affect the pharmacokinetics and pharmacodynamics of anti-cancer drugs impacting the drug response and adverse events. Both germline and somatic alterations can influence drug-induced adverse events and drug response (Chan et al., 2019). Polymorphisms in the *UGT1A1* gene, coding an important enzyme of the metabolic pathway for hepatic bilirubin glucuronidation, are associated with an increased risk for side effects for colorectal cancer and NSCLC patients with irinotecan treatment (Han et al., 2006). A genotyping test for mutations in the *TPMT* (thiopurine *S*-methyltransferase) gene is used to assess the risk for severe myelosuppression with standard dosing of thiopurine drugs in individuals for whom thiopurine therapy is being considered (Dean, 2012). The response rate of cetuximab and panitumumab in patients with colorectal cancer was found to be predicted by the presence of *NRAS* and *BRAF* somatic mutations. Clinical data indicates that anti-EGFR monoclonal antibodies are unlikely to work in individuals whose tumors contain mutations in BRAF-V600E and NRAS exons 2, 3, and 4. Since cetuximab and panitumumab are not recommended for patients whose tumors harbor these mutations, RAS mutation testing is presently required before the start of treatment (van Brummelen et al., 2017). Thus, pharmacogenomics testing can help optimize treatment plans by identifying patients who are more likely to benefit from certain drugs or experience adverse effects.

1.4 CLINICAL GENETIC TESTING TECHNOLOGIES IN PERSONALIZED CANCER THERAPY

A diverse array of technologies has been adopted for molecular profiling of cancer over the years. These technologies include Sanger sequencing, polymerase chain reaction (PCR)-based technologies, immunohistochemistry (IHC), fluorescence in situ hybridization (FISH), and next-generation sequencing (NGS) (El-Deiry et al., 2019). The development of the NGS platforms has shifted the paradigm of cancer genetic testing from single-gene testing to comprehensive genomic profiling which allows the analysis of multiple genomic events in parallel in a manner that is tissue, time, and cost-efficient. The assay technology used in clinical genetic testing depends upon the testing approach in personalized oncology. The testing can be approached via two different strategies: targeted testing for specific mutations and comprehensive methods such as whole-genome sequencing (WGS) or whole-exome sequencing (WES). Quantitative PCR (qPCR), digital droplet PCR (ddPCR), allele-specific PCR, Sanger sequencing, and next-generation sequencing (NGS) are commonly used technologies for targeted testing (Casolino et al., 2024). Such testing can be done for a single gene or using multigene NGS panels. The targeted gene panels could be predefined or custom-designed for a specific set of genes such as *KRAS, EGFR, TP53,* and *BRCA1/2,* to detect clinically actionable mutations, driver mutations, prognostic markers (e.g., *TP53*), or predictive markers for therapy response (e.g., *EGFR* mutations for tyrosine kinase inhibitors). The NGS-based gene panels offer thorough risk assessment with cost-effective findings and easy-to-interpret results. Efficient detection of clinically actionable variants has made them a mainstay in cancer management. WGS and WES are nontargeted comprehensive NGS-based methods. WGS can examine all the classes and signatures of genomic variants across the entire genome. WES is extremely useful for the detection of rare or novel mutations in case of unidentified primary tumors or uncommon cancer types. The classification of variants as germline or somatic becomes critical in the case of WGS or WES. Paired tumor-normal sequencing is often required to distinguish germline variants from tumor-specific somatic mutations. Collectively, these genetic testing approaches (Table 1.3) serve as the cornerstone of individualized cancer treatment, allowing for tailored strategies that considerably enhance patient outcomes.

Table 1.3: Overview of Genetic Testing Methods in Personalized Oncology

Test Type	Description	Cancer Types	Purpose
Gene Panel Sequencing	• Analysis of multiple cancer-related genes simultaneously using next-generation sequencing technology. • Identification of mutations in several genes associated with cancer development and progression.	• Multiple cancers including breast, ovarian, colorectal, lung, and pancreatic cancers	• Diagnosis • Treatment selection • Prognosis • Identification of hereditary cancer syndromes
Whole-Exome Sequencing	• Examine the protein-coding regions (exons) of all genes in the genome. • Comprehensive approach to identify both common and rare mutations that may be missed by targeted gene panels.	• Various cancers, particularly useful in cases with unknown primary tumors or rare cancer types	• Identifying rare or novel mutations • Guiding personalized treatment strategies • Uncovering potential hereditary cancer predispositions
Liquid Biopsy	• Detection of circulating tumor DNA (ctDNA) in blood samples. • Non-invasive technique • Detection and monitoring of cancer-specific genetic alterations without the need for tissue biopsy.	• Various cancers, including lung, breast, colorectal, and prostate cancers	• Early detection of cancer • Monitoring treatment response • Identification of drug resistance mechanisms • Detection of minimal residual disease
BRCA1/BRCA2 Testing (Sanger Sequencing)	• Identifies mutations in the BRCA1 and BRCA2 genes, which are associated with an increased risk of certain cancers. • This test can be performed using blood or saliva samples.	• Primarily breast and ovarian cancers, but also relevant for pancreatic and prostate cancers	• Risk assessment for individuals with a family history of cancer • Guiding preventive measures • Informing treatment decisions, particularly regarding PARP inhibitor therapy
Microsatellite Instability (MSI) Testing	• Detection of defects in DNA mismatch repair mechanisms by examining specific repetitive DNA sequences called microsatellites. • MSI-high tumors often respond well to immunotherapy.	• Colorectal and endometrial cancers, as well as other solid tumors	• Diagnosis of Lynch Syndrome • Determining prognosis • Assessing eligibility for immunotherapy treatments such as checkpoint inhibitors
Fluorescence In Situ Hybridization (FISH)	• Detection of specific DNA sequences or chromosomal abnormalities using fluorescent probes that bind to particular regions of chromosomes. • Identification of gene amplifications, deletions, and translocations.	• Leukemia, lymphoma, breast cancer, lung cancer, and other solid tumors	• Diagnosis of specific cancer subtypes • Prognosis • Guided treatment selection for targeted therapies
Polymerase Chain Reaction (PCR)	• Amplification and detection of specific DNA sequences of interest. • Highly sensitive technique • Identification small amounts of genetic material, making it useful for detecting minimal residual disease.	• Various cancers, including leukemia, lymphoma, and solid tumors	• Diagnosis • Monitoring minimal residual disease after treatment • Detection of specific genetic alterations for guided targeted therapy selection
Chromosomal Microarray	• Identification of large-scale chromosomal changes, including copy number variations (CNVs) and loss of heterozygosity (LOH). • High-resolution view of genomic alterations.	• Various cancers, particularly useful in hematological malignancies and pediatric cancers	• Diagnosis of specific cancer subtypes • Prognosis • Identifying potential therapeutic targets based on chromosomal abnormalities
Next-Generation Sequencing (NGS)	• High-throughput sequencing • Comprehensive genetic profiling of tumors • Detection of genetic alterations, including mutations, insertions, deletions, and gene fusions.	• Various cancers, applicable to both solid tumors and hematological malignancies	• Comprehensive genetic profiling for personalized medicine approaches • Identification of potential targeted therapy options • Uncover novel genetic alterations
Epigenetic Testing	• Analysis of DNA methylation patterns • Epigenetic modifications that can affect gene expression without changing the DNA sequence • Reveal important regulatory changes in cancer cells.	• Various cancers, including colorectal, lung, and breast cancers	• Early detection of cancer • Prognosis • Identification of potential epigenetic therapeutic targets

Note: NGS = Next-Generation Sequencing; IHC = Immunohistochemistry; PCR = Polymerase Chain Reaction; qPCR = Quantitative PCR; ddPCR = Droplet Digital PCR; FISH = Fluorescence In Situ Hybridization; CISH = Chromogenic In Situ Hybridization; MLPA = Multiplex Ligation-dependent Probe Amplification.

1.4.1 PCR-based Technologies

Polymerase chain reaction (PCR) technique is used for the detection of DNA and RNA molecules. It can amplify specific fragments of DNA into billions of copies in a few hours for detection and analysis. A typical PCR reaction involves three major steps: (a) denaturation of the dsDNA template; (b) annealing of primers, i.e., forward and reverse primers; and (c) extension or elongation of the dsDNA molecules. For molecular investigation, reverse transcription PCR transforms RNA templates into complementary DNA (El-Deiry et al., 2019; Zhou et al., 2024). This approach is typically fundamental to genetic testing; however, it is associated with several limitations, such as the preferential amplification of smaller fragments, the generation of chimeric sequences, and challenges in identifying low-abundance or poorly represented sequences. Apart from this, complex DNA mixture analysis through bulk PCR-based techniques provides an averaged signal that compromises on the sensitivity required for detection of rare sequences in such complex DNA mixtures, particularly from biological sources. This limitation is overcome by embracing digital PCR, which allows each target DNA molecule to be isolated into separate compartments before amplification (Perkins et al., 2017). Digital PCR-based techniques, like real-time PCR and digital droplet PCR, allow for efficient detection of single-gene mutations. They are characterized by high sensitivity and are well suited for detection and monitoring of minimal residual disease. They provide fast turnaround times when incorporated into automated systems. However, these methods are limited by their narrow assay scope, typically allowing for the detection of mutations in only one or a few genes, and they have restricted multiplexing capabilities (Casolino et al., 2024; Gezer et al., 2022). The quantitative real-time PCR (qPCR) assay is regarded as the gold standard for the analysis of prognostic and predictive biomarkers due to its quantitative benefits. The utilization of PCR in the diagnostic analysis of gene mutations, such as those in the B-raf proto-oncogene (*BRAF*), *EGFR*, Kirsten rat sarcoma viral oncogene homolog (*KRAS*), neuroblastoma RAS viral oncogene homolog (*NRAS*), and phosphatidylinositol-4,5-bisphosphate 3-kinase catalytic subunit alpha (*PIK3CA*) from blood samples, plays a crucial role in the initial stratification of cancer and the monitoring of disease progression (Bruegl et al., 2017; Cree, 2016; Zhou et al., 2024). In addition, a number of FDA-approved PCR assays screen for *KRAS* mutations in treated and paraffin-embedded tissues. This directs treatment with anti-EGFR antibodies for metastatic colorectal cancer (CRC). Likewise, qPCR assays are also crucial in detecting minimal residual disease in leukemia. For instance, they are employed to quantify the number of BCR-ABL-positive cells after initial chemotherapy or transplantation in acute lymphoblastic leukemia (ALL). Furthermore, PCR technology is also extensively applied to detect aberrant genes and quantify aberrant mRNA in tumors, such as *MYCN* amplification in neuroblastoma. Ligand-targeted PCR is also extremely important in the detection of folate receptor-positive circulating tumor cells, which may serve as a potential diagnostic marker in pancreatic cancer (Bowen & Chung, 2009; H. Cheng et al., 2020; Cree, 2016; Zhou et al., 2024).

1.4.2 Fluorescence In Situ Hybridization (FISH)

Fluorescence in situ hybridization (FISH) is a molecular hybridization method employed in the routine diagnosis of genetic abnormalities. By utilizing fluorescent labels, this technique enables the identification of specific DNA or RNA sequences within tissue sections (in situ) or in circulating tumor cells through the application of labeled complementary DNA, RNA, or modified nucleic acid strand probes. FISH is capable of detecting various genetic alterations, including gene deletions, amplifications, translocations, and fusions (Chrzanowska et al., 2020). Gene fusions are known to occur in epithelial tumors due to genomic rearrangements or aberrations of mRNA processing. FISH technique is extensively utilized for the detection of tumor markers in diagnostics and prediction in various malignancies, including lung cancer, glioma, breast cancer, ovarian cancer, and soft tissue sarcomas, especially for metastasis (Ratan et al., 2017). This widespread application is attributed to its ease of manipulation, rapid hybridization process, and the potential for automation in both the procedural and scoring aspects (Bishop, 2010; Zhou et al., 2024). Comprehensive prognostic and predictive biomarkers, including *ALK*, mesenchymal-epithelial transition factor (*c-MET*), and *ROS1*, are detected using fluorescence in situ hybridization (FISH) (Chrzanowska et al., 2020). The cost-effective nature and durability has established FISH as the gold standard for identifying *ALK* rearrangements in non-small cell lung cancer (NSCLC) (Shackelford et al., 2015). In 2011, the FDA simultaneously approved the new anti-cancer drug crizotinib and the associated *ALK* FISH probe detection kit, emphasizing the central role played by the FISH assay as a facilitator of *ALK*-targeted therapies (Hu et al., 2014). The advances in FISH has led to considerable progress in the diagnosis of hematological malignancies (Bishop, 2010). Multiple myeloma represents a diverse malignancy originating from terminally differentiated B cells. Molecular investigations have revealed that primary translocations occur early in the disease process, followed by a substantial number of secondary translocations as the tumor progresses. FISH is especially adept at examining interphase nuclei and identifying subtle changes in chromosomes, thereby positioning itself in a frontline position as a genetic test for the detection of cytogenetic abnormalities in multiple myeloma (Kuehl & Bergsagel, 2002). Pathological fusion proteins caused by chromosomal rearrangements have profoundly impacted the molecular events involved in leukemia. *BCR/ABL1* translocation is especially prevalent in chronic myeloid leukemia (CML). The fluorescence in situ hybridization (FISH) test is known as the gold standard for the detection of such chromosomal translocations, thereby making it an essential tool for the guidance of targeted therapies in various leukemias (Wertheim et al., 2012). In half of the prostate cancer cases, androgen-regulated *TMPRSS2* and E26 transformation-specific (ETS) family members (*ERG, RTV1, and ETV4*) were detected. Invariably, chromosome rearrangement involves the fusion of *TMPRSS2* to the oncogene ETS-related gene (*ERG*), which leads to the abnormal activation of *ERG*. In recent years, a four-color FISH assay was used for the detection of either *TMPRSS2* or *ERG* rearrangements (Jiang et al., 2012; Ratan et al., 2017). Melanoma is a form of cancer that arises from melanocytes, the cells responsible for producing pigment. The detection of this condition can be effectively achieved using fluorescence in situ hybridization (FISH). For diagnostic purposes, four specific probes are employed, which target the regions 6p25 (*RREB1*), 6q23 (*MYB*), 11q13 (*CCND1*), and the centromere of chromosome 6 (*CEP6*). Additionally, optimal algorithms have been developed to identify positive FISH results based on these probes (Ferrara & De Vanna, 2016). Overexpression of HER2 is identified in approximately 10% to 20% of human breast cancer cases. The HER2 protein, which acts as an active tyrosine kinase, is pivotal in regulating normal cell growth and differentiation. The assessment of HER2 status is vital for the selection of targeted therapies. Presently, fluorescence in situ hybridization (FISH) assays are utilized to evaluate HER2 overexpression, and these assays are deemed essential for the clinical determination of HER2 status (Schlam & Swain, 2021; Slamon et al., 1989). The FISH technique is thus characterized by its high accuracy, clarity, and consistent biomarker data.

1.4.3 Sanger Sequencing

Sanger sequencing is one of most utilized platform mutation detection in various cancer settings. It allows for detailed analysis of all genetic variations present in the sample. In many clinical laboratories direct sequencing of PCR products is performed using this method. Sequencing involves a reaction mixture that includes PCR products, sequencing primers (either forward or reverse), deoxynucleotides (dNTPs), dideoxynucleotides (ddNTPs, generally labeled with different fluorescent dyes), and thermostable DNA polymerase. The process begins with the hybridization of the sequencing primer to the PCR products, followed by elongation by the DNA polymerase during the PCR cycle. During this elongation, ddNTPs are randomly integrated into the DNA strands, leading to the termination of strand elongation at various positions along the sequence. Capillary electrophoresis is subsequently used to separate the DNA strands according to size, with the terminating nucleotides being identified through their associated fluorescent dyes (Sanger et al., 1977; Turner et al., 2023). Widely recognized as the gold standard for mutational analysis, this method is capable of elucidating complete sequences and detecting unknown mutations. However, the disadvantage of this testing platform is the requirement for 40–50% tumor cellularity in the test sample (20–25% mutated allele assuming heterozygosity at the targeted chromosomal site), with tested samples of lower tumor cellularity showing a higher number of false-negative results (Shiau & Tsao, 2017). The principal drawbacks of this technique include its high expense, labor-intensive nature, and limited sensitivity. Specifically, the sensitivity of this method ranges from 10% to 20% for mutations within a wild-type background. Consequently, infrequent mutations, defined as those occurring at rates below 10% in tumor samples, cannot be accurately identified through Sanger sequencing (Ishige et al., 2018). While this method served as the predominant sequencing approach for more than two decades and continues to be utilized, next-generation sequencing (NGS) has emerged as the preferred option for the assessment of multiple genes and variants.

1.4.4 Next-Generation Sequencing (NGS)

The increasing array of molecularly directed treatment modalities has been accompanied by revolutionary advances in next-generation sequencing (NGS) technology, which have been increasingly adopted in the clinical environment. NGS is an ultrahigh-throughput method that efficiently scans and identifies a broad range of DNA mutations in an efficient way. NGS can be used for a variety of different cancer types through samples obtained from blood, solid tissues, and bone marrow. However, for accurate outcomes, meticulous tissue collection and processing are essential. The capacity of NGS to accurately and efficiently identify genetic aberrations across multiple genes has fundamentally transformed the landscape of cancer treatment. Currently, NGS facilitates the concurrent analysis of multiple genes, which aids in the detection of mutations, copy number variations, gene fusions, structural rearrangements, and biomarkers such as tumor mutational burden (TMB) and microsatellite instability (MSI) within a single assay (Casolino et al., 2024; Sabour et al., 2017). For certain advanced cancer types, initial NGS tumor testing is in fact now endorsed by both the American Society of Clinical Oncology (ASCO) and the European Society for Medical Oncology (ESMO) as a standard practice (Chakravarty et al., 2022; Mosele et al., 2020). These guidelines are grounded in robust evidence supporting the anti-tumor effectiveness of therapies linked to genomic biomarkers, with regulatory approval granted for agents targeting specific genomic alterations.

NGS encompasses a variety of deep sequencing technologies that can concurrently identify low-frequency variations across multiple DNA targets. NGS assays may be employed to sequence the entire genome (whole-genome sequencing, WGS) or to focus on specific genomic regions of interest. WGS can identify all types of genomic variants and signatures throughout most of the genome. While more targeted approaches include whole-exome sequencing and targeted gene panels. In these assays, a preliminary step is employed to enrich targeted regions for sequencing, achieved using DNA baits or PCR amplification. The targeted strategy significantly reduces the sequencing workload. Compared to WGS as the whole-exome accounts for only 1% to 2% of the genome, while even a large panel of 500 genes corresponds to just 0.1% of the total genomic content (Casolino et al., 2024). Targeted sequencing is increasingly becoming a cost-effective alternative to the sequential testing of single genes in clinical laboratory settings. The combination of recent genetic findings and substantial improvements in sequencing technology has led to the adoption of simultaneous testing for panels of selected genes associated with hereditary breast and ovarian cancer predisposition (Prapa et al., 2017). Also, the treatment strategies informed by next-generation sequencing (NGS) gene panel tests have found significant success in lung adenocarcinoma, with various genes, including *EGFR, ROS1,* and *ALK,* demonstrating the presence of targetable driver mutations. Therefore, these gene panel tests not only allow us to detect the targetable driver-genes but also mutations conferring drug resistance (Nagahashi et al., 2019). In principle, this panel testing approach enables a more thorough risk assessment by integrating the latest insights on risk variants and may provide risk stratification for individuals who do not fit the conventional testing criteria.

Targeted gene panels are cost-effective and represent the most comprehensive genomic assays currently utilized in clinical settings. Beyond their economic advantages, these assays offer customizable designs that can encompass a variable number of genes (typically ranging from 50 to 500 in clinical applications), the capability to analyze both DNA and RNA, and their applicability to tumor and cell-free nucleic acids. Furthermore, these assays facilitate automated laboratory workflows, feature low reagent costs, optimize tissue utilization, and enable the capture of all significant classes of genomic alterations (Bewicke-Copley et al., 2019). Recent years have seen a growing interest in the analysis of cell-free DNA as a method for genomic profiling in cancer patients. Both cancerous and normal cells release DNA into the bloodstream, and cancer cell DNA, or circulating tumor DNA (ctDNA), is of great value in the identification of tumor cell mutations. The capability of next-generation sequencing (NGS) tests to examine ctDNA through blood tests, also referred to as liquid biopsies, provides a means of monitoring tumor activity and treatment response over time (Lone et al., 2022).

1.5 ADVANTAGES AND CONCERNS OF GENETIC TESTING IN ONCOLOGY

Genetic testing offers multiple advantages in clinical oncology:

a. It ensures that individuals at an increased risk are identified in time to implement the appropriate screening and preventive measures, which can lead to earlier diagnosis and better outcomes.

b. Targeted therapies: Genetic evaluation may identify a specific genetic change fueling the tumor and may be targeted using therapies that will benefit from these weaknesses.

c. Personalized Treatment Plans: Knowing the genetic makeup of a single tumor, doctors can personalize treatment plans for the patient, enhancing effectiveness and reducing harmful side effects.

d. Genetic testing promotes informed decision-making, which provides patients with essential information on cancer risk and the treatments on offer.

The advantages are currently superseded by concerns among clinicians for genetic testing as:

a. Emotional and Psychological Impact: Receiving genetic testing results can have significant emotional and psychological implications, requiring appropriate counseling and support.

b. Cost and Access: Genetic testing can be costly and therefore not accessible to everyone.

c. Ethical Considerations: Thus, the issue of genetic testing raises questions about privacy and discrimination as well as possible misuse of the information.

1.6 CONCLUSION AND FUTURE ROADMAP IN GENETIC TESTING

Cancer diagnosis at an early stage is essential for effective treatment of the disease. There are multiple tests that are used for this diagnosis however there is no single test that can accurately diagnose cancer especially at or near its onset. The doctors therefore use a series of traditional evaluation strategy that starts with patient and family history followed by physical assessments that includes several diagnostic tests. The tests are generally aimed at determining whether the symptoms are actually cancer or just any other infection or disease condition that are mimicking cancer. These diagnostic tests include imaging, laboratory tests including tumor markers, endoscopic examination, surgery with biopsy, and more recently multiple genetic tests. The biggest challenge in bringing the genetic testing to daily testing routine of clinicians used to be the time taken for the tests and the cost. Although the advent of more advanced technologies have reduced the cost and the time taken for the generation of data generation and the delivery of reports, the complexity and clear interpretation of results still keeps clinicians skeptical about the use of these tests. Therefore, currently the biggest challenge especially in a country like India where health insurance doesn't generally cover genetic testing is to bring the clinicians and general public on board by convincing them about the significance of genetic testing in cancer diagnosis.

In this context it may be noted that the current general practice of tests used for cancer diagnosis especially the blood tests and the imaging technology have the advantage of being relatively rapid. They also give you a more definite diagnosis that is more clearly understood by the general public and clinicians who are not well averse with the "ATGC" code of human genes. The intricacies associated with the genetic diversity and the inability in many cases to give a fool proof prediction of the association with diseases is a big drawback of genetic testing. Another limitation in the field is the lack of sufficient genetic variations that are actionable or where a definite therapy can be suggested. The current diagnostic methods provide both the above features in most cases that makes it a preferred choice among clinicians. However, most of these diagnostic methods, in practice, still are unable to predict predisposition to cancer or have much prognostic values in spite of several advances in the field. That is the advantage of genetic testing that needs to be emphasized and brought to public notice more and more so that it gets more accepted especially in managing the predisposition of cancer and other such diseases. Therefore, the newer and more recent trends in genetic testing especially with the advances in Next Generation Sequencing technologies need to be brought into clinical practice.

In this chapter we introduce you to the genetic tests in use for cancer diagnosis as discussed throughout the book and the need to develop more advanced clinical practices and conclude by discussing the limitations and overcoming them to make genetic testing an integral part of the cancer diagnosis field. Cancer genetic testing is evolving at a rapid rate, driven by advancements in technology and expanded knowledge of cancer genomics. Predictive genetic testing, in general, is progressively becoming a central aspect of cancer therapy, directing treatment decisions and allowing personalized approaches. For example, NGS is circumventing the limitations of previous methods and allowing for more comprehensive genomic characterization. Even with the development, the practical application of genomic testing is limited in the context of patients' awareness and acceptability of the complex concepts. As the advances in genetic testing evolve, it is necessary to develop evidence-based models for clinical decision-making application of genetic test results to maximize the potential of personalized cancer treatment. With rapid development of new tests and technologies, the selection of an appropriate genetic test for a patient depends on a number of factors such as the type and stage of cancer, family medical history, and planned treatment. Genetic counseling is usually recommended before and after genetic testing to allow patients to understand test implications and make informed treatment choices.

REFERENCES

Adashek JJ et al. (2020). Cancer genetics and therapeutic opportunities in urologic practice. *Cancers* 12(3), 710.

Al-Shinnag M et al. (2024). Germline potential should not be overlooked for cancer variants identified in tumour-only somatic mutation testing. *Pathology* 56/4:468–472.

André F et al. (2019). Alpelisib for *PIK3CA* -mutated, hormone receptor–positive advanced breast cancer. *New Engl J Med* 380/20:1929–1940.

Barbour JA et al. (2024). ERCC2 mutations alter the genomic distribution pattern of somatic mutations and are independently prognostic in bladder cancer. *Cell Genom* 4/8:100627.

Batist G et al. (2011). Resistance to cancer treatment: The role of somatic genetic events and the challenges for targeted therapies. *Front Pharmacol* 2/59.

Bayliss R et al. (2016). Molecular mechanisms that underpin EML4-ALK driven cancers and their response to targeted drugs. *Cell Molec Life Sci* 73/6.

Bazzichetto C et al. (2019). Pten as a prognostic/predictive biomarker in cancer: An unfulfilled promise? *Cancers* 11/4.

Bedrosian I et al. (2024). Germline testing in patients with breast cancer: ASCO-Society of Surgical Oncology Guideline. *J Clin Oncol* 42/5:584–604.

Bewicke-Copley F et al. (2019). Applications and analysis of targeted genomic sequencing in cancer studies. *Comput Structural Biotechnol J* 17.

Bishop R. (2010). Applications of fluorescence in situ hybridization (FISH) in detecting genetic aberrations of medical significance. *Bioscience Horizons* 3/1.

Bister K. (2015). Discovery of oncogenes: The advent of molecular cancer research. *Proc Nat Acad Sci USA* 112/50:15259–15260.

Boos L, Wicki A. (2024). The molecular tumor board—A key element of precision oncology. *Memo - Mag Eur Med Oncol* 17/3:190–193.

Bouck N, Di Mayorca G. (1976). Somatic mutation as the basis for malignant transformation of BHK cells by chemical carcinogens. *Nature* 264/5588:722–727.

Bowen KA, Chung, DH. (2009). Recent advances in neuroblastoma. *Curr Opinion Pediat* 21/3.

Brady SW et al. (2022). Therapeutic and prognostic insights from the analysis of cancer mutational signatures. *Trends Genet* 38/2:194–208.

Bruegl AS et al. (2017). Importance of PCR-based tumor testing in the evaluation of lynch syndrome-associated endometrial cancer. *Adv Anatomic Pathol* 24/6:372–378.

Canon J et al. (2019). The clinical KRAS(G12C) inhibitor AMG 510 drives anti-tumour immunity. *Nature* 575/7781:217–223.

Casolino R et al. (2024). Interpreting and integrating genomic tests results in clinical cancer care: Overview and practical guidance. *CA* 74/3:264–285.

Catana A et al. (2019). Multi gene panel testing for hereditary breast cancer - Is it ready to be used? *Med Pharmacy Rep* 92/3:220–225.

Chakravarty D et al. (2022). Somatic genomic testing in patients with metastatic or advanced cancer: ASCO provisional clinical opinion. *J Clin Oncol* 40/11.

Chan HT et al. (2019). The roles of common variation and somatic mutation in cancer pharmacogenomics. *Oncol Ther* 7/1:1–32.

Chapman PB et al. (2011). Improved survival with vemurafenib in melanoma with BRAF V600E mutation. *New Engl J Med* 364/26:2507–2516.

Chen X et al. (2022). Mutant p53 in cancer: from molecular mechanism to therapeutic modulation. *Cell Death Dis* 13/11.

Cheng HH et al. (2019). Germline and somatic mutations in prostate cancer for the clinician. *JNCCN* 17/5.

Cheng HH et al. (2020). Ligand-targeted polymerase chain reaction for the detection of folate receptor-positive circulating tumour cells as a potential diagnostic biomarker for pancreatic cancer. *Cell Proliferation* 53/9.

Cheng L et al. (2018). Molecular testing for BRAF mutations to inform melanoma treatment decisions: A move toward precision medicine. *Mod Pathol* 31/1.

Chiang YT et al. (2021). The function of the mutant p53-r175h in cancer. *Cancers* 13/16.

Chrzanowska NM et al. (2020). Use of fluorescence in situ hybridization (FISH) in diagnosis and tailored therapies in solid tumors. *Molecules* 25/8.

Cooper GM et al. (1980). Transforming activity of DNA of chemically transformed and normal cells. *Nature* 284/5755:418–421.

Crawford K, Warren Y. (2023). Management of cancer genetic testing: A brief overview. *Rhode Isl Med J* 106/5:18–23.

Cree IA. (2016). Diagnostic RAS mutation analysis by polymerase chain reaction (PCR). *Biomolec Detect Quantific* 8.

De S, Ganesan S. (2017). Looking beyond drivers and passengers in cancer genome sequencing data. *Ann Oncol* 28/5:938–945.

Dean, L. (2012). Mercaptopurine therapy and TPMT genotype. In Pratt, V., et al. (Eds.), Medical genetics summaries (pp. 229). National Center for Biotechnology Information.

DeLeonardis K et al. (2019). When should tumor genomic profiling prompt consideration of germline testing? *J Oncol Pract* 15/9:465–473.

Douillard JY et al. (2013). Panitumumab–FOLFOX4 treatment and *RAS* mutations in colorectal cancer. *New Engl J Med* 369(11):1023–1034.

Drilon A et al. (2018). Efficacy of larotrectinib in *TRK* fusion–positive cancers in adults and children. *New Engl J Med* 378(8):731–739.

Duesberg PH, Vogt PK. (1970). Differences between the ribonucleic acids of transforming and non-transforming avian tumor viruses. *Proc Nat Acad Sci USA* 67/4:1673–1680.

Ece Solmaz A et al. (2021). Clinical contribution of next-generation sequencing multigene panel testing for BRCA negative high-risk patients with breast cancer. *Clin Breast Cancer* 21/6:e647–e653.

El-Deiry WS et al. (2019). The current state of molecular testing in the treatment of patients with solid tumors, 2019. *CA* 69/4:305–343.

Faguet GB. (2015). A brief history of cancer: Age-old milestones underlying our current knowledge database. *Int J Cancer* 136/9:2022–2036.

Ferrara G, De Vanna AC. (2016). Fluorescence in situ hybridization for melanoma diagnosis: A review and a reappraisal. *Am J Dermatopathol* 38/4.

Frey MK et al. (2022). Cascade testing for hereditary cancer syndromes: Should we move toward direct relative contact? A systematic review and meta-analysis. *J Clin Oncol* 40/35:4129–4143.

Gajos-Michniewicz A, Czyz M. (2024). WNT/β-catenin signaling in hepatocellular carcinoma: The aberrant activation, pathogenic roles, and therapeutic opportunities. *Genes and Diseases* 11/2.

Garber JE, Offit K. (2005). Hereditary cancer predisposition syndromes. *J Clin Oncol* 23/2:276–292.

Garutti M et al. (2023). Hereditary cancer syndromes: A comprehensive review with a visual tool. *Genes* 14/5.

Gezer U et al. (2022). The clinical utility of droplet digital PCR for profiling circulating tumor DNA in breast cancer patients. *Diagnostics* 12/12.

Gomez-Martin C et al. (2013). Level of HER2 gene amplification predicts response and overall survival in her2-positive advanced gastric cancer treated with trastuzumab. *J Clin Oncol* 31/35.

Guan JL et al. (2013). KRAS mutation in patients with lung cancer: A predictor for poor prognosis but not for EGFR-TKIs or chemotherapy. *Ann Surg Oncol* 20/4:1381–1388.

Guha T, Malkin,D. (2017). Inherited TP53 mutations and the Li-fraumeni syndrome. *Cold Spring Harbor Perspectives Med* 7/4.

Guo L et al. (2023). Molecular profiling provides clinical insights into targeted and immunotherapies as well as colorectal cancer prognosis. *Gastroenterol* 165/2:414–428.e7.

Han JY et al. (2006). Comprehensive analysis of UGT1A polymorphisms predictive for pharmacokinetics and treatment outcome in patients with non-small-cell lung cancer treated with irinotecan and cisplatin. *J Clin Oncol* 24/15:2237–2244.

Hu L et al. (2014). Fluorescence in situ hybridization (FISH): An increasingly demanded tool for biomarker research and personalized medicine. *Biomarker Res* 2/1.

Huang LT et al. (2022). Impact of EGFR exon 19 deletion subtypes on clinical outcomes in EGFR-TKI-Treated advanced non-small-cell lung cancer. *Lung Cancer* 166.

Ishige T et al. (2018). Locked nucleic acid technology for highly sensitive detection of somatic mutations in cancer. *Adv Clin Chem* 83.

Jiang H et al. (2012). The utility of fluorescence in situ hybridization analysis in diagnosing myelodysplastic syndromes is limited to cases with karyotype failure. *Leukemia Res* 36/4.

Jorge SEDC et al. (2014). Epidermal growth factor receptor (EGFR) mutations in lung cancer: Preclinical and clinical data. *Braz J Med Biolog Res* 47/11:929–993.

Kaehler M, Cascorbi I. (2019). Germline variants in cancer therapy. *Cancer Drug Resist* 2/1:18–30.

Ke L et al. (2022). The prognostic role of tumor mutation burden on survival of breast cancer: A systematic review and meta-analysis. *BMC Cancer* 22/1.

Kern SE, Winter JM. (2006). Elegance, silence and nonsense in the mutations literature for solid tumors. *Cancer Biol Ther* 5/4:349–359.

Klempner SJ et al. (2020). Tumor mutational burden as a predictive biomarker for response to immune checkpoint inhibitors: A review of current evidence. *The Oncologist* 25/1:e147–e159.

Kontomanolis EN et al. (2020). Role of oncogenes and tumor-suppressor genes in carcinogenesis: A review. *Anticancer Res* 40/11:6009–6015.

Kuehl WM, Bergsagel PL. (2002). Multiple myeloma: Evolving genetic events and host interactions. *Nature Rev Cancer* 2/3.

Kurian AW et al. (2023). Germline genetic testing after cancer diagnosis. *JAMA* 330/1:43–51.

Lee HJ et al. (2014). HER2 heterogeneity affects trastuzumab responses and survival in patients with her2-positive metastatic breast cancer. *Am J Clin Pathol* 142/6.

Li FP, Fraumeni JF. (1969). Soft-tissue sarcomas, breast cancer, and other neoplasms. A familial syndrome? *Ann Intern Med* 71/4:747–752.

Lin KK et al. (2019). BRCA reversion mutations in circulating tumor DNA predict primary and acquired resistance to the PARP inhibitor rucaparib in high-grade ovarian carcinoma. *Cancer Disc* 9/2.

Liu YL, Stadler ZK. (2021). The future of parallel tumor and germline genetic testing: Is there a role for all patients with cancer? *JNCCN* 19/7.

Lone SN et al. (2022). Liquid biopsy: A step closer to transform diagnosis, prognosis and future of cancer treatments. *Molec Cancer* 21/1.

Loriot Y et al. (2019). Erdafitinib in locally advanced or metastatic urothelial carcinoma. *New Engl J Med* 381/4:338–348.

Lynch TJ et al. (2004). Activating mutations in the epidermal growth factor receptor underlying responsiveness of non–small-cell lung cancer to gefitinib. *New Engl J Med* 350/21:2129–2139.

Marcom, P. K. (2017). Breast cancer. In G. S. Ginsburg, H. F. Willard, & S. P. David (Eds.), Genomic and precision medicine: Primary care (3rd ed., pp. 181–190). Elsevier.

Martin GS. (2004). The road to Src. *Oncogene* 23/48,REV. ISS. 7:7910–7917.

Matsuoka T, Yashiro M. (2024). Current status and perspectives of genetic testing in gastrointestinal cancer (Review). *Oncol Lett* 27/1.

Mok TS et al. (2009). Gefitinib or carboplatin–paclitaxel in pulmonary adenocarcinoma. *New Engl J Med* 361/10:947–957.

Mosele F et al. (2020). Recommendations for the use of next-generation sequencing (NGS) for patients with metastatic cancers: A report from the ESMO Precision Medicine Working Group. *Ann Oncol* 31/11.

Nagahashi M et al. (2019). Next generation sequencing-based gene panel tests for the management of solid tumors. *Cancer Sci* 110/1:6–15.

Nalejska E et al. (2014). Prognostic and predictive biomarkers: Tools in personalized oncology. *Molec Diagn Ther* 18/3.

Oaknin A et al (2022). Endometrial cancer: ESMO Clinical Practice Guideline for diagnosis, treatment and follow-up. *Ann Oncol* 33/9:860–877.

Ott, G., et al. (2013). Understanding MYC-driven aggressive B-cell lymphomas: Pathogenesis and classification. Education Program Hematology, 122(24), 3884–3891.

Paik PK et al. (2020). Tepotinib in non–small-cell lung cancer with *MET* Exon 14 skipping mutations. *New Engl J Med* 383/10:931–943.

Pakneshan S et al. (2013). Clinicopathological relevance of BRAF mutations in human cancer. *Pathol* 45/4:346–356.

Pelegrina B et al. (2023). Evaluation of somatic mutations in cervicovaginal samples as a non-invasive method for the detection and molecular classification of endometrial cancer. *EBioMedicine* 94.

Peltomäki P et al. (2023). Lynch syndrome genetics and clinical implications. *Gastroenterol* 164/5:783–799.

Perkins G et al. (2017). Droplet-based digital PCR: application in cancer research. *Adv Clin Chem* 79:43–91.

Petrich AM et al. (2014). MYC-associated and double-hit lymphomas: A review of pathobiology, prognosis, and therapeutic approaches. *Cancer* 120/24.

Poei D et al. (2024). ALK inhibitors in cancer: Mechanisms of resistance and therapeutic management strategies. *Cancer Drug Res* 7/20.

Pon JR, Marra MA. (2015). Driver and passenger mutations in cancer. *Ann Rev Pathol* 10:25–50.

Prapa M et al. (2017). The use of panel testing in familial breast and ovarian cancer. *Clin Med* 17/6.

Ragupathi A et al. (2023). Targeting the BRCA1/2 deficient cancer with PARP inhibitors: Clinical outcomes and mechanistic insights. *Front Cell Development Biol* 11.

Ratan ZA et al. (2017). Application of Fluorescence In Situ Hybridization (FISH) technique for the detection of genetic aberration in medical science. *Cureus* 9/6:e1325.

Reck M et al. (2016). Pembrolizumab versus chemotherapy for PD-L1–positive non–small-cell lung cancer. *New Engl J Med* 375/19:1823–1833.

Robson M et al. (2017). Olaparib for metastatic breast cancer in patients with a germline *BRCA* mutation. *New Engl J Med* 377/6:523–533.

Rooney MM et al. (2023). Genetics of breast cancer: Risk models, who to test, and management options. *Surg Clin N Am* 103/1:35–47.

Ruark E et al. (2013). Mosaic PPM1D mutations are associated with predisposition to breast and ovarian cancer. *Nature* 493/7432:406–410.

Sabour L et al. (2017). Clinical applications of next-generation sequencing in cancer diagnosis. *Pathol Oncol Res* 23/2.

Samowitz WS et al. (2005). Poor survival associated with the BRAF V600E mutation in microsatellite-stable colon cancers. *Cancer Res* 65/14.

Sanger F et al. (1977). DNA sequencing with chain-terminating inhibitors. *Proc Nat Acad Sci USA* 74/12.

Santarpia, M et al. (2017). Osimertinib in the treatment of non-small-cell lung cancer: Design, development and place in therapy. *Lung Cancer Target Ther* 8.

Schlam I, Swain SM. (2021). HER2-positive breast cancer and tyrosine kinase inhibitors: the time is now. *Breast Cancer* 7/1.

Schmidlen TJ et al. (2022). The impact of proband indication for genetic testing on the uptake of cascade testing among relatives. *Front Genet* 13.

Schneider K et al. (1999). *Li-Fraumeni Syndrome*. GeneReviews®. www.ncbi.nlm.nih.gov/books/NBK1311/.

Shackelford RE et al. (2015). ALK-rearrangements and testing methods in non-small cell lung cancer: A review. *Genes Cancer* 5/1–2.

Shaw AT et al. (2013). Crizotinib versus chemotherapy in advanced *ALK* -positive lung cancer. *New Engl J Med* 368/25:2385–2394.

Shaw AT et al. (2014). Crizotinib in *ROS1* -rearranged non–small-cell lung cancer. *New Engl J Med* 371/21:1963–1971.

Shiau, C. J., & Tsao, M. S. (2017). Molecular testing in lung cancer. In H. I. Pass, D. Ball, & G. V. Scagliotti (Eds.), Molecular testing in lung cancer (2nd ed., pp. 164–177.e5). Elsevier. https://doi.org/10.1016/B978-0-323-52357-8.00018-4

Slamon DJ et al. (1989). Studies of the HER-2/neu proto-oncogene in human breast and ovarian cancer. *Science* 244/4905.

Slamon DJ et al. (2001). Use of chemotherapy plus a monoclonal antibody against HER2 for metastatic breast cancer that overexpresses HER2. *New Engl J Med* 344/11:783–792.

Stein EM et al. (2021). Ivosidenib or enasidenib combined with intensive chemotherapy in patients with newly diagnosed AML: A phase 1 study. *Blood* 137/13:1792–1803.

Stoffel EM, Carethers JM. (2020). Current approaches to germline cancer genetic testing. *Ann Rev Med*. 71:85–102.

Subbiah V et al. (2021). Structural basis of acquired resistance to selpercatinib and pralsetinib mediated by non-gatekeeper RET mutations. *Ann Oncol* 32/2:261–268.

Tjota MY et al. (2024). Clinical utility and benefits of comprehensive genomic profiling in cancer. *J Applied Lab Med* 9/1:76–91.

Tsaousis GN et al. (2019). Analysis of hereditary cancer syndromes by using a panel of genes: Novel and multiple pathogenic mutations. *BMC Cancer* 19/1.

Turner NC et al. (2015). Palbociclib in hormone-receptor–positive advanced breast cancer. *New Engl J Med* 373/3:209–219.

Turner SA et al. (2023). The basics of commonly used molecular techniques for diagnosis, and application of molecular testing in cytology. *Diagn Cytopathol* 51/1.

Valtorta E et al. (2013). KRAS gene amplification in colorectal cancer and impact on response to EGFR-targeted therapy. *Int J Cancer* 133/5.

van Brummelen EMJ et al. (2017). BRAF mutations as predictive biomarker for response to anti-EGFR monoclonal antibodies. *The Oncologist, 22*(7):864–872.

Velpeau A. (1854). Traité des maladies du sein et de la région mammaire [Treatise on diseases of the breast and the mammary region]. Victor Masson.

Venables JP et al. (2009). Cancer-associated regulation of alternative splicing. *Nature Structur Molec Biol* 16/6:670–676.

Verdaguer H et al. (2017). Predictive and prognostic biomarkers in personalized gastrointestinal cancer treatment. *J Gastrointest Oncol* 8/3.

Vermaat JS et al. (2012). Primary colorectal cancers and their subsequent hepatic metastases are genetically different: Implications for selection of patients for targeted treatment. *Clin Cancer Res* 18/3.

Vogelstein B et al. (2013). Cancer genome landscapes. *Science* 340/6127:1546–1558.

Weinberg RA. (2008). In retrospect: The chromosome trail. *Nature* 453/7196:725–725.

Wertheim GBW et al. (2012). Molecular-based classification of acute myeloid leukemia and its role in directing rational therapy: Personalized medicine for profoundly promiscuous proliferations. *Molec Diagn Ther* 16/6.

Zhou Y et al. (2024). Tumor biomarkers for diagnosis, prognosis and targeted therapy. *Signal Transduct Target Ther* 9/1:132.

2

Molecular Basis of Cancer

Genetic Alterations and Tumor Development

Samkeliso Takaidza, Nnana M. Molefe, and Patience Chihomvu

2.1 INTRODUCTION

Cancer is a genetic disorder that is defined by the uncontrolled proliferation of abnormal cells, which have the potential to infiltrate healthy tissue and impair its functionality. It is the consequence of the accumulation of genetic and epigenetic alterations in humans. These modifications transpire before the onset of cancer and are observed in both malignant and non-cancerous cells. Environmental factors induce modifications. For instance, genetic abnormalities are primarily induced by chronic inflammation and aging, while epigenetic changes are primarily influenced by mutagenic substances, ultraviolet light, and other factors. Additionally, these malignant cells have the potential to move to distant locations, leading to the development of metastases (Watanabe et al., 2020).

2.2 ACTIVATION OF PROTO-ONCOGENES AND THEIR CONVERSION TO ONCOGENES

2.2.1 Genetic Changes

In a healthy state, proto-oncogenes are proteins encoded by cells that stimulate cell division, inhibit cell differentiation, and halt cell demise. They are the primary regulatory factors of the biological processes of the cell (Dakal et al., 2024). Growth factors (e.g., PDGF), their receptors (e.g., EGFR), signal transducers (e.g., RAS), transcription factors (e.g., MYC), and BCL2, a critical regulator of apoptosis, are all examples of human proto-oncogenes (Brown, 2021). Activated oncogenes can be observed in cancer cells because of modifications to these genes, which can impact the structure of their encoded proteins or their regulatory functions (Kontomanolis et al., 2020). Brown (2021) posits that oncogenes facilitate cancer development by inhibiting apoptosis and operating in opposition to the normal control of cell proliferation. Chromosomal translocation, gene amplification, and point mutations are among the mechanisms by which proto-oncogenes are activated (Kontomanolis et al., 2020).

2.2.2 Chromosomal Reordering

In cancer, proto-oncogenes may be triggered via chromosomal translocations. This chromosomal defect confers a selective growth advantage to some stem or embryonic cells, ultimately expediting the formation of aggressive tumors. In the context of oncogenes, chromosomal translocations can alter the original positions of proto-oncogenes, leading to two effects on gene products. One approach involves the creation of oncogenic fusion proteins, while the other entails the interaction of proto-oncogenes with regulatory regions, leading to the overexpression of proto-oncogenes (Hasty and Montagna, 2014; Pierotti et al., 2022).

The BCR-ABL fusion gene in chronic myeloid leukemia exemplifies proto-oncogene activation induced by chromosomal translocations. The reciprocal translocation between chromosomes 9 and 22 fuses the BCR gene on chromosome 22 with the ABL gene on chromosome 9, resulting in the formation of a hybrid BCR-ABL oncogene. The BCR-ABL fusion protein has constitutive tyrosine kinase activity, resulting in abnormal signaling pathways that enhance leukemic cell proliferation and survival (El-Tanani et al., 2024).

Translocations involving the MYC proto-oncogene frequently occur in many malignancies, such as Burkitt lymphoma. The interplay between MYC and highly active enhancer areas results in aberrant MYC expression, culminating in unregulated cellular proliferation and oncogenesis. The MYC oncogene regulates cell cycle progression, metabolism, and apoptosis, highlighting its function as a cancer promoter (Stine et al., 2015).

2.2.3 Gene Amplification

Gene amplification is a technique for activating proto-oncogenes by augmenting the copy number of their genomic locus. Amplification events may arise from several reasons, such as chromosomal rearrangements, replication mistakes, and selective pressure from the tumor microenvironment. Amplified genes may be structured as extrachromosomal elements that replicate at a singular locus or are dispersed throughout the genome (Wagner and Krontiris, 1988). The correlation

DOI: 10.1201/9781003542162-2

between the two forms of gene amplification observed in cancers, intrachromosomal homogenous and extrachromosomal molecules, remained ambiguous. Various hypotheses regarding the initiation of amplification have been proposed, including complications in DNA replication, telomere dysfunction, and fragile chromosomal areas (Cheng et al., 2016).

The amplification of the human epidermal growth factor receptor 2 (HER2/neu), a proto-oncogene, is being thoroughly examined as a contributor to breast cancer. HER2/neu amplification leads to the overexpression of the HER2 protein, a component of the EGFR family of receptor tyrosine kinases. Elevated HER2 expression activates downstream signaling pathways, hence facilitating cell proliferation and tumor development. HER2-positive breast cancer is a specific molecular subtype marked by aggressive disease characteristics and an unfavorable prognosis (Kontomanolis et al., 2020).

2.2.4 Point Mutation

Point mutations involve single nucleotide alterations in a proto-oncogene's coding or regulatory region (Esteban-Villarrubia et al., 2020), resulting in constitutive activation of its proteins. Point mutations can cause the creation of hyperactive proteins, which promote uncontrolled cell growth and survival (Dakal et al., 2024).

Point mutations decrease RAS proteins' intrinsic GTPase activity, resulting in constitutive activation and persistent signaling via downstream effector pathways like Mitogen-Activated Protein Kinase (MAPK) (Takacs et al., 2020). The MAPK pathway is crucial in key cellular processes, including differentiation, proliferation, survival, autophagy, and apoptosis. Activation of any component in the MAPK cascade (RAS/RAF/MEK/ERK) can trigger downstream signaling, potentially leading to carcinogenesis (Shan et al., 2024).

Mutations in the RAS proto-oncogene family (KRas, HRas, and NRas) are commonly seen in pancreatic, colorectal, and lung malignancies. KRAS mutations, in particular, are observed in approximately 30% of all human malignancies predominantly in lung and gastrointestinal cancers (Meng et al., 2018), 50% of colon carcinomas (Pierotti MA. 2003), and 90–95% of pancreatic cancer cases, specifically pancreatic ductal adenocarcinoma (PDAC), all harboring a point mutation at the G12 codon (Meng et al., 2018). NRAS has been associated with hematologic malignancies, with a prevalence of up to 25% in acute myeloid leukemia and myelodysplastic syndromes. (Pierotti MA. 2003).

2.2.5 Epigenetic Changes

The translation of DNA, or genetic code, into protein sequences, involves more than just the nucleotide sequence itself; it also depends on a complex regulatory network shaped by both genetic and environmental influences. This network, which falls under the field of epigenetics, utilizes chemical modifications to regulate gene activity and governs the expression of the genetic code (Ilango et al., 2020).

Epigenetic modifications refer to heritable alterations in gene activity that occur without altering the DNA sequence. These modifications play a key role in regulating gene expression and governing essential biological processes like cell differentiation and embryogenesis. Substantial evidence supports the role of epigenetic reprogramming as a driving factor behind the dynamic transcriptomic variability observed in cancer (Davalos and Esteller, 2023). Therein, gene expression is regulated by intricate epigenetic mechanisms, specifically through covalent post-translational modifications (PTMs) that alter chromatin structure and accessibility. These include DNA methylation, histone modifications, nucleosome remodeling, and the activity of small non-coding RNAs, summarized in Figure 2.1. When these processes become dysregulated, they disrupt normal gene function, playing a critical role in cancer onset, growth, and progression (Neganova et al., 2022).

2.2.5.1 DNA Methylation

DNA methylation is a mechanism that silences genes by adding a methyl group to the C5 position of cytosines, producing 5-methylcytosine (Davalos and Esteller, 2023). This modification, catalyzed by DNA methyltransferases (DNMTs), influences both gene expression and chromatin structure. In mammals, the DNMT family includes DNMT1, DNMT2, DNMT3A, DNMT3B, and DNMT3L, but only DNMT1, DNMT3A, and DNMT3B are involved in catalyzing DNA methylation. DNMT2 acts as RNA methyltransferases, while DNMT3L modulates the activity of other DNMTs (Castro-Munoz et al., 2023). The ten-eleven translocation (TET) enzymes—TET1, TET2, and TET3—play an essential role in active DNA demethylation by converting 5-methylcytosine into hydroxymethyl cytosine (Ross and Bogdanovic, 2019), formyl cytosine, and carboxyl cytosine (Koivunen and Laukka, 2018). Alterations in DNA methylation patterns are prevalent across nearly all forms

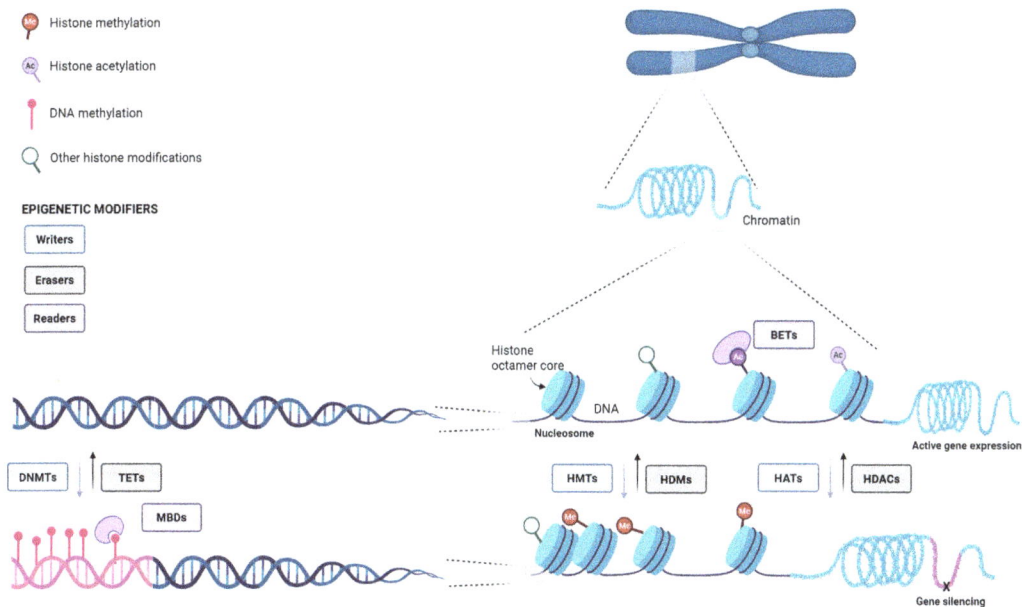

Figure 2.1 Epigenetic modification of chromatin structure. Adapted from Tao et al. (2024). The figure was created with Biorender.com

of hematologic malignancies. These disruptions have become a defining characteristic of various blood cancers, including myelodysplastic syndromes (MDS), acute myeloid leukemia, acute lymphoblastic leukemia, diffuse large B-cell lymphomas, and peripheral T-cell lymphomas. The dysregulation of methylation plays a pivotal role in the pathogenesis, influencing gene expression and contributing to disease onset and progression (Joshi et al., 2022).

2.2.5.2 Histone Modification

2.2.5.2.1 Histone Acetylation

Histone acetylation is facilitated by histone acetyltransferases (HATs), which transfer an acetyl group from acetyl-CoA to the amino group of lysine residues on the histone tails. Conversely, the removal of these acetyl groups is catalyzed by histone deacetylases (HDACs), restoring the histones to their deacetylated state (Ramazi et al., 2020). The structural change resulting from histone acetylation reduces negative and positive charge interactions between DNA and histone tails, respectively, and promotes chromatin decompaction, allowing regulatory proteins and transcription machinery to access the gene sequences (Castro-Munoz et al., 2023). HATs are classified into the following three families: the GNAT (Gcn5, PCAF, Hat1), MYST (MOZ/Morf, Ybf2, Sas2, Tip60), and CBP/P300 family (p300/CBP, Taf1). These transferases also acetylate other proteins, such as p53, STAT3, and GATA; and they have biological functions that include regulating protein stability, enhancing DNA binding affinity, and facilitating protein-protein interactions (Park and Han, 2019). Alterations in the genes and functional dysregulation of the HAT family of transferases are closely associated with cancer development. Different HAT family members exhibit distinct mutations in tumors and play varying roles throughout cancer progression, influencing stages from the initiation and growth of malignant tumors to their metastasis. Mutations in p300/CBP genes have been linked to various types of leukemia and B-cell non-Hodgkin lymphoma, while GCN5 is upregulated in several cancers, including human glioma, colorectal cancer, breast cancer, and lung carcinoma (Neganova et al., 2022). Abnormal acetylation patterns of histone lysine residues, particularly the reduction of acetylation at lysine 16 of histone H4 (H4K16ac), have been identified as a frequent characteristic of human cancers (Park and Han, 2019).

2.2.5.2.2 Histone Methylation

Histone methylation involves the addition and removal of a methyl group to arginine or lysine residues on histone tails, using S-adenosylmethionine (SAM) as the methyl donor (Qin et al., 2020). Histone methylation transferases are divided into three families: the SET-domain enzymes, the

Dot1-like proteins which target lysine residues (KMTs), and the N-methyltransferases (PRMTs), which methylate arginine residues. Histone Demethylation Transferases on the other hand are divided into the amine oxidases family and the Jumanji C (JmjC)-domain dioxygenases (Gong and Miller, 2019). SAM is converted into S-adenosylhomocysteine (SAH during methylation), suppressing methyltransferase activity. Therefore, methyltransferases are affected by changes in the levels of SAM and SAH within the cell (Michalak et al., 2019).

Methylation changes are widespread in cancer genomes, affecting thousands of promoters and many histone and DNA modification genes. While few metabolic enzymes are frequently mutated in cancer, each mutation in these enzymes influences methylation (Su et al., 2016). Many KMTs and KDMTs are overexpressed in cancer, with studies showing abnormal global histone lysine methylation in several cancer cell lines (McGrath and Trojer, 2015).

2.2.5.3 Non-Coding Ribonucleic Acid Interference

Non-coding ribonucleic acids (ncRNAs) are a class of RNA transcripts that do not encode proteins, in contrast to mRNAs. They are often viewed as by-products of protein transcription with minimal biological roles. MicroRNA (miRNA), small interfering RNA (siRNA), piwi-interacting RNA (piRNA), and long non-coding RNA (lncRNA) are some of the most extensively studied regulatory ncRNAs involved in controlling gene expression at both transcriptional and post-transcriptional levels (Li, 2021).

Research shows that ncRNAs play a crucial role in cancer initiation and progression (Wang et al., 2019). lncRNAs in particular are recognized as playing roles in nearly all the hallmarks of cancer, including sustained proliferation, replicative immortality, evasion of growth suppressors, angiogenesis, resistance to apoptosis, and metastasis (Li, 2021). However, the mechanisms through which lncRNA modifications influence gene regulation, and the proteins involved in regulating both remain unclear (Kazimierczyk and Wrzesinski, 2021).

2.2.6 Microsatellite Instability (MSI)

Microsatellites (MSs), also referred to as Short Tandem Repeats (STRs) or Simple Sequence Repeats (SSRs), are made up of 1–6 nucleotide repeating units; with distribution patterns ranging from 15 to 65 nucleotide tandem repeats within small satellite DNA, located near the chromosome end (Li et al., 2020). They are distributed predominantly in non-coding regions of the eukaryotic genome (Yang et al., 2019) and account for 1–3% of the human genome (Bagshaw, 2017). They are frequently positioned adjacent to coding sequences, and may also be located in other regions, such as introns (Li et al., 2020).

MSs frequently undergo insertion or deletion of repeat units due to errors by DNA polymerase during replication; however, the MMR system is typically effective in rectifying these errors to maintain genome integrity. The mismatch repair (MMR) mechanism is a system preserved through evolution, essential for safeguarding DNA integrity and cellular homeostasis (Gilson et al., 2021).

Deactivation of MMR genes caused by genetic and epigenetic changes leads to MMR defects, resulting in spontaneous, genome-wide mutations that primarily impact the integrity of MSs, leading to microsatellite instability (MSI); and increasing the risk of developing cancer (Gilson et al., 2021).

2.3 UNDERSTANDING THE ROLES OF ONCOGENES IN CANCER DEVELOPMENT

Oncogenes can be triggered through point mutations, gene amplification, and chromosomal rearrangements. These genetic abnormalities result in the persistent activation of signaling pathways that facilitate cell proliferation, suppress apoptosis, and augment other malignant characteristics like as invasion and metastasis. Understanding the role of oncogenes in cancer progression is crucial for the advancement of targeted treatments. Researchers and physicians can discover and suppress specific oncogenes associated with various tumors to develop more effective treatments with fewer adverse effects than traditional chemotherapy. Oncogenes are essential in the conversion of healthy cells into malignant cells, and their study is crucial for the development of new cancer treatments.

2.3.1 Unchecked Cell Proliferation and Dysregulation of the Cell Cycle

Controlled cell proliferation is achieved through the strict regulation of the cell cycle (Figure 2.2). Cancer is characterized by the dysregulation of the cell cycle machinery, which results in uncontrolled proliferation (Cavalu et al., 2024). This cycle is composed of four distinct phases: G1 (gap 1), S (synthesis), G2 (gap 2), and M (mitosis). The fidelity of cell division is guaranteed by the specific checkpoints and regulatory proteins that govern each phase.

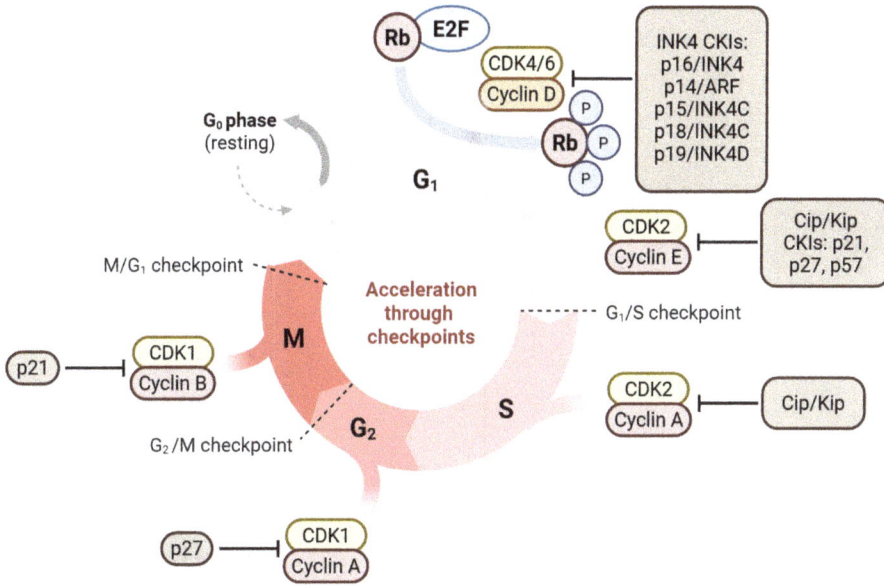

Figure 2.2 An overview of the cell cycle regulation: A representation of the main cdk/cyclin complexes with their major regulators. Adapted from Vermeulen et al. (2003). The figure was created with Biorender.com

2.3.1.1 The Role of Cell Cycle Regulators

Cyclins, cyclin-dependent kinases (CDKs), and tumor-suppressor proteins are among the most significant regulators of the cell cycle. Cyclins are a collection of proteins that exhibit periodic expression and controlled degradation, resulting in fluctuations in their levels throughout the cell cycle. Cyclins activate and direct CDKs to specific substrate sets that facilitate cell cycle progression by interacting with CDKs, as illustrated in Figure 2.2.

Out of the numerous members of the mammalian cyclin family, only a small number, including cyclins A (A1 and A2), B, D (D1, D2, and D3), and E (E1 and E2), are recognized as playing critical roles in the progression of the cell cycle. CDK is a member of a family of serine/threonine protein kinases that are proline-dependent and are essential for the regulation of cell cycle progression. CDKs cyclically engage in phosphorylation activities by interacting with their regulatory subunits (cyclins). The precise and orderly progression of events that are essential for the cell cycle is guaranteed by this phosphorylation, which targets a specific set of molecules. The cell cycle is regulated by only a subset of the 20 members of the CDKs (CDK1, CDK2, CDK4, and CDK6), which number 28 and 29. Cyclins and CDKs establish complexes that propel the cell through distinct phases of the cycle. For example, the transition from the G1 to S phase is dependent on the cyclin D-CDK4/6 complex (Cavula et al., 2024).

Tumor-suppressor proteins, including retinoblastoma protein (Rb) and p53, function as brakes to prevent unregulated cell division. In response to DNA damage, p53, which is frequently referred to as the "guardian of the genome," can induce apoptosis or cell cycle arrest (Figure 2.3). The p53 gene is a prominent example of a tumor suppressor that is frequently altered in human malignancies. P53 is a transcription factor that induces the production of proteins that limit cell proliferation and induce cell apoptosis in response to DNA damage. It is essential for the preservation of the G1 to S cell cycle checkpoint. The DNA damage response, which is responsible for preventing cell cycle progression, will be impeded by disabling of p53 genetic mutations. Despite the presence of DNA damage, a cell continues to divide during this process (Chen et al., 2020a).

When pRb activity is inhibited, the genes required for progression into the S phase of the cell cycle are not expressed (Figure 2.4). Thus, the inactivation of pRb results in uncontrolled cellular proliferation. This technique applies to all tumor suppressors; genetic alterations in the gene lead to carcinogenesis, impairing the regulatory protein's capacity to inhibit cell growth. The predominant genetic alterations that cause the inactivation of pRb are frameshifts or deletions in the RB1 gene, resulting in the premature introduction of a stop codon and the synthesis of a defective protein.

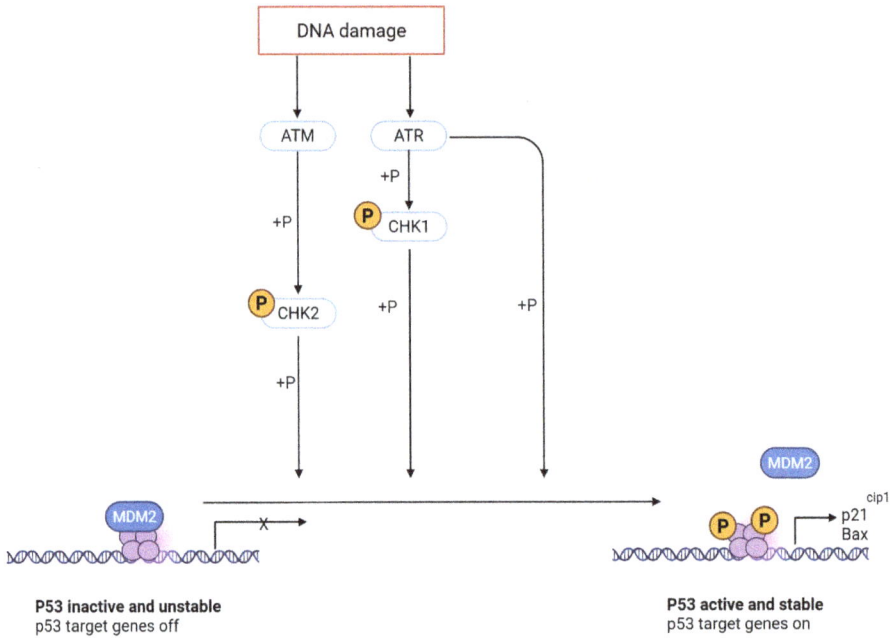

Figure 2.3 Summary of the P53 pathway. DNA damage and other cellular stresses trigger sensor proteins such as ATM (ataxia-telangiectasia mutated) and ATR (ataxia-telangiectasia mutated and Rad3-related kinase), which phosphorylate P53, leading to stabilization. P53 is mainly regulated by MDM2, which is a P53 target, thus forming a negative feedback loop. Adapted from Hernández Borrero and El-Deiry (2021). The figure was created by Biorender.com

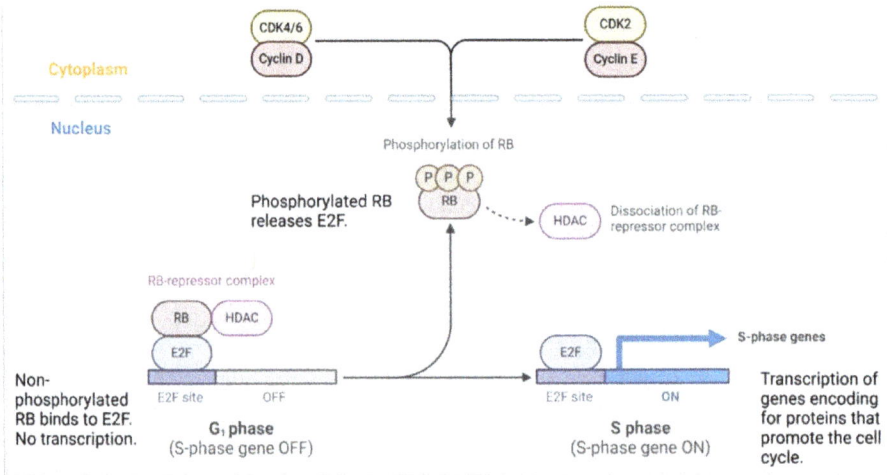

Figure 2.4 The pRB pathway: E2F family of transcription factors coordinates the transcription of genes that are required for cell cycle progression. When bound to pRb, E2F-mediated transcriptional activity is reduced, and cell cycle progression is prevented. Adapted from Munro et al. (2012). The figure was created by Biorender.com

At times, pRb expression may remain intact, although the functionality of its operational pathway is compromised due to the inactivity of other pathway components (Dakal et al. 2024). Tumor-suppressor genes, including TP53 (which encodes p53) and RB1 (which encodes Rb), when rendered inactive by mutations, forfeit their capacity to impede the cell cycle in reaction to DNA damage or other stressors. Mutations in a single allele within a cell can inhibit the function of the

P53 protein, as all tetramers will incorporate at least one mutant P53 protein. Mutations of the P53 tumor-suppressor gene are consequently widespread. The retinoblastoma protein functions as a monomer, resulting in residual mutations. Loss of heterozygosity may result from intermediate deficiencies, chromosomal deletions, or aberrant mitotic divisions, and is believed to indicate the loss of one or more tumor-suppressor genes (Kontomanolis et al., 2020).

Changes in the expression or activity of cyclins and CDK inhibitors, as well as mutations in genes encoding CDKs or their regulators, can disrupt the normal progression of the cell cycle and result in uncontrolled cell division. Unchecked progression of the cell cycle can be achieved through the over-expression of cyclins, including cyclin D, or CDKs. This overexpression may be the consequence of increased transcriptional activity or gene amplification (Almalki, 2023). In cancer cells, proteins that inhibit cyclin-CDK complexes, including p21 and p27, can be downregulated or mutated. This loss eliminates critical safeguards that prevent uncontrolled proliferation. Uncontrolled cell division and the development of cancer can result from the dysregulation of cyclin expression and activity. For instance, the uncontrolled proliferation of cancer cells can result from the overexpression of cyclin D, which is a prevalent characteristic of numerous cancer types (Almalki, 2023).

2.3.1.2 Consequences of Dysregulation

The dysregulation of the cell cycle results in various malignant characteristics, including uncon-trolled proliferation, wherein cells divide incessantly, forming tumors; genomic instability, char-acterized by the absence of adequate checkpoints that permit the continuation of division in cells with DNA damage, culminating in mutations and chromosomal abnormalities; and resistance to apoptosis, whereby cancer cells frequently evade programmed cell death, enabling their survival and proliferation despite damage or stress (Kontomanolis et al., 2020; Alkmalki, 2023).

Comprehending the processes of cell cycle dysregulation holds considerable therapeutic signifi-cance. Targeted therapies seek to reestablish the normal regulation of the cell cycle or capitalize on the weaknesses of cancer cells. For instance, CDK inhibitors such as palbociclib inhibit CDK4/6, hence arresting the cell cycle in neoplastic cells, while checkpoint inhibitors can reactivate tumor-suppressor mechanisms, facilitating cell cycle arrest or apoptosis in neoplastic cells (Almalki, 2023).

Uncontrolled cell proliferation and cell cycle dysregulation are fundamental to cancer progres-sion. By clarifying these systems, researchers can create targeted treatments that provide more effective and less hazardous therapy alternatives for cancer patients.

2.3.2 Genomic Instability and Metabolic Reprogramming

Cancer is characterized by a series of complex biological processes, among which genomic insta-bility and metabolic reprogramming are pivotal. These processes not only drive the initiation and progression of cancer but also contribute to its heterogeneity and resistance to therapy.

2.3.2.1 Genomic Instability

Genomic instability is a characteristic of cancer that results in an escalation of genetic changes, hence facilitating the attainment of extra capacities necessary for carcinogenesis and develop-ment (Moon et al., 2019). Genomic instability denotes a range of DNA modifications, from single nucleotide variations to entire chromosome mutations, and is generally classified into three groups according to the extent of genetic disruption. Nucleotide instability (NIN) is defined by an elevated occurrence of base substitutions, deletions, and insertions of one or a few nucleotides; microsatellite instability (MIN or MSI) arises from deficiencies in mismatch repair genes, resulting in the expansion and contraction of short nucleotide repeats known as microsatellites; chromo-somal instability (CIN) represents the most common type of genomic instability, causing altera-tions in both chromosome number and structure. Although instability is a hallmark of nearly all human malignancies, cancer genomes exhibit significant variation in both the extent and nature of genomic instability present. The instability phenotype significantly affects patient prognosis and therapy, particularly in the selection of therapeutic drugs (Pikor et al., 2013).

2.3.2.1.1 Mechanisms of Genomic Instability

Genomic instability plays a critical role in cancer development and progression. Defects in DNA repair mechanisms, particularly mutations in genes like BRCA1/2, lead to the accumulation of DNA damage. This is compounded by replication stress, where errors during DNA replication can result in mutations and chromosomal abnormalities. Additionally, chromosomal instability, char-acterized by structural alterations such as translocations, deletions, and amplifications, further facilitates cancer growth (Huang and Zhou, 2021).

The implications of genomic instability are substantial. The accumulation of mutations can activate oncogenes and silence tumor-suppressor genes, resulting in cancerous cells. Moreover, genomic instability contributes to tumor heterogeneity, creating a variety of neoplastic cells with distinct genetic profiles. This heterogeneity is a key factor in treatment resistance and disease advancement, as it allows for the selection of resistant clones under therapeutic pressure. Thus, genomic instability not only initiates cancer but also promotes its evolution and adaptation, posing significant challenges for effective treatment (Moon et al., 2019).

2.3.2.2 Metabolic Reprogramming

Metabolic reprogramming denotes the capacity of cancer cells to alter their metabolism, enhancing the uptake and utilization of carbohydrates, lipids, and proteins to facilitate a pro-tumorigenic response while acquiring and sustaining malignant characteristics. Numerous elements influence metabolic reprogramming: oncogenes, growth factors, hypoxia-inducible factors, and the impairment of tumor-suppressor genes. These modifications induce changes in cellular metabolism, particularly glucose, whose absorption rate significantly escalates (Warburg effect) in cancer. Metabolic reprogramming enables cancer cells to acclimate to significant alterations in the tumor microenvironment. Tumors develop chemoresistance, residual disease, and relapse in response to standard antineoplastic treatments. Its significance remains incompletely elucidated; however, it is regarded as a prospective therapeutic target in cancer treatment (Xu et al., 2023; Navarro et al., 2022; Yoshida, 2015).

2.3.2.2.1 Mechanisms of Metabolic Reprogramming

Oncogene activation plays a crucial role in the metabolic reprogramming of cancer cells. Oncogenes like MYC and RAS are known to induce metabolic alterations that support the rapid proliferation of these cells. These changes are further influenced by the tumor microenvironment, where conditions such as hypoxia and nutrient scarcity drive additional metabolic adaptations. In addition, epigenetic modifications contribute to the regulation of metabolic genes. Alterations in DNA methylation and histone modifications can lead to changes in gene expression, which in turn affect cellular metabolism (Xu et al., 2023). The implications of metabolic reprogramming in cancer are significant:

Glycolysis Dependency: Cancer cells often rely on glycolysis for ATP synthesis, even when oxygen is available, a phenomenon known as the Warburg effect.

Metabolite Accumulation: The build-up of metabolites like lactate can create an environment that promotes tumor growth and helps cancer cells evade the immune system.

Therapeutic Resistance: The ability of cancer cells to adapt their metabolism allows them to survive under harsh conditions, contributing to resistance against various treatments.

These insights into cancer metabolism highlight potential therapeutic interventions, such as targeting specific metabolic pathways that are crucial for cancer cell survival and proliferation.

2.3.2.2.2 Interaction between Genomic Instability and Metabolic Reprogramming

The interaction between genomic instability and metabolic reprogramming establishes a detrimental cycle that facilitates cancer advancement. Genomic instability can induce mutations in metabolic genes, hence augmenting the metabolic flexibility of cancer cells. Conversely, metabolic reprogramming can produce reactive oxygen species (ROS) and other by-products that induce DNA damage, hence worsening genomic instability. Comprehending the mechanics and ramifications of genomic instability and metabolic reprogramming is essential for formulating successful cancer treatments. Targeting these mechanisms may affect the survival and multiplication of cancer cells, presenting new therapy opportunities. Advancements in research indicate that medicines targeting both genomic instability and metabolic reprogramming may enhance cancer outcomes (Xu et al., 2023).

2.3.3 Tumor Microenvironment Modification and Immune Evasion

The tumor microenvironment (TME) is a complex and dynamic milieu that interacts with tumor cells and is crucial for cancer dissemination. The tumor microenvironment (TME) has several cellular and acellular constituents, including neoplastic cells, stromal cells (mesenchymal stem cells and fibroblasts), immune cells (macrophages, dendritic cells, T cells, and B cells), extracellular matrix (ECM), and various signaling chemicals. These components are not independent; instead, they engage in constant and complex interactions that profoundly affect tumor behavior, encompassing its development, longevity, and capacity to metastasize to other areas of the body (El-Tanani et al., 2024).

Tumors can utilize multiple ways to resist immune system responses, including the limiting of antigen recognition, immune system suppression, and the production of T-cell exhaustion. Moreover, cancers obstruct or evade the immune system by either limiting the nutrients available to immune cells or by collecting certain metabolites and signaling molecules inside the tumor microenvironment (Kim and Cho, 2022).

TME utilizes the establishment of an immunosuppressive environment as a crucial strategy for immune evasion. This occurs through the recruitment of regulatory T cells (Tregs) and myeloid-derived suppressor cells (MDSCs), which inhibit the functional activities of cytotoxic T cells and natural killer (NK) cells (Kalia et al., 2024). The tumor microenvironment (TME) secretes many immunosuppressive cytokines, including TGF-β and IL-10, which inhibit the immune response and promote tumor development. Immune checkpoint molecules, such as PD-L1 on tumor cells and PD-1 on T cells, exist in the tumor microenvironment to facilitate immune evasion. The combination of these drugs inhibits T-cell function, leading to T-cell exhaustion and reduced immunological responses to malignancies. Moreover, the tumor microenvironment might modify the processes of antigen presentation, thereby diminishing the recognition of cancer cells by the immune system. This approach may entail the suppression of major histocompatibility complex (MHC) molecules in cancer cells, hence hindering the presentation of tumor antigens and reducing T-cell recognition (El-Tanani et al., 2024).

These mechanisms collaboratively enable the tumor microenvironment to create a protective barrier around cancer cells, allowing them to evade immune detection and destruction. Thus, this poses significant challenges to cancer immunotherapy strategies aimed at reactivating the immune response against malignancies.

2.3.4 Apoptosis and Cellular Immortality Inhibition

Cancer cells possess two essential traits that facilitate their unregulated proliferation and persistence: the suppression of apoptosis (programmed cell death) and the attainment of cellular immortality. Comprehending these processes is crucial for formulating successful cancer treatments.

2.3.4.1 Apoptosis

Apoptosis destroys unwanted, excessive, and damaged cells to maintain tissue homeostasis. Individual cells undergo energy-dependent apoptosis. Apoptosis dysregulation causes neurodegenerative illnesses that entail excessive apoptosis, as well as cancer, which is characterized by cell accumulation and apoptosis evasion. There are two types of apoptosis: intrinsic and extrinsic. Cysteine aspartyl-specific proteases, or "caspases," are the ultimate effectors of apoptosis, breaking down many proteins and killing cells through both pathways. Death receptors from the tumor necrosis factor (TNF) superfamily, including Fas (Apo/CD95), TNF Receptor 1 (TNFR1), TRAIL receptors, and others, can activate the extrinsic route by attaching to their respective ligands. The B-cell lymphoma (BCL-2) protein family controls the intrinsic (mitochondrial) pathway, which is activated by internal stress sensors in response to cellular difficulties such as food restriction, DNA damage, hypoxia, and so on.

Multiple mechanisms are employed by cancer cells to elude cell death, one of which is the dysregulation of the intrinsic apoptosis pathway. Numerous malignancies demonstrate an increase in anti-apoptotic BCL-2 proteins and a decrease in pro-apoptotic BH3 proteins. The fusion of the BCL-2 gene locus with the immunoglobulin heavy chain locus on the chromosome was the result of the chromosomal translocation associated with follicular lymphoma. The variable heavy chain genes were reciprocally translocated to chromosome 18. In numerous solid tumors and hematological malignancies, there has been an increase in the expression of BCL-2. Numerous methods have been employed to identify elevated levels of BCL-xL and MCL-1, which have been shown to promote carcinogenesis. Numerous malignancies activate pathways that stabilize MCL-1, a protein that is highly unstable and characterized by rapid turnover because of proteasomal degradation. Conversely, the downregulation of pro-apoptotic proteins functions as an additional mechanism to prevent the initiation of apoptosis. In numerous malignancies, the loss of the p53 tumor suppressor has been observed, which increases the expression of pro-apoptotic BH3-only proteins, including PUMA, BID, and NOXA. In numerous malignancies, the pro-apoptotic effectors BAX and BAK have been observed to be downregulated (Sharma et al., 2019).

2.3.4.2 Cellular Immortality

Cancer cells can sustain stable telomere length, therefore evading senescence and apoptosis, and attaining biological immortality. Preliminary studies have revealed two biological mechanisms associated with the maintenance of telomeric length: the transcriptional activation of the telomerase enzyme and the alternative lengthening of telomeres (ALT). The former is found in almost 90% of cancer cells, while the latter comprises the remaining percentage (de Bardet et al., 2023). As a result, cancer cells will persist in dividing, hence facilitating tumor proliferation. The processes that regulate telomere length may also contribute to genomic instability, hence promoting cancer progression.

The suppression of apoptosis and the attainment of cellular immortality are essential to cancer genesis and progression. By comprehending these processes, researchers can formulate tailored medicines that reinstate apoptotic pathways or obstruct the mechanisms that grant immortality to cancer cells. These medicines show potential for enhancing cancer therapy efficacy and alleviating the burden of the disease.

2.3.5 Cancer Stem Cell Invasion, Metastasis, and Maintenance

Cancer stem cells (CSCs) are acknowledged as the principal catalysts of tumor genesis, progression of epithelial-mesenchymal transition (EMT), and metastasis (Loh and Ma, 2024). CSCs, derived from hematologic and solid malignancies, exhibit quiescence, pluripotency, and self-renewal akin to normal stem cells, hence promoting tumor heterogeneity and progression. Cancer stem cells transition from differentiated cancer cells through a dynamic interaction with the tumor microenvironment and intricate signaling pathways, leading to therapeutic resistance and disease recurrence (Dakal et al., 2020).

Epithelial-mesenchymal transition (EMT) is a process in which epithelial cells gain mesenchymal characteristics, hence augmenting their migratory and invasive powers. Cancer stem cells frequently undergo EMT, facilitating their detachment from the main tumor, invasion of adjacent tissues, and entry into the bloodstream. Essential regulators of EMT are transcription factors including Snail, Slug, and Twist, which inhibit epithelial indicators (e.g., E-cadherin) and enhance mesenchymal markers (e.g., N-cadherin, vimentin). The tumor microenvironment, comprising stromal cells, immune cells, and extracellular matrix components, facilitates cancer stem cell invasion and metastasis. Cancer-associated fibroblasts (CAFs) release substances that facilitate the migration and invasion of cancer stem cells (CSCs).

CSCs facilitate angiogenesis, the development of new blood vessels, by releasing pro-angiogenic molecules such as VEGF2. This process delivers nutrients and oxygen to the tumor while also facilitating the entry of cancer stem cells into the bloodstream, enabling metastasis to distant organs. Multiple signaling pathways, such as Wnt/β-catenin, Notch, and Hedgehog, are essential for preserving cancer stem cell characteristics. These mechanisms govern the self-renewal, differentiation, and survival of cancer stem cells (CSCs). Dysregulation of these pathways may result in the proliferation of the cancer stem cell population and facilitate tumor growth and therapeutic resistance (Chu et al., 2024).

CSCs inhabit specialized microenvironments termed niches, which deliver signals that preserve their stemness. These niches are frequently situated in hypoxic areas of the tumor, where diminished oxygen levels contribute to the maintenance of CSC characteristics. The interplay between cancer stem cells and their microenvironments encompasses several cell types and extracellular matrix constituents that facilitate cancer stem cell viability and self-renewal. Cancer stem cells demonstrate resistance to standard treatments, including chemotherapy and radiotherapy, owing to their proficient DNA repair capabilities, dormant status, and the production of drug efflux pumps. This resistance facilitates tumor recurrence and spread, as cancer stem cells can endure treatment and reconstitute the tumor (Dakal et al., 2024).

Cancer stem cells have critical roles in tumor invasion, metastasis, and maintenance. Their capacity to undergo EMT, interact with the TME, and maintain angiogenesis helps them spread to distant organs. Furthermore, the persistence of CSCs via signaling pathways and habitats, combined with their resistance to therapy, emphasizes the importance of tailored treatments that precisely target these cells. By focusing on CSCs, researchers hope to develop more effective medicines that can prevent metastasis and lower the likelihood of cancer recurrence.

2.4 CLINICAL IMPLICATIONS OF ONCOGENE ACTIVATION

The clinical implications of oncogene activation in cancer research are crucial for understanding how certain genes can contribute to the growth and spread of cancer cells (MacConaill and Garraway, 2010). Oncogenes are altered versions of normal genes known as proto-oncogenes, which regulate cellular growth and division (Shortt and Johnstone, 2012). Activation of these genes can lead to uncontrolled cell proliferation and bypass standard regulatory mechanisms.

The process usually leads to the development of tumors that can advance from non-cancerous to malignant states (Zhou et al., 2024). Additionally, specific mutations in oncogenes can act as indicators for different types of cancers. For instance, the presence of BCR-ABL fusion genes is a sign of chronic myeloid leukemia (Abdulmawjood et al., 2021). Additionally, the level and nature of oncogene activation can also offer insights into the prognosis. For example, overexpression of HERS2 in breast cancer has been linked to the progression of the disease (Swain et al., 2023; Cheng, 2024).

Oncogene activation profiles can determine the use of targeted therapies tailored for patients. These therapies are designed specifically to inhibit the activity of oncogenes (Min and Lee, 2022). For instance, medications such as imatinib are crafted to target the BCR-ABL tyrosine kinase in individuals with leukemia. Targeted therapies can lead to improved response rates and reduced side effects compared to traditional methods like chemotherapy (Braun et al., 2020). Additionally, activation of oncogenes can lead to resistance against standard cancer treatments, and research into oncogene activation can help identify mechanisms of resistance, which in turn can help researchers and clinicians modify treatment plans, such as combining therapies or developing second-generation inhibitors (Liu et al., 2024).

The presence of specific activated oncogenes can serve as biomarkers for the diagnosis of diverse types of cancers. Identifying oncogene mutations in high-risk individuals can facilitate early detection and intervention (Zhou et al., 2024). Moreover, some oncogene mutations are hereditary, necessitating genetic counselling and screening of family members (Singh et al., 2023). Additionally, oncogene activation patterns can inform about the cancer's aggressiveness and progression. Moreover, quantitative measurement of oncogene activation can help detect Minimal Residual Disease (MRD) after treatment (Tyner et al., 2022; Zhou et al., 2024). Therefore, monitoring the effectiveness of therapy and potential relapse is possible in cancer patients. Additionally, ongoing monitoring allows for adjustments in treatment protocols (Graham et al., 2014).

2.4.1 BRAF Therapy Targeting in Cancer

Targeting BRA and cancer treatment to treat cancer have been a focus of study and medical advancement since mutations in the BRA gene have an impact on the V600E mutation linked to types of cancer. The BRA gene produces a protein kinase that plays a role in the MAP/ERK signaling pathway controlling cell growth and division. Recent studies have categorized BRA mutations into three groups based on their functions (Li et al., 2015; Imani et al., 2024). Class 1, V600 mutations are marked by high kinase activity, and they show MEK/ERK signaling activation as RAS-independent monomers. Class 2 mutations also involve intermediate kinase activity and exhibit RAS-independent activation of MEK/ERK signaling in a dimer with BRAF (Graham et al., 2014). Meanwhile, class 3 mutations show reduced kinase activity and rely on RAS for signaling activation (Dankner et al., 2018). Class 3 mutations are more likely associated with long-term survival than class 1 and class 2 mutations (Schirripa et al., 2019). Moreover, patients with BRAF mutations may respond to treatments based on their mutation class. Patients with classes 2 and 3 BRAF mutations do not show a response to RAF inhibitors. However, class 3 mutants depend on RAS and may benefit from EGFR treatments (Dankner et al., 2018; Özgü et al., 2024).

Mutation in the BRAF gene, particularly the V600E mutation, causes activation of pathways that lead to uncontrolled cell proliferation and survival in the context of mutation studies concerning cancer development, like metastatic melanoma. Studies indicate that around half of melanoma cases are linked to BRAF mutations, which are more prevalent in people occasionally or chronically exposed to the sun. Moreover, BRAF-mutated melanomas exhibit more aggressive behavior than wild-type (WT) melanomas. In patients with advanced-stage tumors like stage IV melanoma, there is a chance of cancer spreading to the brain and leading to reduced survival rates (Czarnecka et al., 2020; Castellani et al., 2023). Over the past 10 years in studies and clinical trials, late-stage melanoma treatment options have been explored extensively to improve effectiveness while minimizing side effects. The recent application of checkpoint inhibitors in treating melanoma has shown promising outcomes in prognosis enhancement (Rotte et al., 2015; Boutros et al., 2024).

Nevertheless, 60% of patients faced toxicity due to abnormal immune system activation, leading to damage to healthy tissues. Similarly, to this discovery is the progress in handling melanoma through medications that can block molecular targets (Castellani et al., 2023). As mentioned earlier, melanoma patients with mutations in oncogenes affect around 70% of control pathways in tumor advancement and, subsequently, the rather aggressive characteristics for therapeutic intervention with specific drug-sensitive mutations. Targeted therapy focuses on using substances, like molecules or antibodies, to block the abnormal proteins identified in the study by Castellani et al. (2023). Some examples of targeted BRAFi drugs include dabrafenib, encorafenib and vemurafenib (PLX4032), which specifically interact with mutated BRAF proteins at their ATP-binding site and deactivate them, thus stopping ERK phosphorylation and cell growth in cells with mutations. Vemurafenib was given the green light by the FDA in August 2011 to treat melanoma that cannot be surgically removed (Castellani et al., 2023). Vemurafenib was developed as a low-molecular-weight molecule which inhibits the mutated serine-threonine kinase BRAF, and it selectively binds to the ATP-binding site of BRAF V600E kinase and hence inhibits the MAPK pathway, leading to cellular apoptosis (Garbe and Eigentler, 2018). Clinical trials showed positive results, but despite the initial therapeutic response observed in most patients, the early resistant relapse remains the central limit of this therapeutic strategy (Garbe and Eigentler, 2018). In 2013, the FDA gave approval for Dabrafenib as a BRAFi drug option, which is almost 20 times more specific for BRAF V600E mutants in a variety of cancer cell types, with a lower IC50 level for greater effectiveness in comparison with other BRAFis (Bowyer et al., 2015). Additionally, Encorafenib was among the BRAFi medications to receive FDA approval and functions as an ATP-competitive RAF serine/threonine kinase inhibitor. This medication has proven more effective in treating metastatic melanoma than vemurafenib (Rose, 2019; Anaya et al., 2025).

In individuals diagnosed with advanced melanomas carrying the BRAF V600 mutation, utilizing the three combinations of BRAFi alongside MEKi may lead to better clinical results than using BRAFi alone. For instance, vemurafenib combined with cobimetinib outperforms vemurafenib; dabrafenib and trametinib surpass dabrafenib alone; encorafenib paired with binimetinib shows better outcomes than encorafenib alone (Long et al., 2019). (Figure 2.5)

2.4.1.1 Colorectal Cancer

Colorectal cancer ranks as the second most common form of cancer in women and third most in men globally, with around 1.8 million new cases and close to 880,800 fatalities in 2018 (Morris and Bekail-Saab, 2020). Approximately 10% of colorectal cancers carry BRAF mutations (Caputo et al., 2019; Sun et al., 2022), making it vital to focus on addressing these mutations due to their unfavorable impact on prognosis in colorectal cancer (CRC) (Potocki et al., 2023). The BRAF V600E mutation is crucial in developing CRC cases and has been a critical target for various treatment approaches (Clarke and Kopetz, 2015).

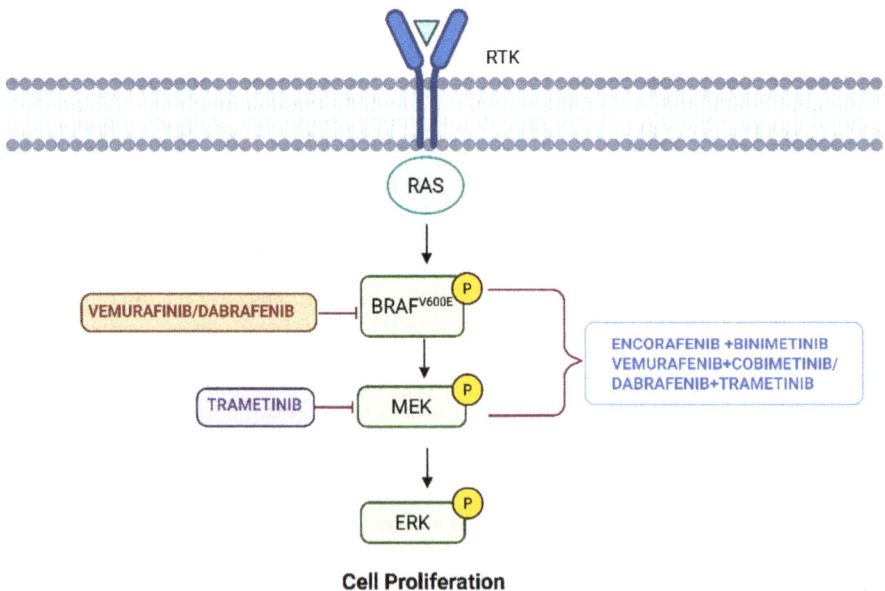

Figure 2.5 Targeted therapies for metastatic melanoma. Activation of receptor tyrosine kinases (RTKs) triggers the MAPK signaling pathway, leading to uncontrolled cell proliferation. BRAF inhibitors (vemurafenib, dabrafenib) selectively block BRAF V600E activity, while the MEK inhibitor (trametinib) prevents downstream signaling. Combination therapies (encorafenib + binimetinib, vemurafenib + cobimetinib, or dabrafenib + trametinib) effectively inhibit both BRAF and MEK, enhancing treatment efficacy (from Castellani et al., 2023, under Creative Commons Attribution licence). The figure was created by Biorender.com

Two meta-analyses to date have investigated how using that target EGFR may impact the treatment of cancer in BRAF-mutated mCRC. While these studies hinted at an improvement in survival rates with EGFR therapy for progression-free survival (PFS) as well as overall survival (OS), they did not find a clear statistical significance in the results (Rowland et al., 2015; Pietrantonio et al., 2015). Previously, in the VOLFI trial (also known as AIO KRK0109), a randomized phase II trial was carried out to explore the benefits of adding panitumumab to chemotherapy with FOLFOXIRI for patients with BRAF-mutated mCRC. The results showed that the overall response rate (ORR) for patients receiving FOLFOXIRI plus panitumumab was 86% higher than the 22% ORR in patients receiving FOLFOXIRI alone. Despite the ORRs, the progression-free survival (PFS) was modest. The PFS was 6.5 and 6.1 months for the FOLFOXIRI plus panitumumab and FOLFOXIRI-alone arms, respectively (Modest et al., 2019).

Monotherapy with BRAF inhibitors in mCRC is less promising than melanoma. For example, the efficacy of encorafenib as a monotherapy for 18 mCRC patients with BRAF V600E–mutation was tested in a phase I dose-escalation study. Unfortunately, this yielded no responses among the patients. A stable disease status was achieved for 12 patients, with a PFS of 4.0 months (Gomez-Roca et al., 2014). Another study on 21 patients with BRAF-mutated mCRC, using vemurafenib treatment, showed that one patient responded to the treatment. The study also revealed that seven patients had stable disease as the best response, and the median PFS was 2.1 months (Kopetz et al., 2015).

Furthermore, a study involving ten patients with mCRC who were treated with vemurafenib monotherapy for BRAF V600E–mutated cancers did not show any positive response to the treatment. In both in vitro and in vivo studies, it has been found that the lack of response was due to the quick reactivation of ERK through the EGFR feedback activation mechanism. This led researchers to believe that combining BRAF inhibitors and anti-EGFR antibody medications could enhance the effectiveness expected in mCRC cases. Therefore, a combination of vemurafenib and cetuximab was attempted in another cohort. However, out of the 27 patients involved in the study, only one showed improvement (Hyman et al., 2015). Similarly, a study testing dabrafenib in patients with various solid tumors showed a partial response in only 1 of 11 patients with BRAFV600E-mutant colorectal cancer (Falchook et al., 2012).

The limited effectiveness of using single-agent BRAF inhibitors in treating BRAFV600E-mutant mCRC in comparison to BRAFV600E-mutant melanoma and other types of tumors may be because, in cancer specifically, when BRAF is inhibited, it triggers a quick feedback activation of EGFR, permitting sustained MAPK activation and continued cell growth (Prahallad et al., 2012, Corcoran et al., 2012). The lack of effectiveness of monotherapy with BRAF and EGFR inhibitors to treat BRAFV600E-mutant colorectal cancer has driven a multitargeted approach to treatment (Kopetz et al., 2015; Piercey et al., 2024). The advantages of this approach become more evident when both BRAF and EGFR are employed together. Inhibitors of BRAF cause feedback activation of EGFR in mutant BRAFV600E colorectal cancer, leading to continued cell proliferation, whereas EGFR-mediated MAPK pathway reactivation leads to resistance to BRAF inhibition (Prahallad et al., 2012; Corcoran et al., 2012). Consequently, combining BRAF inhibitors and anti-EGFR agents may overcome this feedback loop (Prahallad et al., 2012; Corcoran et al., 2012). In a study where 142 participants were involved and 20 patients received both dabrafenib and the anti-EGFR agent, panitumumab, for their treatment against EGFR-related issues, it was found that the positive response rate was noted at 10% in this group. The median PFS and overall survival (OS) were reported to be approximately 3.5 and 13.2 months, respectively (Corcoran et al., 2018).

Research and clinical advancements in targeting BRAF mutations in colorectal cancer show promise for further research in the field. The approval of therapies targeting BRAF mutations along with EGFR for cancers with BRAF V600E mutations, alongside the investigation of combination therapies and novel approaches, provide optimism for enhancing outcomes in this challenging subset of CRC. Ongoing research and clinical trials will contribute to advancing our knowledge and enhancing the management of cancer BRAF-mutant colorectal cancer.

2.4.2 Amplification of N-myc in Neuroblastoma

The amplification of N-myc (also referred to as MYCN) in cases of neuroblastoma is a recognized indicator linked to a poor prognosis and rapid advancement of the disease severity level in individuals affected by it during childhood years. Neuroblastoma (NB), the most common extracranial solid malignancy among children and adolescents, is a rapidly progressive, fatal tumor in over 50% of diagnosed cases. In contrast, progress in treatment outcomes for high-risk patients has been slow compared to pediatric cancers, leading to overall survival rates (Castleberry, 1997). The increase in activity of the MYCN gene results in the overexpression of the N-Myc oncoprotein, which plays a vital role in neuroblastoma development (Matthay et al., 2016; Weiss et al., 1997). N-Myc interacts with another protein called basic helix-loop–loop–helix zipper protein, Max, through its basic helix-loop–loop–helix zipper domain, to form a transcription factor that attaches to DNA sequences known as Myc-responsive enhancer box (E-box). The binding of this component triggers the activation of genes for cellular functions, such as cell growth, proliferation, metabolism, apoptosis, and differentiation (Dang, 2012; Eilers and Eisenman, 2008; Schütz et al., 2022). The N-Myc oncoprotein is perceived as a difficult target because it lacks active sites for ligands to attach to and has not yet crystallized (Soucek and Evan, 2010; Beltran, 2014). Thus, rather than targeting N-Myc directly, targeting downstream factors vital for N-Myc's oncogenic effects is an attractive approach for treating MYCN-amplified neuroblastoma (Putra et al., 2021). RNA helicases fall into six superfamilies; among them are the DEAD-box helicases known for their involvement in ATP binding and hydrolysis, intramolecular rearrangements, and their interactions with RNA interactions (Sloan and Bohnsack, 2018; Cai et al., 2017). The DEAD-box RNA helicase protein (DDX21) is involved in interacting with different types of species of RNA and RNA polymerase I- and II-transcribed genes. It helps release the positive transcription elongation factor b (P-TEFb) from the 7SK ribonucleoproteins through a helicase-driven process and supports the transcription of target genes (Calo et al., 2015). DDX21 plays a role in untangling and unwinding the R loops and overcomes the R-loop-mediated stalling of RNA polymerases. By resolving estrogen-induced R loops on estrogen-responsive genes in breast cancer cells, DDX21 promotes transcription elongation (Song et al., 2017). N-Myc and c-Myc oncoproteins are widely recognized for their role in promoting tumor formation by attaching to Myc-responsive E-boxes located at the promotors of target genes to initiate gene transcription (Eilers and Eisenman, 2008; Dang, 2012). Another study by Putra et al. identified two Myc-responsive E-boxes were identified within the promotor region of the DDX21 gene; their ChIP experiments confirmed the binding of N-Myc to the DDX21 gene promoter. Reducing the levels of N-Myc through knockdown techniques led to a decrease in both mRNA and protein levels of DDX21. In studies conducted with human neuroblastoma tissues, a strong connection between increased levels of DDX21 and N-Myc expression leads to a bleak prognosis for patients regardless of standard prognostic markers (Putra et al., 2021). As a result of this finding, they hypothesized that DDX21 and CEP55 are potential therapeutic targets for MYCN-amplified neuroblastoma. The development of small molecule inhibitors targeting DDX21 was proposed by implementing helicase targeting approaches to those used for DDX3 and DDX41 inhibitors (Putra et al., 2021).

Another study by Maeda H. (2010) revealed that specific siRNA-targeted MYCN, known as siMYCN, could potentially be utilized in treating neuroblastoma through the systemic administration of the siRNA encapsulated in a nanoparticle formulation. Neuroblastoma tumors are known for being highly vascularized and possessing endothelium that could facilitate the entry of nanoparticles into the tumor from the bloodstream (Maeda, 2010). The study demonstrated suppression of MYCN in vitro in neuroblastoma cells without causing significant harm to the cells. Receptor-targeted nano (RTNs) address a challenge in creating siRNA cancer treatments by evading liver clearance and accumulating in the tumor due to a leaky tumor/endothelial barrier. These RTNs also possess integrin-targeting and fusogenic characteristics that facilitate efficient transfection of the target tumor cells. Anionic receptor-targeted nano complexes (RTNs) were shown to possess efficiency and specificity to their cationic counterparts while providing lower systemic and cellular toxicity levels. In vivo, these RTNs effectively penetrate the tumor site with little off-target biodistribution and deliver genetic material to tumor cells in an integrin-mediated fashion. Administering siMYCN through this method led to tumor growth suppression and prolonged the lifespan of the mice. These nano complexes enhanced nucleic acid delivery and could provide improved non-viral vectors to deliver gene therapies for a variety of disorders (Tagalakis et al., 2021).

Inactivation of β1-integrin by FNIII14 leads to proteasomal degradation in N-Myc of neuroblastoma cells with MYCN amplification. A study by Sasada et al. (2019) highlighted the significance of inactivating β1-integrins by FNIII14 for targeting Myc proteins. Since integrin-mediated cell adhesion to the ECM is essential for fundamental cell functions, including survival, proliferation, differentiation, and gene expression, β1-integrin inactivation by FNIII14 may exhibit cytotoxic solid effects on normal cells. However, tissue cells adhere to various ECM components using several membrane receptors, such as the β2-6 subfamily of integrins and transmembrane proteoglycans. The study showed that β1-integrin inactivation by FNIII14 is unable to induce cell detachment but does induce de-adhesion, which is defined as the process involving the transition of the cell from a strongly adherent state to a state of intermediate adherence (Sasada et al., 2019)

2.4.3 MiR-1224: A Potential Biomarker and Therapeutic Target

MiR-1224 is a microRNA that controls gene expression by interacting with target messenger RNAs (mRNAs). Numerous studies have highlighted the potential of miR-1224 as both a marker and a promising target, showing its potential as a biomarker and a therapeutic target in different types of cancers, such as hepatocellular carcinoma (HCC) and gastric cancer (GC). One study found that decreased levels of miR-1224 in individuals with HCC were closely linked to unfavorable clinical characteristics and overall prognosis. Their findings revealed a positive feedback loop linked miR-1224 and CREB, where miR-1224 inhibited tumor growth by suppressing the CREB/YAP pathway and was repressed by CREB/EZH2-mediated transcriptional inhibition. Therefore, this indicates that targeting the miR-1224/CREB pathway could be a promising therapeutic strategy for HCC (Yang et al., 2021).

Moreover, miR-1224 can act as a prognostic biomarker and inhibit the progression of GC by targeting SATB1. Furthermore, the overexpression of miR-1224 inhibits β-catenin and c-myc in miR-1224-overexpression cells, proving its therapeutic potential for GC patients (Han et al., 2021). In vivo experiments further showed that miR-1224 could inhibit the growth of tumor cells (Yang et al., 2021). Another study revealed that LINC00665 expression was upregulated in prostate cancer (PC) tissues. Furthermore, LINC00665 upregulation indicated an unsatisfactory prognosis. They showed that LINC00665 could activate SND1 expression via sponging miR-1224-5p. Then, upregulated SND1 expression led to enhanced proliferation, migration and invasion of PC cells (Chen et al., 2020b).

2.4.4 Tyrosine Kinase Blockers in Targeted Cancer Therapies

Tyrosine kinases are intracellular enzymes that mediate the tyrosine phosphorylation of downstream molecules. These kinases are crucial for transmitting signals through cell surface receptors, like growth factor receptors, adhesion receptors, immunoreceptors, and cytokine receptors. Due to their involvement in signaling pathways and their significance in disease treatment strategies, tyrosine kinases have emerged as targets for therapeutic intervention across different medical conditions. For instance, small molecule tyrosine kinase inhibitors have contributed significantly to the pharmacological control of several diseases, including various malignant processes and immune-mediated diseases such as autoimmune and inflammatory conditions. Tyrosine kinase inhibitors (TKIs) are now essential in targeted cancer therapy (Gadina, 2014). Many TKIs are designed to inhibit the catalytic activity of the target kinase by blocking the ATP-binding site. Therefore, this can prevent cellular targets' phosphorylation in cell proliferation (Yamaoka et al., 2018; Crisci et al., 2019). However, due to the structural conservation of the ATP-binding site, many TKIs have inhibitory activity against a broader range of protein kinases, with the potential to affect multiple signaling pathways—the so-called off-target activities (Liu and Kurzrock, 2014). In total, there are 10 groups of non-receptor tyrosine kinase families, for example, Src-family kinases, Janus kinases (also known as Jak-family kinases), Syk tyrosine kinase, and the Btk kinase family (Szilveszter et al., 2019).

The first drug in this class is imatinib mesylate (IMAT), developed specifically for addressing BCR-ABL-associated leukemia and introduced in 2001 (Cohen et al., 2002). More than 40 TKIs have received approval for cancer treatment (Pottier et al., 2020). In the context of breast cancer treatment, HER2-targeted TKIs can trigger therapy-induced senescence. This phenomenon underscores cancer cells' reactions to TKI therapy and emphasizes the necessity for comprehensive treatment strategies (Singh et al., 2022). The way lapatinib works involves triggering senescence marked by increased SA-β-gal activity and increased levels of p15 and p27 expression. Lapatinib has a lasting senescence effect, even after six months of exposure.

In contrast, removing lapatinib from cells in senescence allows them to start growing while still responding well to lapatinib treatment. Their study provided new perspectives on how lapatinib acts and how resistance to lapatinib develops. They also suggested new therapeutic strategies to improve the response to HER2-targeted therapies (McDermott et al., 2019).

2.4.5 Trastuzumab (Herceptin) Development and Efficacy

Breast cancer is the most common cancer among women and the second most frequently newly diagnosed cancer worldwide (Kolak et al., 2017). Herceptin, or Trastuzumab, is a monoclonal antibody designed to target the HER2 receptor that tends to be overexpressed in different types of breast cancers (Nayar et al., 2019). The initial course of action for treating metastatic HER2-positive breast cancer typically involves a combination therapy, including pertuzumab along with Trastuzumab plus taxane (Swain et al., 2020). A recent study by Ozaki et al., 2022 revealed that using a combination of Trastuzumab and fulvestrant to treat HR + HER2+ metastatic breast cancer showed promising results in clinical effectiveness. This study helped shed some light on the effectiveness of Trastuzumab and fulvestrant combination therapy as control data for further development of anti-HER2 agents and hormone therapy (Ozaki et al., 2022)

Trastuzumab is a humanized type of IgG1 monoclonal antibody. In breast cancer cell lines, show that these types of antibodies target the HER2 receptor and can help stop the signals that instruct the tumor cells to proliferate, resulting in cell death and causing changes such as stopping tumor growth, reducing levels of HER2 receptors, reversing resistance to cytokines, restoring E-cadherin expression, and decreasing the production of vascular endothelial growth factor (Sliwkowski et al., 1999; Hudis, 2007).

Its development marked a significant advancement in targeted cancer therapy, particularly for HER2-positive breast cancer patients. Here are critical insights into its development and efficacy. The HER2 (ErbB2) receptor tyrosine kinase is a member of the epidermal growth factor receptor family of transmembrane receptors. These receptors, which also include HER3 (ErbB3) and HER4 (ErbB4), are known to play critical roles in both development and cancer (Yarden and Sliwkowski, 2001). Due to HER2 significance in the development of breast cancer pathogenesis and the accessibility of the extracellular portion of HER2, it was identified as a potential candidate for targeted antibody therapy. The humanized HER2 antibody, Trastuzumab (Herceptin), was approved by the Food and Drug Administration in 1998 for use in treating metastatic breast cancer. The drug has shown positive outcomes and clinical benefits when combined with cytotoxic chemotherapy as first-line or adjuvant therapy (Slamon et al., 2001; Smith et al., 2007). Although the mechanisms for response to Trastuzumab remain unclear, its clinical benefit is a result of interference with signal transduction pathways, impairment of extracellular domain (ECD) cleavage, inhibition of DNA repair, reduction angiogenesis, cell cycle arrest, and antibody-mediated cellular cytotoxicity. Various strategies are being pursued to enhance Trastuzumab's efficacy and address resistance.

REFERENCES

Abdulmawjood B et al. 2021. Genetic biomarkers in chronic myeloid leukemia: What have we learned so far? *Int J Molec Sci*, 22(22):12516.

Almalki WH et al. 2023. Beyond the genome: lncRNAs as regulators of the PI3K/AKT pathway in lung cancer. *Pathol Res Pract*, 251:154852.

Anaya YA et al. 2025. Small molecule B-RAF inhibitors as anti-cancer therapeutics: advances in discovery, development, and mechanistic insights. *Int J Mol Sci*, 26:2676.

Bagshaw ATM. 2017. Functional mechanisms of microsatellite DNA in eukaryotic genomes. *Genome Biol Evolution*, 9(9):2428–2443.

Beltran H. 2014. The N-myc oncogene: maximizing its targets, regulation, and therapeutic potential. *Molec Cancer Res*, 12:815–822.

Boutros A et al. 2024. The treatment of advanced melanoma: current approaches and new challenges. *Crit Rev Oncol Hematol*, 196:104276.

Bowyer S et al. 2015. Dabrafenib and its use in the treatment of metastatic melanoma. *Melanoma Manage*, 2:199–208.

Braun TP et al. 2020. Response and resistance to BCR-ABL1-targeted therapies. *Cancer Cell*, 37(4):530–542.

Brown G. 2021. Oncogenes, proto-oncogenes, and lineage restriction of cancer stem cells. *Int J Mol Sci*, 22(18):9667.

Cai W et al. 2017. Wanted DEAD/H or alive: helicases winding up in cancers. *JNCI J Natl Cancer Inst*, 109(6):djw278.

Calo E et al. 2015. RNA helicase DDX21 coordinates transcription and ribosomal RNA processing. *Nature*, 518:249–253.

Caputo F et al. 2019. BRAF-mutated colorectal cancer: clinical and molecular insights. *Int J Molec Sci,* 20(21):5369.

Castellani G et al. 2023. BRAF mutations in melanoma: Biological aspects, therapeutic implications, and circulating biomarkers. *Cancers,* 15(16):4026.

Castleberry RP. 1997. Biology and treatment of neuroblastoma. *Pediat Clin N Am,* 44:919–937.

Castro-Munoz LJ et al. 2023. Modulating epigenetic modifications for cancer therapy (Review). *Oncol Rep,* 49(3):1–23.

Cavalu, S. et al. 2024. Cell cycle machinery in oncology: A comprehensive review of therapeutic targets. *FASEB,* 38(11): e23734.

Chen L et al. 2020(a). Regulating tumor suppressor genes: Post-translational modifications. *Signal Transduct Target Ther,* 5(1):90.

Chen W et al. 2020(b). LncRNA LINC00665 promotes prostate cancer progression via miR–1224-5p/SND1 axis. *Oncol Target Ther,* 13:2527–2535.

Cheng Z et al. 2016. Knockdown of EHF inhibited the proliferation, invasion and tumorigenesis of ovarian cancer cells. *Mol Carcinog,* 55(6):1048–1059.

Cheng X et al. 2024. A comprehensive review of HER2 in cancer biology and therapeutics. *Genes (Basel),* 15(7):903.

Chu X et al. 2024. Cancer stem cells: advances in knowledge and implications for cancer therapy. *Signal Transduct Target Ther,* 9(1):170.

Clarke CN, Kopetz ES. 2015. BRAF mutant colorectal cancer as a distinct subset of colorectal cancer: Clinical characteristics, clinical behavior, and response to targeted therapies. *J Gastrointest Oncol,* 6:660–667.

Cohen MH et al. 2002. Approval summary for imatinib mesylate capsules in the treatment of chronic myelogenous leukemia. *Clin Cancer Res,* 8:935–942.

Corcoran RB et al. 2012. EGFR-mediated re-activation of MAPK signaling contributes to insensitivity of BRAF mutant colorectal cancers to RAF inhibition with vemurafenib. *Cancer Disc,* 2:227–235.

Corcoran RB et al. 2018. Combined BRAF, EGFR, and MEK inhibition in patients with BRAF(V600E)-mutant colorectal cancer. *Cancer Disc,* 8:428–443.

Crisci S et al. 2019. Overview of current targeted anti-cancer drugs for therapy in onco-hematology. *Medicina,* 55.

Czarnecka AM et al. 2020. Targeted therapy in melanoma and mechanisms of resistance. *Int J Molec Sci,* 21(13):4576.

Dakal TC et al. 2020. Mechanistic basis of co-stimulatory CD40–CD40L ligation mediated regulation of immune responses in cancer and autoimmune disorders. *Immunobiology,* 225(2):151899.

Dakal TC et al. 2024. Oncogenes and tumor suppressor genes: Functions and roles in cancers. *MedComm,* 5(6):e582.

Dang CV. 2012. MYC on the path to cancer. *Cell,* 149:22–35.

Dankner M et al. 2018. Classifying BRAF alterations in cancer: New rational therapeutic strategies for actionable mutations. *Oncogene,* 37:3183–3199.

Davalos V, Esteller M. 2023. Cancer epigenetics in clinical practice. *CA*, 73(4):376–424.

de Bardet JC et al.2023. Cell immortalization: In vivo molecular bases and in vitro techniques for obtention. *BioTech*, 12:14.

Eilers M, Eisenman RN. 2008. Myc's broad reach. *Genes Develop*, 22:2755–66.

El-Tanani M et al. 2024. The complex connection between obesity and cancer: Signaling pathways and therapeutic implications. *Nutr Cancer*, 76(8):683–706.

Esteban-Villarrubia J et al. 2020. Tyrosine kinase receptors in oncology. *Int J Molec Sci*, 21(22):8529.

Falchook GS et al. 2012. Dabrafenib in patients with melanoma, untreated brain metastases, and other solid tumors: A phase 1 dose-escalation trial. *Lancet*, 379:1893–901.

Gadina M. 2014. Advances in kinase inhibition: Treating rheumatic diseases and beyond. *Curr Opinion Rheumatol*, 26:237–243.

Garbe C, Eigentler TK. 2018. Vemurafenib. *Recent Results Cancer Res*, 211:77–89.

Gomez-Roca C et al. 2014. Encorafenib (LGX818), an oral BRAF inhibitor, in patients (pts) with BRAF V600E metastatic colorectal cancer (mCRC): Results of dose expansion in an open-label, phase 1 study. *Ann Oncol*, 25:iv182.

Graham LJ et al. 2014. Current approaches and challenges in monitoring treatment responses in breast cancer. *J Cancer*, 5:58–68.

Gilson P et al. 2021. Detection of microsatellite instability: State of the art and future applications in circulating tumor DNA (ctDNA). *Cancers*, 13(7):1491.

Gong F, Miller KM. 2019. Histone methylation and the DNA damage response. *Mutat Res Rev Mutation Res*, 780:37–47.

Han GD et al. 2021. MiR-1224 Acts as a prognostic biomarker and inhibits the progression of gastric cancer by targeting SATB1. *Front Oncol*, 11:748896.

Hasty P, Montagna C. 2014. Chromosomal Rearrangements in Cancer: Detection and potential causal mechanisms. *Molecular & Cellular Oncology*, 1(1):e29904.

Hernández Borrero LJ et al. 2021. Tumor suppressor p53: biology, signaling pathways, and therapeutic targeting. *Biochim Biophys Acta Rev Cancer*, 1876(1):188556.

Huang R, Zhou PK. 2021. DNA damage repair: historical perspectives, mechanistic pathways and clinical translation for targeted cancer therapy. *Signal Transduct Target Ther*, 6:254.

Hudis CA. 2007. Trastuzumab--mechanism of action and use in clinical practice. *New Engl J Med*, 357:39–51.

Hyman DM et al. 2015. Vemurafenib in multiple nonmelanoma cancers with BRAF V600 mutations. *New Engl J Med* 373:726–36.

Ilango S et al. 2020. Epigenetic alterations in cancer. *Front Biosci-Landmark*, 25(6):1058–1109.

Imani S et al. 2024. The evolution of BRAF-targeted therapies in melanoma: overcoming hurdles and unleashing novel strategies. *Front Oncol*, 14:1504142.

Joshi K et al. 2022. Mechanisms that regulate the activities of TET proteins. *Cellul Molec Life Sci*, 79(7):363.

Kazimierczyk M, Wrzesinski J. 2021. Long non-coding RNA epigenetics. *Int J Molec Sci* 22(11):1–19.

Kalia M et al. 2024. Tumor microenvironment regulates immune checkpoints: Emerging need of combinatorial therapies. *Curr Tissue Microenviron Rep*, 5(1):1–11.

Kim SK, Cho SW. 2022. The evasion mechanisms of cancer immunity and drug intervention in the tumor microenvironment. *Front Pharmacol*, 13:1–16.

Koivunen P, Laukka T. 2018. The TET enzymes. *Cellul Molec Life Sci*, 75(8):1339–1348.

Kolak A et al. 2017. Primary and secondary prevention of breast cancer. *Ann Agricult Environm Med*, 24:549–553.

Kontomanolis EN et al. 2020. Role of oncogenes and tumor-suppressor genes in carcinogenesis: A review. *Anticancer Res*, 40(11):6009–6015.

Kopetz S et al. 2015. Phase II pilot study of vemurafenib in patients with metastatic BRAF-mutated colorectal cancer. *J Clin Oncol*, 33:4032–4038.

Liu B et al. 2024. Exploring treatment options in cancer: tumor treatment strategies. *Signal Transduct Target Ther*, 9(1):175.

Li J et al. 2015. The BRAF V600E mutation predicts poor survival outcome in patients with papillary thyroid carcinoma: a meta analysis. *Int J Clin Exp Med*, 8(12):22246.

Li K et al. 2020. Microsatellite instability: A review of what the oncologist should know. *Cancer Cell Int*, 20(1):16.

Li Y. (2021). Modern epigenetics methods in biological research. *Methods*, 187:104–113.

Liu S, Kurzrock R. 2014. Toxicity of targeted therapy: Implications for response and impact of genetic polymorphisms. *Cancer Treat Rev*, 40:883–891.

Loh JJ, Ma S. 2024. Hallmarks of cancer stemness. *Cell Stem Cell*, 31(5):617–639.

Long GV et al. 2019. Neoadjuvant dabrafenib combined with trametinib for resectable, stage IIIB-C, BRAF(V600) mutation-positive melanoma (NeoCombi): A single-arm, open-label, single-centre, phase 2 trial. *Lancet Oncol*, 20:961–971.

MacConaill LE, Garraway LA. 2010. Clinical implications of the cancer genome. *J Clin Oncol*, 28:5219–28.

Maeda H. 2010. Tumor-selective delivery of macromolecular drugs via the EPR effect: Background and future prospects. *Bioconjug Chem*, 21:797–802.

Matthay KK et al. 2016. Neuroblastoma. *Nature Rev Dis Primers*, 2:16078.

McDermott MSJ et al. 2019. HER2-targeted tyrosine kinase inhibitors cause therapy-induced-senescence in breast cancer cells. *Cancers*, 11:197.

McGrath, J., & Trojer, P. (2015). Targeting histone lysine methylation in cancer. *Pharmacol Therapeut*, 150:1–22.

Meng Q et al. 2018. KRAS RENAISSANCE(S) in tumor infiltrating B cells in pancreatic cancer. *Front Oncol*, 8:384.

Michalak EM et al. 2019. The roles of DNA, RNA and histone methylation in ageing and cancer. *Nature Rev Molec Cell Biol*, 20(10):573–589.

Min HY, Lee HY. 2022. Molecular targeted therapy for anticancer treatment. *Experim Molec Med*, 54:1670–1694.

Modest DP et al. 2019. FOLFOXIRI plus panitumumab as first-line treatment of RAS wild-type metastatic colorectal cancer: The randomized, open-label, phase II VOLFI study (AIO KRK0109). *J Clin Oncol*, 37:3401–3411.

Moon JJ et al. 2019. Role of genomic instability in human carcinogenesis. *Experim Biol Med*, 244(3):227–240.

Morris VK, Bekail-Saab T. 2020. Improvements in clinical outcomes for BRAFV600E-mutant metastatic colorectal cancer. *Clinl Cancer Res*, 26:4435–4441.

Munro S et al. 2012. Diversity within the pRb pathway: is there a code of conduct? *Oncogene*, 31:4343–4352.

Navarro C et al. 2022. Metabolic reprogramming in cancer cells: Emerging molecular mechanisms and novel therapeutic approaches. *Pharmaceut*, 19;14(6):1303.

Nayar U et al. 2019. Acquired HER2 mutations in ER(+) metastatic breast cancer confer resistance to estrogen receptor-directed therapies. *Nature Genet*, 51:207–216.

Neganova ME et al. 2022. Histone modifications in epigenetic regulation of cancer: Perspectives and achieved progress. *Semin Cancer Biol*, 83:452–471.

Ozaki Y et al. 2022. Trastuzumab and fulvestrant combination therapy for women with advanced breast cancer positive for hormone receptor and human epidermal growth factor receptor 2: A retrospective single-center study. *BMC Cancer*, 22:36.

Özgu E et al. 2024. Therapeutic vulnerabilities and pan-cancer landscape of BRAF class III mutations in epithelial solid tumors. *BJC Reports*, 2:77.

Park JW, Han JW. 2019. Targeting epigenetics for cancer therapy. *Arch Pharmaceut Res*, 42(2):159–170.

Pierotti MA. 2003. Mechanisms of oncogene activation. In: *Holland-Frei Cancer Medicine*. 6th edn. BC Decker.

Piercey O et al. 2024. BRAFV600E-mutant metastatic colorectal cancer: current evidence, future directions, and research priorities. *Clin Colorectal Cancer*, 23:215–229.

Pierotti MA, Sozzi G, Croce CM. Mechanisms of oncogene activation. In: Kufe DW, Pollock RE, Weichselbaum RR, Bast RC Jr, Gansler TS, Holland JF, Frei E III, editors. Holland-Frei Cancer Medicine. 6th ed. Hamilton (ON): BC Decker Inc.; 2003. Chapter 6. Available from: https://www.ncbi.nlm.nih.gov/books/NBK13272/

Pietrantonio F et al. 2015. Predictive role of BRAF mutations in patients with advanced colorectal cancer receiving cetuximab and panitumumab: A meta-analysis. *Eur J Cancer*, 51:587–594.

Pikor L et al. 2013. The detection and implication of genome instability in cancer. *Cancer Metast Rev*, 32(3–4):341–52.

Potocki PM et al. 2023. Clinical characterization of targetable mutations (BRAF V600E and KRAS G12C) in advanced colorectal cancer-A nation-wide study. *Int J Molec Sci*, 24(9073):1–17.

Pottier C et al. 2020. Tyrosine kinase inhibitors in cancer: Breakthrough and challenges of targeted therapy. *Cancers*, 12:731:1–17.

Prahallad A et al. 2012. Unresponsiveness of colon cancer to BRAF(V600E) inhibition through feedback activation of EGFR. *Nature*, 483:100–103.

Putra V et al. 2021. The RNA-helicase DDX21 upregulates CEP55 expression and promotes neuro-blastoma. *Molec Oncol*, 15:1162–1179.

Qin J et al. 2020. Histone modifications and their role in colorectal cancer (Review). *Pathol Oncol Res*, 26(4):2023–2033.

Ramazi S et al. 2020. Evaluation of post-translational modifications in histone proteins: A review on histone modification defects in developmental and neurological disorders. *J Biosci*, 45(1):135.

Rose AAN. 2019. Encorafenib and binimetinib for the treatment of BRAF V600E/K-mutated mela-noma. *Drugs Today (Barc)*, 55:247–264.

Ross SE, Bogdanovic O. 2019. TET enzymes, DNA demethylation and pluripotency. *Biochem Soc Trans*, 47(3):875–885.

Rotte A et al. 2015. Immunotherapy of melanoma: present options and future promises. *Cancer Metast Rev*, 34:115–128.

Rowland A et al. 2015. Meta-analysis of BRAF mutation as a predictive biomarker of benefit from anti-EGFR monoclonal antibody therapy for RAS wild-type metastatic colorectal cancer. *Br J Cancer*, 112:1888–94.

Sasada M et al. 2019. Inactivation of beta1 integrin induces proteasomal degradation of Myc oncop-roteins. *Oncotarget*, 10:4960–4972.

Schirripa M et al. 2019. Class 1, 2, and 3 BRAF-mutated metastatic colorectal cancer: A detailed clinical, pathologic, and molecular characterization. *Clin Cancer Res*, 25:3954–3961.

Schütz S et al. 2022. The disordered MAX N-terminus modulates DNA binding of the transcrip-tion factor *MYC:MAX*. *J Mol Biol*, 434:167833.

Shan KS et al. 2024. Molecular targeting of the BRAF proto-oncogene/mitogen-activated protein kinase (MAPK) pathway across cancers. *Int J Molec Sci*, 25(1):624.

Sharma P et al. 2019. Epigenetics and oxidative stress: A twin-edged sword in spermatogenesis. *Andrologia*, 51(11):e13432.

Shortt J, Johnstone R.W. 2012. Oncogenes in cell survival and cell death. *Cold Spring Harbor Perspect Biol*, 4 (12):1–10.

Singh DD et al. 2022. Clinical updates on tyrosine kinase inhibitors in HER2-positive breast cancer. *Front Pharmacol*, 13.

Singh DN., et al. 2023. Genetic testing for successful cancer treatment. *Cureus*, 15:e49889.

Slamon DJ et al. 2001. Use of chemotherapy plus a monoclonal antibody against HER2 for meta-static breast cancer that overexpresses HER2. New *Engl J Med*, 344:783–792.

Sliwkowski MX et al. 1999. Nonclinical studies addressing the mechanism of action of trastu-zumab (Herceptin). *Semin Oncol*, 26:60–70.

Sloan KE, Bohnsack MT. 2018. Unravelling the mechanisms of RNA helicase regulation. *Trends Biochem Sci*, 43:237–250.

Smith I et al. 2007. 2-year follow-up of trastuzumab after adjuvant chemotherapy in HER2-positive breast cancer: A randomised controlled trial. *Lancet*, 369:29–36.

Song C et al. 2017. SIRT7 and the DEAD-box helicase DDX21 cooperate to resolve genomic R loops and safeguard genome stability. *Genes Developm*, 31:370–1381.

Soucek L, Evan GI. 2010. The ups and downs of Myc biology. *Curr Opinion Genet Developm*, 20:91–95.

Su X et al. 2016. Metabolic control of methylation and acetylation. *Curr Opinion Chem Biol*, 30:52–60.

Sun C et al. 2022. Treatment of advanced BRAF-mutated colorectal cancer: where we are and where we are going. *Clin Colorect Cancer*, 21:71–79.

Swain SM et al. 2020. Pertuzumab, trastuzumab, and docetaxel for HER2-positive metastatic breast cancer (CLEOPATRA): End-of-study results from a double-blind, randomised, placebo-controlled, phase 3 study. *Lancet Oncol*, 21:519–530.

Swain SM et al. 2023. Targeting HER2-positive breast cancer: Advances and future directions. *Nature Rev Drug Disc*, 22:101–126.

Szilveszter KP et al. 2019. Tyrosine kinases in autoimmune and inflammatory skin diseases. *Front Immunol*, 10(1862):1–21.

Tagalakis AD et al. 2021. Integrin-targeted, short interfering RNA nanocomplexes for neuroblastoma tumor-specific delivery achieve MYCN silencing with improved survival. *Advanced Funct Mat* 31:2104843.

Takacs T et al. 2020. The effects of mutant Ras proteins on the cell signalome. *Cancer Metast Rev*, 39(4):1051–1065.

Tyner, JW et al. 2022. Understanding drug sensitivity and tackling resistance in cancer. *Cancer Res*, 82:1448–1460.

Vermeulen K et al. 2003. The cell cycle: a review of regulation, deregulation and therapeutic targets in cancer. *Cell Prolif*, 36(3):131–149.

Wagner RF, Krontiris TG. 1988. Oncogenes and human malignancy. *Adv Dermatol*, 3:277–292.

Wang J et al. 2019. ncRNA-encoded peptides or proteins and cancer. *Molec Ther*, 27(10):1718–1725.

Watanabe M et al. 2020. Recent progress in multidisciplinary treatment for patients with esophageal cancer. *Surgery Today*, 50(1):12–20.

Weiss, WA et al. 1997. Targeted expression of MYCN causes neuroblastoma in transgenic mice. *Embo J*, 16:2985–2995.

Xu X et al. 2023. Metabolic reprogramming and epigenetic modifications in cancer: from the impacts and mechanisms to the treatment potential. *Experim Molec Med*, 55:1357–1370.

Yamaoka T et al. 2018. Receptor tyrosine kinase-targeted cancer therapy. *Int J Molec Sci*, 6;19(11):3491.

Yang G et al. 2019. Correlations between microsatellite instability and the biological behaviour of tumors. *J Cancer Res Clin Oncol*, 145(12):2891–2899.

Yang S et al. 2021. Epigenetically modulated miR-1224 suppresses the proliferation of HCC through CREB-mediated activation of YAP signaling pathway. *Molec Ther - Nucleic Acids*, 23:944–958.

Yarden Y, Sliwkowski MX. 2001. Untangling the ErbB signalling network. *Nature Rev Molec Cell Biol*, 2:127–137.

Yoshida GJ. 2015. Metabolic reprogramming: the emerging concept and associated therapeutic strategies. *J Experim Clin Cancer Res*, 6(34):111.

Zhou Y et al. 2024. Tumor biomarkers for diagnosis, prognosis and targeted therapy. *Signal Transduct Target Ther*, 9:132.

3

Fundamentals of Cancer Genetics

Lata Kumari, Dipansh Katoch, Gangandeep Singh, Arshiya Sood, and Neelam Thakur

ABBREVIATIONS

Acronym	Full Form
TME	Tumor microenvironment
RNA	Ribonucleic acid
TECs	Tumor endothelial cells
CNVs	Copy number variations
BRCA	Breast cancer gene
UV	Ultraviolet radiations
DNA	Deoxyribonucleic acid
PTEN	Phosphate and tensin homolog
HER2	Human epidermal growth factor receptor 2
ECs	Endothelial cells
TSG	Tumor suppressor gene
CML	Chronic myelogenous leukemia
MYC	Myelocytomatosis oncogene
TAMs	Tumor-associated macrophages
Mb	Mega base
UTR	Untranslated region
RAS	Rat sarcoma
KRAS	Kirsten rat sarcoma
PG	Protooncogene
Rb	Retinoblastoma
ECM	Extracellular matrix
CAF	Cancer-associated fibroblasts
ERK	Extracellular signal regulated kinase
piRNA	PIWI-interacting RNA
PD-1	Programmed cell death protein 1
EMT	Epithelial-mesenchymal transition
snoRNA	Small nucleolar RNA
ROS	Reactive oxygen species
PI3K	Phosphatidylinositol 3-kinase
VEGF	Vascular endothelial growth factor
MCED	Multi cancer early detection
PTM	Post-translational modifications
ADP	Adenosine diphosphate
HDAC	Histone deacetylase
HAT	Histone acetylase transferase
SUMO	Small ubiquitin-like modifiers
AKT	Ak strain transforming
circRNA	Circular RNA
lncRNA	Long nuclear RNA
ceRNA	Competitive endogenous RNA
miRNA	Micro nuclear RNA
PAH	Polycyclic aromatic hydrocarbons
ctDNA	Circulating tumor DNA

DOI: 10.1201/9781003542162-3

RT	Radiation therapy
MDR	Multi drug resistance
PTT	Photothermal therapy
NPs	Nanoparticles
PDT	Photo dynamic therapy

3.1 INTRODUCTION

Cancer refers to a collection of diseases marked by the unregulated proliferation and growth of cells within the body (Chandraprasad et al., 2022; Matthews et al., 2022). These cells lead to the development of tumors, which can be benign or malignant. Through the process of metastasis, cells from a primary tumor might travel to another organ and develop into a secondary tumor in a malignant tumor (Fares et al., 2020). The biological processes involved in metastasis begin with the potential of tumor cells to invade the mucosa and penetrate deeper tissues. From there, the cells spread via blood, lymphatics, or direct infiltration of nearby structures. Once established in distant organs, the cells proliferate and colonize them (Gerstberger et al., 2023). Cancer is a leading cause of death worldwide (Siegel et al., 2023). Normal cell to cancer cell transformation necessitates a number of epigenetic and genomic changes in important cellular mechanisms, which are known as hallmarks of cancer (Qing et al., 2020).

3.1.1 Overview of Cancer Genetics

Cancer genetics is the study of genetic changes that play a key role in the initiation and advancement of cancer. This mainly includes genes that are crucial for regulating cell division and growth, like proto-oncogenes (PG) and tumor suppressor genes (TSG). Proto-oncogenes are responsible for normal cell division and growth, and TSG maintains homeostasis during DNA replication and cell division (Ostroverkhova et al., 2023). Gain of function mutations in an oncogene and loss-of-function mutations in a TSG both lead to abnormal expression and uncontrollable growth and division of cells (You & Jones, 2012). DNA repair genes are responsible for fixing the mutations that either occurred during replication or were caused by external sources or endogenous damage, and mutations in DNA repair genes are associated with causing cancer (Lahtz & Pfeifer, 2011). Continuous interaction between tumor microenvironment (TME) and tumor cells also contributes significantly to the initiation and progression of tumors. The TME is composed of a variety of immune cells, endothelial cells, cancer-associated fibroblasts (CAFs), pericytes, and additional cell types (Arneth, 2020). Also, the significance of epigenetic changes in cancer has been highlighted in recent research (Pathak et al., 2023). Epigenetic changes mostly include nucleosome remodeling, non-coding RNAs, DNA methylation, and post-translational modifications of histones (You & Jones, 2012). These changes control gene expression by changing chromatin dynamics and structure without changing the DNA sequence, which ultimately contribute to the emergence and evolution of cancer (Sandoval & Esteller, 2012).

3.1.2 Importance of Understanding Cancer Genetics

Personalized medicine: The knowledge of specific genetic mutations responsible for causing cancer is very helpful in developing personalized medicines and targeted therapies for a patient. As an example, patients with HER2-positive breast cancer have much better results now that targeted treatments like trastuzumab have been developed in response to the findings related to gene amplification of HER2 in some breast tumors (Derakhshani et al., 2020).

Early detection and prevention: This can be achieved by identifying individuals with inherited cancer-causing genetic alterations. Enhanced screening, preventive procedures, or chemoprevention are among options for lowering the likelihood of developing ovarian and breast cancers in people who have the BRCA1 or BRCA2 mutations.

Prognosis and risk stratification: Tumor genetic profiling can reveal important details regarding the disease's prognosis. While some genetic changes could indicate a worse prognosis, others are linked to more aggressive tumors. Patient risk stratification, therapeutic decision-making, and overall result improvement are all aided by this data.

Understanding cancer biology: One way to get to the bottom of cancer is to study the genetic alterations that causes it. A great understanding of cancer development, evolution, and resistance to treatment, along with the discovery of new therapeutic targets, can result from studying these genetic changes.

Drug resistance: Over time, cancer cells may develop resistance to therapies, usually due to genetic changes that render them resistant to the treatment's effects. To improve the long-term effectiveness of cancer treatments, understanding the genetic pathways is essential for identifying the cause for drug resistance. Only then can new tactics be created to either overcome or avoid resistance.

3.2 DNA STRUCTURE AND FUNCTION

3.2.1 Structure of DNA

Genetic material of living organisms is present in the form of nucleic acid inside the nucleus or in cytoplasm. Nucleic acid is composed of polynucleotides and is of two types, RNA (ribonucleic acid) and DNA (deoxyribonucleic acid).

Most of the organisms have DNA as their genetic material. Watson and Crick first gave the structure of DNA (Pray, 2008). DNA is a double helical structure formed of two polynucleotide chains coiled around each other in an antiparallel manner. The two strands run in antiparallel direction of each other with one strand oriented from 5' to 3', while the other runs from 3' to 5' and these strands are joined together by hydrogen bonds. Nucleotides are the building blocks of DNA that repeat throughout each strand. A nucleotide consists of three components: a ribose sugar, nitrogenous bases, and a phosphate group.

Sugar: The sugar found in DNA is 2'-deoxy- D- ribose sugar which is a pentose sugar.

Nitrogenous bases: These are heterocyclic aromatic molecules and are divided into two categories; Purines and pyrimidines. Purines are nine membered rings and are further of two types; Guanine (G) and Adenine (A). Pyrimidines are 6- membered ring structures and are of three types; Thymine (T), Cytosine (C), and Uracil (U). DNA contains four nitrogenous bases: adenine, guanine, cytosine and thymine, and uracil is found in RNA in place of thymine. These nitrogenous bases are responsible for the linking of two DNA stands together by forming the hydrogen bonds between complementary bases. Adenine forms two hydrogen bonds with thymine, while guanine pairs with cytosine through three hydrogen bonds. These nitrogenous bases are joined to 1' carbon of sugar by a glycosidic bond.

The phosphate group: Joined to sugar by the phosphodiester linkage. The alternating pentose residue and phosphate form the backbone of the DNA. The phosphate group of one nucleotide is joined to sugar of next nucleotide and form a phosphodiester linkage. DNA is found in three forms: A-DNA, B-DNA, and Z-DNA, with Z-DNA being the only left-handed form (Pray, 2008).

3.2.2 Functions of DNA

Storage of genetic information: DNA stores genetic information in the form of nucleotides which code for a specific protein which is very important for growth, functioning, development, and reproduction of organisms.

Replication: It is an important process of cell division and this mechanism ensures the precise transmission of genetic information to daughter cells during cell division.

Protein synthesis: Coding region of DNA is responsible for formation of protein through transcription and then translation and non-coding region is also responsible for the regulation of protein expression.

Control of gene expression: DNA not only contains genetic information but also contributes to the regulation of when and how genes are expressed.

Mutation and evolution: Mutations are changes in the DNA sequence that can occur due to errors during replication or environmental factors. While many mutations are neutral or harmful, some can confer advantages that may lead to evolutionary changes over generations.

Repair mechanisms: DNA possesses inherent mechanisms for repair to maintain its integrity. Various enzymes recognize and correct errors or damage caused by environmental factors such as UV radiation or chemical exposure.

Transmission of hereditary information: DNA is responsible for passing genetic traits from one generation to another through reproduction. In sexually reproducing organisms, half of the DNA comes from each parent, ensuring genetic diversity (Figure 3.1).

3.2.3 Genetic Mutations and Their Types

Genetic mutations are changes in the DNA sequence that can impact an organism's characteristics and functions. These changes can occur at various scales, from small changes affecting a single nucleotide to large-scale alterations involving entire chromosomes. Different types of mutations are discussed below (Clancy, 2008; Stenson et al., 2020):

3.2.3.1 Point Mutations

In Point mutations there is a change in a single nucleotide that can affect protein expression. They are induced by mistakes in DNA replication or modification of DNA by some other means, like UV radiation. They are further divided into 3 types:

Silent Mutations: In this type of mutations, insertion of a nucleotide leads to formation of a new codon that codes for the same amino acid as the original one. Example: If the codon ACU is mutated to ACC, both codons code for threonine. This mutation is also considered silent as it does not alter the protein's amino acid sequence.

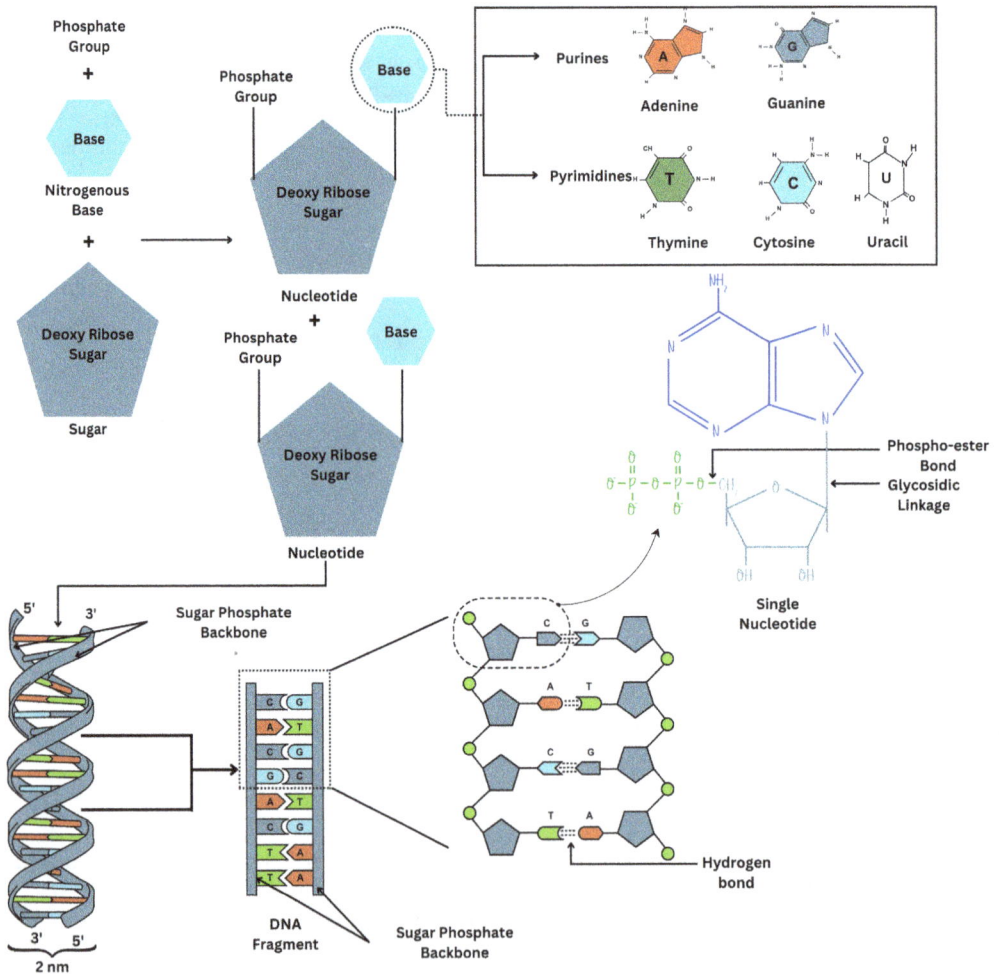

Figure 3.1 Structure of DNA showing ribose sugar, nitrogenous bases, phosphate group, and different types of bonds.

Missense Mutations: In this type of mutation, the substitution of a nucleotide leads to formation of a codon that codes for a different amino acid, which will alter the protein's function. Example: The P53 gene, which encodes the p53 protein, carries missense mutations. These mutations can affect the protein's ability to regulate the cell cycle and induce apoptosis, leading to tumorigenesis (Olivier et al., 2010).

Nonsense Mutations: In this type of mutations, insertion of a new base pair results in the formation of a stop codon which will lead to premature termination of protein synthesis. The truncated protein may lack essential functional domains necessary for its activity, leading to loss of tumor suppressor functions or gain of oncogenic properties. Example: Nonsense mutations in genes like BRCA1 can disrupt its role in DNA repair mechanisms, significantly increasing breast and ovarian cancer risk (Saleem et al., 2020).

3.2.3.2 Frame Shift Mutation

Here one or more DNA bases are added or deleted (not in multiples of three), which will lead to a complete loss of function of proteins by altering the reading frame of the gene. This type of mutation changes how subsequent codons are read during translation, often resulting in completely different and usually nonfunctional proteins. Example: Frameshift mutations in the PTEN gene can lead to loss of its tumor-suppressing function, contributing to various cancers including prostate cancer (Jurca et al., 2023).

3.2.3.3 Chromosomal Rearrangements

These involve alterations in the structure or number of chromosomes, which can result in a range of genetic disorders when a region of a chromosome is inverted, deleted, duplicated, or translocated, leading to altered proteins that can have oncogenic properties. Cri-du-chat syndrome (deletion), some cancers (duplications), and Opitz-Kaveggia syndrome (inversion) are some examples (Stenson et al., 2020). The translocation between chromosomes 9 and 22 leads to the formation of the BCR-ABL fusion protein that is a hallmark of chronic myelogenous leukemia (CML). This fusion protein has constitutive tyrosine kinase activity that drives cell proliferation (Soverini et al., 2011).

3.2.3.4 Gene Amplifications

The process of increasing the copy numbers of a specific gene is called gene amplification. Overexpression of oncogenes can lead to increased signaling for cell growth and division. Example: The MYC oncogene is frequently amplified in various cancers, leading to enhanced cellular proliferation and survival signals (Hutter et al., 2017).

3.2.3.5 Germline Mutations

The mutations that are passed from parents to offspring and are present in egg or sperm cells significantly enhance a person's risk for specific malignancies. Examples: Mutations in the BRCA1 and BRCA2 genes significantly elevate the likelihood of developing breast and ovarian cancers. Individuals with these mutations often undergo increased surveillance or preventative surgeries (Saleem et al., 2020).

3.2.3.6 Somatic Mutations

Unlike germline mutations, which are passed down through generations, somatic mutations develop over the course of an individual's life. Somatic mutations caused by environmental factors (such as tobacco smoke or ultraviolet radiation) or errors during DNA replication are the primary cause of most malignancies. Examples: Lung cancer often involves multiple somatic mutations across various genes due to exposure to carcinogens in tobacco smoke (Kobayashi & Mitsudomi, 2016).

3.2.3.7 Non-Coding Indels

A significant discovery has been made regarding small insertions or deletions (indels) in non-coding regions of the genome. Traditionally, mutations were primarily studied in coding regions, but recent findings suggest that indels in non-coding DNA can also play a crucial role in cancer. These mutations, which range from one to 50 nucleotides, occur frequently in various cancers, including liver, stomach, and thyroid cancers. They cluster in genes critical for organ function and may influence gene regulation, thereby affecting normal cell development and potentially leading to cancer progression (Imielinski et al., 2017).

3.2.3.8 Chromoanagenesis

It is currently known that 80–90% of cancer genomes have large-scale genomic rearrangements. These changes can be numerical or structural and can disable tumor suppressor genes through loss or disruption. On the other hand, they can activate proto-oncogenes through amplification, translocation, or the creation of oncogenic fusions (Taylor et al., 2018). It has been linked to poor prognosis in several cancers, indicating its role in promoting tumor heterogeneity and resistance to therapy.

3.2.3.8.1 Types of Chromoanagenesis

Chromothripsis: It is the best studied and the most frequent large-scale genomic rearrangement. Chromothripsis is the breaking of a single or more chromosomes into many fragments of 0.1–10.1Mb size succeeded by random re-ligation. Under this process, some fragments, especially chromothripsis can lead to multiple mutations across a single chromosome and has been seen in a variety of cancers, including gliomas and sarcomas (Krupina et al., 2024).

Chromoanasynthesis: This type of mutation results from replication-based mechanisms along with microhomology-mediated switching of templates or serial fork stalling. Chromoanasynthesis, a localized process, occurs in the germline cells and lead to gain or loss of certain chromosomal parts and was found in about 5% of tumors (Cortés-Ciriano et al., 2020).

Chromoplexy: Chromoplexy is defined by chromosomal rearrangements that are mostly balanced translocations. It was first noted in prostate cancer, but it was later found in sarcomas, carcinomas, and found in approximately 10% of tumors. In chromoplexy, several intrachromosomal and interchromosomal translocations, and deletions occurs simultaneously in five or more chromosomes (Baca et al., 2013).

3.2.3.9 Copy Number Variations (CNVs)

CNVs denote a phenomenon whereby genome regions are either duplicated or removed with varied numbers of such repetitions amongst genomes of different individuals (Feuk et al., 2006). Various mutational processes, which includes those linked to DNA repair, replication, and recombination, produce CNVs. Cancer can also be induced by germline and somatic CNVs (Shlien & Malkin, 2009). Germline CNVs are hereditary and are handed down via generations, and somatic CNVs are mainly non hereditary and are only found in particular cells (Oketch et al., 2024). Example: HER2 amplification and overexpression in breast cancer is responsible for proliferation in cancer cells (Van Bockstal et al., 2020).

3.2.3.10 Nonstop Extension Mutations

These are also called stop-lost, or read-through mutations. Nonstop extension mutations alter the stop codon into a sense codon, which further continues to translate the 3′UTR of succeeding open reading frame until the arrival of the next stop codon, which results in the elongation of protein at the C-terminus (Ghosh et al., 2024).

3.3 GENES RESPONSIBLE FOR CANCER DEVELOPMENT

3.3.1 Proto-oncogenes

Proto-oncogenes, important regulatory components of biological functions, can act as growth factors, transcription factors, and signal transducers are mainly responsible for monitoring normal cell proliferation and differentiation (Derelanko, 2014). A gain of function mutation leads to the activation of proto-oncogenes into oncogenes, which results in uncontrollable cell multiplication and has a significant impact on cancer progression (Gariglio, 2012). These mutations may act by changing the structure of proteins encoded by proto-oncogenes or by deregulating protein expression (Jan & Chaudhry, 2019). The protooncogene gets activated by the following mechanism:

Chromosomal translocation: Proto-oncogenes can be activated by chromosomal translocation of these genes from a non-transcribable locus to a neighboring transcribable locus. Example: chromosomal translocation of the MYC gene family is associated with Burkitt's lymphoma. C-MYC, L-MYC, and N-MYC, which constitutes the MYC gene family, are nuclear phosphoproteins encoded by cellular proto-oncogenes located on chromosomes 8, 1, and 2, respectively. The MYC gene family is responsible for cell proliferation, transformation, immortalization, and dedifferentiation (Hutter et al., 2017).

Point mutation of a proto-oncogenes: Alteration of only one nucleotide through insertion, deletion, or duplication is responsible for this type of mutation. Example: The family members of the RAS gene belong to a category of regulatory GTPases, and when this gene is activated, it leads to activation of another protein that subsequently helps in cellular growth, differentiation, and survival. A point mutation in this gene permanently activates it, resulting in overexpression of the gene even when no proper signal is there. In pancreatic cancer, missense point mutation leads to KRAS (protein21) gene activation, which results in substitution of aspartate or valine in place of glycine, leading to protein activation (Nenclares & Harrington, 2020).

Gene amplification: It involves the incorporation of numerous duplicates of an oncogene, leading to enhanced production of oncoprotein. Example: Cyclin D is associated with cell cycle regulation and progression of several transcription factors. Gene amplification leads to upregulation of this gene. Uncontrolled synthesis of cyclin D has an effect on the amount of cyclin D-cdk4 complex formation, which derives the cell from the G^0/S checkpoint, even when growth factors are not present.

3.3.2 Tumor Suppressive Genes

In normal cells, TSGs are crucial for cell proliferation, differentiation, and cancer prevention. Loss-of-function mutation leads to the activation of this gene, which leads to uncontrolled cell division responsible for causing cancer. It is a recessive type of mutation where both the copies of TSG must be inactivated for a cancer cell to grow or endure (Nenclares & Harrington, 2020).

3.3.2.1 Types of TSGs
3.3.2.1.1 Caretaker Genes

These genes do not suppress proliferation directly but function to promote genetic stability. Basically, they encode the products that stabilize the genome. Inactivation of caretaker genes is equivalent to exposing cells to mutations.

3.3.2.1.2 Gatekeeper Genes

These genes directly hinder cell growth or induce cell death. In the presence of gatekeeper genes, mutations in other genes do not lead to ongoing growth imbalances. When caretaker genes are mutated, the probability of mutation in gatekeeper genes also increases as DNA repair pathway mechanisms are damaged.

3.3.2.1.3 Landscape Genes

Landscape genes basically encode gene products that control the environment in which a cell grows. Stromal cell abnormalities arising from faulty landscape gene products could lead to abnormal cell growth on the epithelium and lead to cancer of that gene.

Examples: P53 gene and retinoblastoma 1 protein (RB1)—the P53 gene, also called as the "guardian of the human genome," is located at the 17th chromosome and is responsible for inhibition of tumor formation in normal cells.

Retinoblastoma protein—retinoblastoma is a cancer that starts in the retina and mainly occurs when RB1 gene is mutated. It is the most frequent type of eye cancer among children and has the potential to spread to other areas also. The RB1 gene is also known as the "master regulator of the cell cycle." The normal activity of RB1 gene helps in the prevention of excessive cycle progression as well as maintaining its differentiation to inhibit the formation of tumors. The function of retinoblastoma in cell cycle is primarily controlled by the E2F family of transcription factors (Ayyanan et al., 2006; Jan & Chaudhry, 2019).

3.4 TUMOR MICROENVIRONMENT (TME) IN CANCER

The cancer is a complex amalgamation that involves a diverse pool of non-cancerous cells. It is established that genetic changes might be essential for the initiation and development of cancer, but they are not adequate. This complex interplay of cancer becomes evident when observing solid tumors under a microscope, which unfolds the highly organized system of the tumor microenvironment (TME), comprising of cancer cells enveloped by different non-malignant cell types which include non-cancerous cells, blood vessels, cancer-associated fibroblasts (CAFs), pericytes, extracellular matrix (ECM), immune cells, endothelial cells (ECs), signaling molecules, and some other types of cell, which varies depending on the tissue, such as adipocytes and neurons (Q. Wang et al., 2023). Earlier, all of these host cells were considered as onlookers of tumorigenesis.

3.4.1 Interaction between TME and Tumor Cells

This interaction is a two-way process where tumor cells alter their microenvironment and contrarily the environment influences tumor behavior. These interactions involve various signaling pathways and cellular mechanisms that may promote or inhibit tumor progression.

3.4.1.1 Stromal Cells

The cells like fibroblasts, mesenchymal stem cells and endothelial cells, establish a fostering environment for the development of cancer. The cancer cells activate CAFs and aid in the development of tumors by stimulating the synthesis of blood vessels, altering the extracellular matrix and releasing growth factors (Lan et al., 2021). Endothelial cells have a vital role in angiogenesis in tumors where they cater essential nutrients and oxygen for tumor development and create a path for cancer cell dissemination. Involvement of stromal cells in the tumor microenvironment is complicated as they either support or hinder tumor growth which is influenced by the circumstances and this dual role poses a challenge for targeted therapies.

3.4.1.2 Immune Cells

The TME comprises of immune cells like dendritic cells, T-cells, macrophages and B cells which have dual roles. They have the ability to both attack and eliminate cancer cells as well as get manipulated to facilitate the growth of tumors. The tumor-associated macrophages can be predisposed by the TME to take on a phenotype that assists tumor growth by suppressing immune responses and promotes angiogenesis and tissue remodel (Zhang et al., 2020). In TME the immune cell landscape is a topic of comprehensive research where studies demonstrate the tumor-suppressing and tumor-promoting functions of different immune cells. Recent research has established the concept of immune checkpoint blockade which presents promising treatment options. However, the effectiveness of such therapies varies and immune cells in certain cases can contribute to treatment resistance (Kubli et al., 2021).

3.4.1.3 Endothelial Cells

The vascular system is lined by endothelial cells and they have crucial roles in controlling the start, advancement and proliferation of tumors. A set of different lineages of endothelial cells have been identified by using single-cell RNA sequencing as the TME evolves spatially and temporally. There are subcategories of endothelial cells which have the ability to either encourage or hinder the progression of tumors to an invasive stage. The activated tumor endothelial cells (TECs) secrete cytokines which can activate the tumor cell receptors or suppress the anti-tumor immune response by reducing the cytotoxic reactions of immune cells.

3.4.1.4 Extracellular Matrix (ECM)

ECM is a crucial component in TME as it not only offers configurational support but also controls cell behavior using both biochemical and mechanical signals. Cancer cells can modify the ECM to progress tumor development and improve its ability to migrate and invade. Recent findings have indicated that changes in the composition and rigidness of the ECM can influence the characteristics of cancer cells i.e. it includes the initiation of EMT which is a vital process for metastasis and reveals how ECM reconstruction can construct pathways for cancer cell movement and shelter the tumor cells (Table 3.1).

3.4.2 Role of TME in Cancer Initiation and Progression

Tumorigenesis is not merely a result of genetic mutations within cells but is influenced by the surrounding stromal components that support malignant transformation and TME plays a critical part in the initiation and development of cancer.

3.4.2.1 Tumor Initiation

A main player in tumor initiation is the subpopulation of cells called cancer stem cells. These cells possess the ability to drive tumor formation and self-renewal. They communicate with surrounding immune cells to hinder immune surveillance in the early phases of tumor development which suppresses immune responses through various mechanisms ensuring their own survival and the establishment of tumors.

During tumor initiation cancer cells can downregulate immunogenic markers or alter their antigen expression capabilities. The concept of "cancer immunoediting" describes how tumors evolve

Table 3.1: Tumor Microenvironment Components and Their Role in Tumor Growth and Development

Component	Description	Role in Cancer Progression and Therapy Response	Affected Elements
Tumor Cells	Malignant cells that proliferate uncontrollably	Drive tumor growth and metastasis; interact with TME components to evade immune detection	Primary tumor site, metastatic sites
Stromal Cells	Includes CAFs, endothelial cells and others	Provide structural support, secrete growth factors and modulate immune responses	Tumor stroma, surrounding tissues
Immune Cells	Comprises macrophages, T-cells and other immune cells	Either anti-tumorigenic or pro-tumorigenic	TME, lymph nodes
Extracellular Matrix (ECM)	An interlinkage of proteins and carbohydrates surrounding cells	Gives structural support and biochemical signals; altered ECM can promote tumor invasion and metastasis	Tumor stroma, surrounding tissues
Cytokines and Chemokines	Soluble factors secreted by various cells in the TME	Mediate communication between cells; can promote inflammation and immune evasion	TME, systemic circulation
Metabolic Factors	Includes metabolites produced by tumor and stromal cells	Influence tumor growth and therapy resistance	Tumor site, distant organs affected by metastasis

Source: Giraldo et al. (2019), Q. Wang et al. (2023).

to carry out an invasion into immune responses by selecting for less immunogenic variants. This process helps them to escape detection by the immune system which is vital for their survival and proliferation.

3.4.2.2 *Cancer Cell Proliferation*

The TME has a significant role in supporting proliferation of cancer cell. Tumor-associated macrophages (TAMs), particularly the ones polarized to the M2 phenotype, promote tumor growth and suppress effective anti-tumor immunity. Several signaling pathways are responsible for encouraging the proliferation and growth of cancer cells within the TME. These include the ERK and PI3K/AKT pathways which are initiated by the response of various growth factors present in the TME and enables tumor growth.

3.4.2.3 *Immune Evasion*

The TME plays a vital role in facilitating immune evasion which is essential for letting cancer cells to succeed and proliferate, fooling the immune surveillance of the body. The TME has various ways to enable immune evasion such as establishing an environment that suppresses the immune system, generating checkpoint molecules that impede functions of T-cell and altering antigen presentation to reduce the detection of cancer cells. Immune evasion within the TME uses a sophisticated approach that diminishes the ability of the immune system to effectively identify and confiscate cancer cells.

3.4.3 Role of TME in Metastasis

Metastasis is a chief cause of deaths resulting from cancer. Studies have shown that tumor metastasis is a consequence of sequential events rather than spontaneous circumstances. Primary tumorigenic sites and potential metastatic sites interact in complex ways where TME facilitates the metastatic process by forming a supportive atmosphere for the tumor cells to travel through the bloodstream and colonize new tissues.

3.4.3.1 *Pre-Metastatic Niche Formation*

This refers to the preparation of distant organs by the primary tumor even before cancer cells arrive. Tumor cells release extracellular vesicles and exosomes that carry signaling molecules and modify the distant tissue environment to make it more favorable for metastasis which includes recruitment of supportive stromal cells and remodeling the ECM to facilitate the colonization of metastatic cells (H. Wang et al., 2021).

3.4.3.2 *Angiogenesis*

The metastatic cells need development of new blood vessels to access the bloodstream and disseminate. The angiogenic factors like VEGF help tumor cells invade the vascular system. This process is vital for providing oxygen and nutrients to tumors, making it easier for cancer cells to enter the bloodstream (Lugano et al., 2020).

3.4.3.3 *Epithelial-Mesenchymal Transition (EMT)*

The EMT is crucial for epithelial cancer cells to gain mesenchymal properties which increases their ability to move and invade. Invasion and migration are essential stages in the spread of cancer cells. These stages are controlled by an intricate network of signaling pathways, such as growth factors cytokines, that oversee the breakdown of the ECM and the development of a mobile and invasive phenotype through EMT.

3.4.4 Role of TME in Cancer Therapy

Immunotherapy boosts the immune response of body against tumors through several strategies with immune checkpoint inhibitors being among the most prominent. These agents such as those targeting PD-1/PD-L1 work by blocking proteins that inhibit T-cell activation. This action reduces T-cell exhaustion and enhances anti-tumor responses. Immune system can attack and recognize cancer cells more effectively by reactivating T- cells therapies (Kumar et al., 2023). Clinical applications of checkpoint inhibitors have shown noteworthy success in various cancers, which include melanoma and lung cancer. They can be used alone or in combination with other therapies to improve outcomes. Also combining the checkpoint inhibitors with chemotherapy has proven fruitful remedy for non-small cell lung cancer that leads to improved survival rates compared to chemotherapy alone.

Combination therapies involve using two or more treatment modalities to target cancer more effectively. The principle behind this approach is that different agents can act on distinct pathways which reduces the likelihood of resistance and enhancing therapeutic effects. For instance, combining chemotherapy with immunotherapy can improve overall treatment efficacy by attacking the tumor from multiple angles (Jin et al., 2023). This strategy includes combinations of chemotherapy and immunotherapy which enhance immune activation while simultaneously reducing tumor burden. The targeted therapy combinations involve using drugs that target specific mutations within cancer cells alongside immunotherapies. Combinations like nivolumab (a checkpoint inhibitor) with ipilimumab (another immunotherapy) have been approved for advanced melanoma (Jin et al., 2023). The benefits of combination therapies include deeper and more durable responses compared to monotherapy as well as the potential for lower doses of individual drugs which can reduce toxicity while maintaining efficacy.

Research is increasingly focusing on targeting specific elements of the TME, such as stromal cells and signaling pathways which reshapes the immune landscape favorably. The inhibiting factors like TGF-β can alter the TME to promote anti-tumor immunity. Strategies may include stromal modulation by targeting immune-suppressive cells or cancer-associated fibroblasts in the TME which can improve the effectiveness of immunotherapies (Tajaldini et al., 2023). The pathway inhibition aims to block mechanisms that tumors use to evade immune detection or promote growth which creates a more hostile environment for cancer cells.

Delivery systems for nanoparticles are developed to minimize systemic toxicity while delivering therapeutic medicines straight to tumor locations. These systems can enclose drugs which allow for targeted release in the tumor sites and enhancing drug efficacy against resistant tumors. Targeted delivery through nanoparticles can be engineered to recognize specific markers on tumor cells ensuring that therapeutic agents are preferably delivered where needed. This approach also helps reduce side effects by concentrating treatment at the tumor site leading to improved patient tolerance and compliance (Mukhtar et al., 2020; Parveen et al., 2023). Research into nanoparticle systems is ongoing with promising results in preclinical studies showing enhanced efficacy in various cancer types. These systems hold potential for integrating multiple therapeutic agents into a single delivery vehicle which will further improve treatment outcomes.

3.5 EPIGENETIC ALTERATIONS IN CANCER

Epigenetics refers to the study of heritable alterations in gene expression that do not arise from changes to the DNA sequence itself. This field has gained prominence in cancer research as studies have pointed towards the epigenetic modifications, especially the DNA methylation, playing a crucial role in the initiation and advancement of several cancers. In contrast to genetic mutations which alter the DNA sequence permanently the epigenetic modifications are reversible and can be impacted by lifestyle choices, environmental influences and medical treatments (Feng & De Carvalho, 2022; Pathak et al., 2023; Skourti & Dhillon, 2022).

3.5.1 DNA Methylation

DNA methylation works by adding the methyl group to the cytosine residues of DNA and it usually happens in relation to CpG dinucleotides. This alteration may contribute to carcinogenesis by activating oncogenes and suppressing tumor suppressor genes (TSGs)(Pathak et al., 2023). Hypermethylation of TSGs is a common characteristic of several malignancies which include ovarian, lung, and breast tumors which have been found to exhibit deviant patterns of DNA methylation. DNA methylation plays a very important role as an early diagnostic indicator for cancer has also been highlighted suggesting its potential utility in cancer screening and prevention strategies.

3.5.1.1 Therapeutic Implications of Targeting DNA Methylation

Given the reversible nature of epigenetic modifications targeting DNA methylation presents a promising therapeutic strategy. Several epigenetic drugs like DNA methyltransferase inhibitors (i.e., decitabine and azacitidine) have been developed and are currently used in clinical settings particularly for hematological malignancies. These agents aim to restore normal gene expression patterns by reversing aberrant methylation thereby reactivating silenced TSGs and enhancing the efficacy of conventional therapies.

3.5.2 Histone Post-Translational Modifications

Post-translational modifications in histones are essential for controlling chromatin shape, gene expression and other biological functions. These changes include phosphorylation, acetylation, ubiquitination, sumoylation, methylation, ADP ribosylation and biotinylation which all are dynamic and reversible allowing cells to adapt to environmental stimuli and maintain homeostasis (Table 3.2).

3.5.2.1 Acetylation

Histone acetylation is mostly linked to transcriptional activity. Histone acetyltransferases (HATs) catalyse the binding of acetyl groups to residues of lysine on histones which counterbalances the positive charge on histones resulting in a more relaxed chromatin shape that promotes access to transcription machinery (Cavalieri, 2021; Ramazi et al., 2020). Conversely histone deacetylases (HDACs) remove these acetyl groups which results in compaction of chromatin and transcriptional repression. Dysregulation of acetylation patterns have been implicated in various cancers which highlights the potential of HATs and HDACs as restorative targets.

Table 3.2: Histone Post-Translational Modifications and Their Site of Modification and Functional Implications

Modification Type	Amino Acid	Functional Implications
Acetylation	Lysine	Associated with transcriptional activation; neutralizes positive charge reducing histone-DNA interaction.
Methylation	Lysine, Arginine	Either activate or inhibit transcription depending on the specific residue and context.
Phosphorylation	Serine, Threonine, Tyrosine	Often involved in signaling pathways; can influence gene expression and chromatin dynamics
Ubiquitination	Lysine	Associated with protein degradation and transcriptional regulation; can affect chromatin structure
Sumoylation	Lysine	Modulates protein interactions and stability; involved in DNA repair and transcriptional regulation.
Biotinylation	Lysine	Associated with gene repression
Ribosylation	Serine, threonine, tyrosine, glutamate, aspartate, lysine, arginine, histidine	Involved in DNA repair and cellular stress responses; modifies chromatin structure

Source: Cavalieri (2021), Ramazi et al. (2020).

3.5.2.2 Methylation

Histone methylation adds methyl groups onto arginine or lysine residues which either stimulate or inhibit the process of transcription (Cavalieri, 2021; Ramazi et al., 2020). While trimethylation of H3K27 is linked to transcriptional inhibition, H3K4 trimethylation is often linked to active transcription. The enzymes responsible for these modifications include histone methyltransferases and demethylases which are critical in maintaining cellular identity and function. Aberrant patterns of methylation are frequently observed that contributes to altered gene expression profiles that promote tumorigenesis.

3.5.2.3 Phosphorylation

Usually occurring on threonine, serine, and tyrosine residues, histone phosphorylation is frequently linked to transcriptional control and DNA damage repair. Phosphorylation can change how histones and DNA interact which affects the accessibility and structure of the chromatin. The H2AX phosphorylation is a determining component of double-strand breaks found in DNA. The histone phosphorylation dysregulation is found to be associated with cancer progression that emphasizes its importance in maintaining genomic stability.

3.5.2.4 Ubiquitination

Ubiquitination involves the attachment of ubiquitin molecules to residues of lysine on histones H2A/H2B and is linked with several cellular processes which includes DNA repair, transcriptional regulation, and chromatin remodeling. The part of ubiquitination in cancer is intricate as it may function both as a tumor suppressor and an oncogenic signal depending on the stimuli. The mono-ubiquitination on H2B is linked to transcriptional elongation and is essential for proper gene expression. The enzymes involved in ubiquitination including E3 ligases and deubiquitinating enzymes are potential therapeutic targets in cancer treatment.

3.5.2.5 Sumoylation

Histones that have small ubiquitin-like modifier (SUMO) proteins attached to them affect a number of biological functions such as DNA repair and transcriptional control. Similar to ubiquitination sumoylation can modulate protein interactions and stability which can impact chromatin dynamics. Although the exact function of sumoylation in cancer is yet unknown it is thought to have a part in the control of tumor suppressor and oncogene genes.

3.5.2.6 Biotinylation

The attachment of biotin to certain residues of lysine on histones is a relatively less understood modification. It is suggested that biotinylation may impact gene expression and chromatin structure but its precise role in cancer biology remains to be discovered.

3.5.2.7 ADP Ribosylation

DNA repair and chromatin remodeling are two biological processes that are linked to ADP ribosylation which is the attachment of ADP-ribose moieties to histones. This modification may have an effect on how histones interact with DNA and other proteins thus influencing gene expression. ADP ribosylation role in cancer is a developing area of research with its potential implications for therapeutic strategies.

3.5.3 Noncoding RNAs

Particularly in the setting of cancer, noncoding RNAs (ncRNAs) have become important modulators of gene expression and cellular functions. The ncRNAs are important for many biological processes which include gene regulation, chromatin remodeling and cellular signaling pathways but do not translate into proteins like protein-coding RNAs do.

Noncoding RNAs can be broadly classified based on their length and function. Transcripts which include more than 200 nucleotides are called long noncoding RNAs (lncRNAs) whereas miRNAs which are normally about 22 nucleotides long are considered as small noncoding RNAs (Mattick et al., 2023). Small nucleolar RNAs (snoRNAs), circular RNAs (circRNAs) and PIWI-interacting RNAs (piRNAs) are some other noncoding RNAs. Every class of ncRNA has unique regulatory functions and modes of action in cellular processes, especially cancer.

3.5.3.1 Long Non-Coding RNAs in Cancer

Numerous facets of cancer biology such as carcinogenesis, metastasis, and medication resistance have been linked to lncRNAs. It has been demonstrated that lncRNA H19 affects insulin-like growth factor signaling and cell proliferation which suggests that it may be an oncogene (Mattick et al., 2023). Since lncRNA dysregulation is frequently linked to a poor prognosis for cancer patients it may be possible to use these molecules as biomarkers for detection and as targets for treatment. Research has shown that lncRNAs can function as sponging miRNAs, competitive endogenous RNAs (ceRNAs), and controlling target gene expression in the process. For instance, the lncRNA HCG11 targets GFI1 and sponging miR-942-5p to prevent proliferation and metastasis in cervical cancer (Zhang et al., 2020).

3.5.3.2 MicroRNAs and Their Regulatory Functions

MicroRNAs are another class of non-coding RNAs which play a vital role in regulating the gene expression post-transcriptionally. Usually, they get attached to the 3′ untranslated regions (UTRs) of target mRNAs which results in translational suppression or mRNA destruction. Dysregulation of miRNAs has been associated to numerous malignancies where they act as oncogenes or tumor suppressors (Syeda et al., 2020). The expression of key genes involved in cell division, cell death and metastasis can be altered by miRNAs which can impact the course of cancer and its response to therapy (Hussen et al., 2021). The role of miRNAs in drug resistance has also been extensively studied. Certain miRNAs can provide resistance to chemotherapeutic agents by aiming the genes that are involved in drug metabolism and apoptosis (Hussen et al., 2021). Understanding the specific miRNA profiles associated with drug resistance may provide an insight into overcoming therapeutic challenges in cancer treatment.

Non-coding RNAs are involved in various cancer-related signaling pathways that includes the Wnt/β-catenin pathway which is crucial for the division and differentiation of cells. The DDX3, a DEAD-box RNA helicase has been shown to interact with non-coding RNAs to activate Wnt signaling which promotes cancer progression (Lin et al., 2020). Ongoing research in the landscape of non-coding RNAs in cancer is continually evolving with identifying novel lncRNAs and miRNAs that can serve as diagnostic and therapeutic targets. The integration of ncRNA profiling in precision oncology offers a promise to improve cancer diagnostics and treatment strategies.

3.6 ENVIRONMENTAL FACTORS IN CANCER

A wide range of environmental factors can be responsible for the development of cancer. These factors include physical, chemical, and biological elements that collaborate with an individual's genetic predisposition in return influencing cancer risk or its progression (Patierno, 2019). These environmental factors are categorized as modifiable and non-modifiable. Lifestyle choices such as diet, physical activity and exposure to carcinogens are modifiable factors while the genetic predispositions and age are non-modifiable ones (Iwasaki et al., 2023; Olakowski & Bułdak, 2022; Sankpal et al., 2012).

3.6.1 Physical Factors

Physical factors usually avoid any direct or indirect chemical reaction and are a selective variation of carcinogens that promotes carcinogenesis by their physical characteristics. These include agents such as mechanical trauma, ionizing radiation and ultraviolet (UV) radiation which can directly damage DNA and increase cancer risk or progression. Generally, exposure to these types of elements is environmental or based on occupation. In mechanical trauma the basic physical architecture of the extracellular matrix is disrupted which promotes oncogene expression. Chronic mechanical stress such as that experienced by individuals in certain occupations can lead to persistent inflammation and cellular turnover which increases the chances of genetic mutations and cancer development. Ionising radiations include X-rays, medical imaging and nuclear fallout, the free radicals formed by these radiations are connected to various cancers like leukemia and thyroid cancer (Mohan & Chopra, 2022). Leukemia and thyroid cancer are among the radiation-induced cancers that are more likely to occur in some populations exposed to nuclear fallout or medical imaging treatments. The latency period for radiation-induced cancers can vary with some cancers manifesting years or even decades after exposure which highlights the long-term implications of ionizing radiation on public health. Another known risk factor for malignancies is UV exposure from the sun mainly for melanoma and non-melanoma skin cancers. The danger of developing skin cancer is particularly pronounced in individuals with fair skin, ones with a history of sunburns or those who engage in outdoor occupations without proper sun protection.

3.6.2 Chemical Factors

Chemical carcinogens are elements that cause cancer through direct damage to DNA or by inducing changes that trigger vital oncogene or tumor suppressor genes. They are the most diverse set of carcinogenic agents that come from various sources like industrial processes, agricultural practices, and consumer products. Skin and lung cancers are intimately associated with molecules called polycyclic aromatic hydrocarbons (PAHs) which are produced when organic material burns incompletely. After entering the body PAHs may be metabolically activated producing reactive intermediates that attach to DNA and cause mutagenic alterations that could start the development of cancer. Tobacco smoke, grilled foods, and vehicle pollution are among the major sources of PAHs (Cani et al., 2023; Ravanbakhsh et al., 2023). Heavy metals like arsenic, cadmium, and chromium have been linked to various cancers, majorly lung and bladder cancer. Exposure to these metals often occurs through contaminated water, occupational settings, or industrial emissions. Reactive oxygen species (ROS) are frequently produced during heavy metal-induced carcinogenesis, resulting in oxidative strain, DNA damage, and interference with cellular signaling pathways (Cani et al., 2023). Certain pesticides and insecticides like DDT and glyphosate have also shown association with cancer risk in agricultural workers or people living in the treated residential areas (Leonel et al., 2021; Pluth et al., 2019). These pesticides cause endocrine disruption, genotoxicity, and the induction of inflammatory responses which contributes to the carcinogenic process.

3.6.3 Biological Carcinogens

Bacteria, parasites, and viruses, are some of the biological carcinogens that can cause cancer. The mechanisms by which these agents induce cancer often involve chronic inflammation, immune suppression, or direct genetic alteration. Certain strains of HPV lead to expression of viral oncogenes which are known to cause cervical cancer and also engage in other anogenital cancers. These oncogenes disrupt the normal regulatory functions of tumor suppressor proteins like p53 and retinoblastoma (Rb) which results in uncontrolled cellular proliferation and genomic instability. Vaccination programs are being implemented to reduce the incidence of HPV-related cancers (Ashique et al., 2023). Chronic infection with viruses like Hepatitis B and C can lead to fibrosis, cirrhosis, and ultimately liver cancer. Public health initiatives aimed at vaccination and screening have been crucial in reducing the burden of these infections (Goossens & Hoshida, 2015; Xu et al., 2014). Helicobacter pylori is associated with gastric cancer and is believed to induce cancer through chronic inflammation and alterations in gastric mucosa. Intestinal metaplasia, atrophic gastritis, and dysplasia are all possible outcomes of the ongoing inflammatory response and they are all indications of stomach cancer (Yang et al., 2021) (Figure 3.2).

3.7 TECHNOLOGIES FOR EARLY CANCER DETECTION

Early cancer detection technologies have evolved significantly over the years, incorporating various methodologies to improve sensitivity and specificity. These technologies can be broadly categorized into imaging techniques, liquid biopsies, and emerging molecular assays. The conventional mainstays for cancer screening have been imaging methods including ultrasound and magnetic resonance imaging (MRI) (Aldhaeebi et al., 2020). However, these methods often face challenges such as high false-positive rates and the potential for over-diagnosis which can lead to unnecessary interventions (Jatoi, 2021).

Recent advances in liquid biopsy technologies have introduced a promising alternative for early cancer detection. Circulating tumor DNA (ctDNA) and other biomarkers in the blood are analyzed by liquid biopsies, which offer a minimally invasive method for identifying cancer at earlier stages. Studies indicate that multi-cancer early detection (MCED) tests utilizing ctDNA can achieve low false-positive rates while detecting multiple cancer types simultaneously (Bredno et al., 2021; Liu et al., 2020). A new finding demonstrated a less than 1% false-positive rate in various types of cancer by using methylation signatures in cell-free DNA (Liu et al., 2020). This contrasts with traditional imaging methods, where the cumulative false-positive rates can significantly increase when multiple tests are combined (Bredno et al., 2021).

Optical biosensors have gained noteworthy importance in the area of cancer detection as a non-invasive alternative due to their ability to provide rapid and specific analysis of biomarkers associated with various malignancies. These biosensors utilize light-based detection methods like

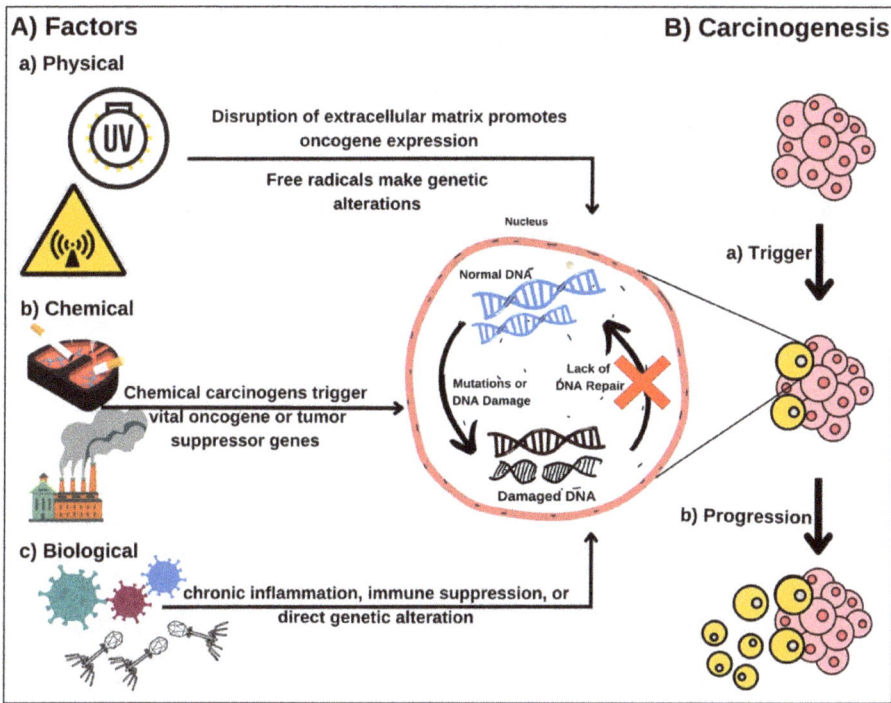

Figure 3.2 Different environmental factors and their mechanisms: (A) Environmental factors. (a) Physical, (b) Chemical, (c) Biological. (B) Mechanism of carcinogenesis (a) Primary trigger and (b) Progression.

fluorescence and surface plasmon resonance to identify cancer-related proteins and nucleic acids in biological samples. The silicon nanowire biosensors have demonstrated remarkable sensitivity that enables the detection of cancer biomarkers at concentrations as low as femtomolar levels, which is crucial for early diagnosis (Ivanov et al., 2021; Smith et al., 2020).

Moreover, integrating advanced technologies such as microfluidics and artificial intelligence (AI) has further enhanced cancer screening capabilities. Microfluidic devices allow for manipulating small fluid volumes which facilitates the detection of cancer biomarkers with high precision (Noor et al., 2023). AI algorithms can analyze complex datasets to identify patterns associated with cancer risk, thus improving early detection rates. The use of next-generation sequencing in liquid biopsies has enhanced the sensitivity of detecting early-stage cancers, but challenges remain regarding the reliability of these tests at the initial stages of cancer (Connal et al., 2023).

3.8 CANCER THERAPIES

The Cancer therapies have evolved significantly over the years, with methods such as chemotherapy, radiation therapy, and surgery being the crucial ones for treatment strategies. Each approach follows a distinct mechanism of action and has its benefits and limits that must be considered when adapting treatment to individual patient needs.

3.8.1 Traditional Cancer Therapies

3.8.1.1 Chemotherapy

It is one of the most widely used traditional cancer therapies, where cytotoxic chemicals are used to kill quickly dividing cancer cells. Chemotherapy's effectiveness can vary according to the type of tumor and personal factors of an affected individual. A recent study found that the date of initiating chemotherapy sessions significantly affects survival outcomes in patients with colon cancer, suggesting that earlier initiation may correspond with improved survival rates (Taieb & Gallois, 2020). The line of action for chemotherapy involves various strategies, including the disruption of DNA synthesis, intervention in mitosis, and inducing apoptosis in cancer cells. However, the non-selective nature of these agents affects normal cells as well, leading to a range of side effects.

The most draining side effect is chemotherapy-induced nausea and vomiting, which significantly impairs a patient's quality of life and makes it hard to keep up with treatment protocols. Some factors like a patient's nutritional status and the presence of coexisting conditions impact the tolerance and effectiveness of chemotherapy, where malnourished patients experience higher rates of treatment-related toxicities (Li et al., 2024).

3.8.1.2 Radiation Therapy

It is a cornerstone of cancer treatment utilized in approximately 50% of patients during their disease course, either as a primary mode of treatment or in conjunction with chemotherapy and surgery. The induction of DNA damage and destruction of cancer cells is caused by the application of these high-powered radiations. The historical context of radiation therapy dates back to the late 19th century following the discovery of X-rays and has evolved significantly with advancements in technology and understanding of radiobiology.

The efficiency of radiation therapy often varies based on several aspects, including the type of cancer, specific radiation technique employed, and biological characteristics of the tumor. Melanoma is often resistant to radiation, which makes it a challenging target for traditional RT protocols (Kaur et al., 2023). Despite its benefits, radiation therapy is not without side effects. Acute and chronic adverse effects can significantly impact patients' quality of life. Common acute effects include fatigue, skin reactions and mucositis while long-term effects may involve fibrosis and secondary malignancies (Ingole et al., 2024).

3.8.1.3 Surgery

This remains a fundamental approach for many solid tumors often serving as the first line of treatment. Surgery does not only remove the tumor but also potentially enhance the effectiveness of subsequent therapies. Recent studies have shown that the timing of adjuvant chemotherapy following surgery can significantly affect patient outcomes with immediate initiation being more beneficial (Kaur et al., 2023). Also, the surgical interventions can modulate the immune responses which may influence the effectiveness of subsequent chemotherapy.

3.8.2 Emerging Cancer Therapies
3.8.2.1 Targeted Nanocarriers

Targeted nanocarriers represent a promising innovation in cancer therapy addressing the limitations of traditional treatment modalities such as chemotherapy and radiotherapy. Conventional therapies often suffer from issues like poor bioavailability, high toxicity and the development of multidrug resistance (MDR) (Duan et al., 2023). Nanocarriers which includes solid lipid nanoparticles (NPs), liposomes and polymeric NPs have been engineered to improve drug delivery by enhancing the stability and solubility of therapeutic agents thereby increasing their therapeutic indices (Parveen et al., 2023). Recent studies pointed out the potential of carbohydrate-functionalized liposomes as effective nanocarriers in cancer therapy. These liposomes can selectively target cancer cells, thereby reducing systemic toxicity and enhancing drug accumulation at the tumor site (Rekha Mol & Mohamed Hatha, 2023). Integrating functional polymers into nanocarrier systems has led to the establishment of non-invasive photothermal therapy (PTT) platforms which combine imaging and therapeutic capabilities which improves targeted therapy (Wu et al., 2021). The combination of photodynamic therapy (PDT) with chemotherapy using pH-responsive copolymer nanocarriers has shown promising results in enhancing anticancer effects demonstrating the versatility of nanocarrier systems in delivering multiple therapeutic modalities (Y. Wu et al., 2022). The ability of these nanocarriers to provide a controlled release and targeted delivery is crucial in overcoming the challenges posed by tumor diverseness and complex tumor microenvironment.

3.8.2.2 Macrophage Targeting

Macrophages play a dual role in progression of cancer behaving as tumor promoters and suppressors based on their polarization. A new approach to cancer treatment is targeting macrophages especially to increase the effectiveness of immunotherapy. Recent advancements in engineered antibodies and nanocarriers have focused on harnessing macrophages to deliver therapeutic agents directly to tumors (Mantovani et al., 2022). The recent evolution of macrophage-targeting strategies involves the use of engineered nanoparticles that selectively bind to macrophages which facilitates the delivery of chemotherapeutic agents or immunotherapeutic. This approach not only increases drug accumulation at the tumor location but also affects macrophages innate immunological capabilities to encourage the killing of tumor cells (Mukhtar et al., 2020). Therapeutic bacteria as vectors for drug delivery has shown potential in targeting macrophages thereby improving the therapeutic outcomes in various cancer models. Furthermore, combining these macrophage-targeting strategies with other treatment methods like checkpoint inhibitors have been proposed to overcome the immunosuppressive tumor microenvironment which will enhance the overall effectiveness of cancer immunotherapy (Mantovani et al., 2022).

3.9 FUTURE DIRECTIONS IN CANCER RESEARCH

Future directions in cancer research are increasingly characterized by the integration of advanced technologies, interdisciplinary collaboration, and a focus on personalized medicine. The convergence of big data analytics, machine learning (ML) and computational systems biology is confident to revolutionize oncology research.

One promising avenue is the enhancement of community-based participatory research (CBPR) initiatives. These initiatives emphasize collaboration between academic institutions and community organizations to address healthcare disparities and improve participation in cancer research among diverse populations. The importance of engaging community partners to develop and implement innovative outreach strategies that can bolster awareness and participation in biomedical research ultimately aims to reduce cancer disparities (Barrett et al., 2020).

The exploration of plant-based therapies and natural elements is gaining traction as researchers seek to identify non-toxic alternatives to conventional treatments. Compounds derived from medicinal plants such as thymol and various polyphenols have demonstrated apoptotic effects on cancer cells and are being investigated for their potential as supplementary therapies (Khan et al., 2022). This approach not only addresses the need for safer treatment options but also influences the rich biodiversity of natural products to discover novel anticancer agents.

Machine learning is revolutionizing cancer research by enhancing predictive modeling and decision-making processes. The ability of ML algorithms to handle complex non-linear relationships in data makes them particularly suited for cancer prognosis and risk assessment. The use of a multimodal deep learning technique that combines genetic and histological data which enhances disease prognosis and finds new biomarkers (Chen et al., 2022). The implementation of computational systems in cancer research is facilitating the development of innovative clinical decision support tools. Recent research highlighted that big data analytics can enhance clinical workflows by providing actionable insights derived from large datasets which ultimately improves patient care (Dash et al., 2019).

Finally, the significance of medical physics in tumor treatment cannot be understated. Innovations in radiotherapy which includes carbon ion therapy, are creating a new approach for more inclusive and effective treatment options that minimize damage to surrounding healthy tissues while maximizing tumor control (Ramazi et al., 2020). The future of cancer treatment will likely involve a multidisciplinary approach that combines the strengths of various therapeutic techniques guided by a deeper understanding of cancer biology and patient-specific factors.

3.10 CONCLUSION

In conclusion, the intricate interplay of genetic mutations, tumor microenvironment interactions, and epigenetic modifications underscores the complexity of cancer initiation and progression. This chapter highlights the critical role of TSG and proto-oncogenes in growth and proliferation of cells, emphasizing how their mutations lead to uncontrolled division. Additionally, the tumor microenvironment, composed of various cellular components, significantly influences tumor behavior and metastasis. The exploration of epigenetic changes further enriches our understanding by illustrating how gene expression can be altered without changes to the DNA sequence itself. As we explore these multifaceted factors, it becomes evident that a comprehensive understanding is critical for development of effective cancer diagnosis, prevention, and treatment modalities. The discussion of both traditional and emerging therapies, including targeted nanocarriers and macrophage-targeting approaches, reflects the ongoing evolution in cancer treatment paradigms. By integrating knowledge from genetics, epigenetics, and TME, we can pave the path for innovative strategies that enhance patient outcomes and address the challenges posed by cancer's complexity.

REFERENCES

Aldhaeebi MA et al. (2020). Review of microwaves techniques for breast cancer detection. *Sensors (Switzerland)* 20/8.

Arneth B. (2020). Tumor microenvironment. *Medicina (Lithuania)* 56/1.

Ashique S et al. (2023). HPV pathogenesis, various types of vaccines, safety concern, prophylactic and therapeutic applications to control cervical cancer, and future perspective. *VirusDisease* 34/2.

Ayyanan A et al. (2006). Increased Wnt signaling triggers oncogenic conversion of human breast epithelial cells by a Notch-dependent mechanism. *Proc Nat Acad Sci USA* 103/10.

Baca SC et al. (2013). Punctuated evolution of prostate cancer genomes. *Cell* 153/3.

Barrett NJ et al. (2020). Factors associated with biomedical research participation within community-based samples across 3 National Cancer Institute–designated cancer centers. *Cancer* 126/5.

Bredno J et al. (2021). Clinical correlates of circulating cell-free DNA tumor fraction. *PLoS One* 16/8.

Cani M et al. (2023). How does environmental and occupational exposure contribute to carcinogenesis in genitourinary and lung cancers? *Cancers* 15/10.

Cavalieri V. (2021). The expanding constellation of histone post-translational modifications in the epigenetic landscape. *Genes* 12/10.

Chandraprasad MS et al. (2022). Introduction to cancer and treatment approaches. In Swamy MK et al., eds, Paclitaxel: Sources, Chemistry, Anticancer Action, and Current Biotechnology, Academic Press, Chicago:1–27.

Chen RJ et al. (2022). Pan-cancer integrative histology-genomic analysis via multimodal deep learning. *Cancer Cell* 40/8.

Clancy S. (2008). Genetic mutation | Learn science at scitable. *Nature Education* 1/1.

Connal S et al. (2023). Liquid biopsies: the future of cancer early detection. *J Translat Med* 21/1.

Cortés-Ciriano I et al. (2020). Comprehensive analysis of chromothripsis in 2,658 human cancers using whole-genome sequencing. *Nature Genet* 52/3.

Dash S et al. (2019). Big data in healthcare: Management, analysis and future prospects. *J Big Data* 6/1.

Derakhshani A et al. (2020). Overcoming trastuzumab resistance in HER2-positive breast cancer using combination therapy. *J Cellul Physiol* 235/4.

Derelanko MJ. (2014). Carcinogenesis. In Derelanko MJ, Auletta CS, eds, Handbook of Toxicology: Third Edn., CRC Press, Boca Raton.

Duan C et al. (2023). Overcoming cancer Multi-drug Resistance (MDR): Reasons, mechanisms, nanotherapeutic solutions, and challenges. *Biomed Pharmacother* 162.

Fares J et al. (2020). Molecular principles of metastasis: A hallmark of cancer revisited. *Signal Transduct Target Ther* 5/1.

Feng S, De Carvalho DD. (2022). Clinical advances in targeting epigenetics for cancer therapy. *FEBS J* 289/5.

Feuk L et al. (2006). Structural variation in the human genome. *Nature Rev Genet* 7/2.

Gariglio P. (2011). Oncogenes and tumor suppressor genes. In Camacho J, ed., Cancer Biology and the Nuclear Envelope: Recent Advances May Elucidate Past Paradoxes, 64–82. Bentham Science Publishers, Sharjah, UAE.

Gerstberger S et al. (2023). Metastasis. *Cell* 186/8:1564–1579.

Ghosh A et al. (2024). Suppressive cancer nonstop extension mutations increase C-terminal hydrophobicity and disrupt evolutionarily conserved amino acid patterns. *Nature Commun* 15/1:9209.

Giraldo NA et al. (2019). The clinical role of the TME in solid cancer. *Br J Cancer* 120/1.

Goossens, N, Hoshida Y. (2015). Hepatitis C virus-induced hepatocellular carcinoma. *Clin Molec Hepatol* 21/2.

Hussen BM et al. (2021). MicroRNA: A signature for cancer progression. *Biomed Pharmacother* 138.

Hutter S et al. (2017). Modeling and targeting MYC genes in childhood brain tumors. *Genes* 8/4.

Imielinski M et al. (2017). Insertions and deletions target lineage-defining genes in human cancers. *Cell* 168/3:460–472.e14.

Ingole S et al. (2024). Toxic effects of cancer therapies. In: *Public Health and Toxicology Issues in Drug Research, Volume 2: Toxicity and Toxicodynamics*, 2, 353–379. https://doi.org/10.1016/B978-0-443-15842-1.00004-1.

Ivanov YD et al. (2021). Use of silicon nanowire sensors for early cancer diagnosis. *Molecules* 26/12.

Iwasaki M et al. (2023). Exposure to environmental chemicals and cancer risk: Epidemiological evidence from Japanese studies. *Genes Environm* 45/1.

Jan R, Chaudhry GES. (2019). Understanding apoptosis and apoptotic pathways targeted cancer therapeutics. *Adv Pharm Bull* 9/2:205–218.

Jatoi I. (2021). Are advancements in screening technology contributing to breast cancer over-diagnosis? *Curr Opinion Oncol* 33/6.

Jin H et al. (2023). Rational combinations of targeted cancer therapies: Background, advances and challenges. *Nature Rev Drug Disc* 22/3.

Jurca CM et al. (2023). A new frameshift mutation of PTEN gene associated with Cowden syndrome—Case report and brief review of the literature. *Genes* 14/10.

Kaur R et al. (2023). Cancer treatment therapies: Traditional to modern approaches to combat cancers. *Molec Biol Rep* 50/11.

Khan AW et al. (2022). Role of plant-derived active constituents in cancer treatment and their mechanisms of action. *Cells* 11/8.

Kobayashi Y, Mitsudomi T. (2016). Not all epidermal growth factor receptor mutations in lung cancer are created equal: Perspectives for individualized treatment strategy. *Cancer Sci* 107/9:1179–1186.

Krupina K et al. (2024). Scrambling the genome in cancer: Causes and consequences of complex chromosome rearrangements. *Nature Rev Genet* 25/3:196–210.

Kubli SP et al. (2021). Beyond immune checkpoint blockade: Emerging immunological strategies. *Nature Rev Drug Disc* 20/12.

Kumar S et al. (2023). Targeting PD-1/PD-L1 in cancer immunotherapy: An effective strategy for treatment of triple-negative breast cancer (TNBC) patients. *Genes Dis* 10/4.

Lahtz C, Pfeifer GP. (2011). Epigenetic changes of DNA repair genes in cancer. *J Molec Cell Biol* 3/1:51–58.

Lan T et al. (2021). Mesenchymal stem/stromal cells in cancer therapy. *J Hematol Oncol* 14/1.

Leonel ACLDS et al. (2021). The pesticides use and the risk for head and neck cancer: A review of case-control studies. *Medicina Oral Patologia Oral y Cirugia Bucal* 26/1.

Li N et al. (2024). Influence of malnutrition according to the glim criteria on the chemotherapy toxicities in patients with advanced lung cancer. *Support Care Cancer* 32/6.

Lin S et al. (2020). Roles of Wnt/β-catenin signaling pathway regulatory long non-coding RNAs in the pathogenesis of non-small cell lung cancer. *Cancer Manage Res* 12.

Liu MC et al. (2020). Sensitive and specific multi-cancer detection and localization using methylation signatures in cell-free DNA. *Ann Oncol* 31(6).

Lugano R et al. (2020). Tumor angiogenesis: Causes, consequences, challenges and opportunities. *Cellul Molec Life Sci* 77/9.

Mantovani A et al. (2022). Macrophages as tools and targets in cancer therapy. *Nature Rev Drug Disc* 21/11.

Matthews HK et al. (2022). Cell cycle control in cancer. *Nat Rev Mol Cell Biol* 23/1:74–88.

Mattick JS et al. (2023). Long non-coding RNAs: Definitions, functions, challenges and recommendations. *Nature Rev Molec Cell Biol* 24/6.

Mohan S, Chopra V. (2022). Biological effects of radiation. In: Dhoble S et al., eds, *Radiation Dosimetry Phosphors: Synthesis, Mechanisms, Properties and Analysis*. Woodhead.

Mukhtar M et al. (2020). Drug delivery to macrophages: A review of nano-therapeutics targeted approach for inflammatory disorders and cancer. *Expert Opinion Drug Deliv* 17/9.

Nenclares P, Harrington KJ. (2020). The biology of cancer. *Medicine* 48/2:67–72.

Noor J et al. (2023). Microfluidic technology, artificial intelligence, and biosensors as advanced technologies in cancer screening: A review article. *Cureus* 15/5:e39634.

Oketch DJA et al. (2024). Copy number variations in pancreatic cancer: From biological significance to clinical utility. *Int J Molec Sci* 25/1.

Olakowski M, Bułdak Ł. (2022). Modifiable and non-modifiable risk factors for the development of non-hereditary pancreatic Cancer. *Medicina (Lithuania)* 58/8.

Olivier, M., Hollstein, M., & Hainaut, P. (2010). TP53 mutations in human cancers: Origins, consequences, and clinical use. *Cold Spring Harbor Perspect Biol* 2/1.

Ostroverkhova D et al. (2023). Cancer driver mutations: Predictions and reality. *Trends Molec Med* 29/7:554–566.

Parveen S et al. (2023). Lipid polymer hybrid nanoparticles as potent vehicles for drug delivery in cancer therapeutics. *Med Drug Disc* 20.

Pathak, A et al. (2023). Epigenetics and cancer: A comprehensive review. *Asia Pacific J Cancer Biol* 8/1:75–89.

Patierno SR. (2019). Environmental factors. In Niederhuber JE, ed., Abeloff's Clinical Oncology, 6th ed., Elsevier, Amsterdam:139–153.e2.

Pluth TB et al. (2019). Pesticide exposure and cancer: An integrative literature review. *Saúde Em Debate* 43/122.

Pray LA. (2008). Discovery of DNA double helix: Watson and Crick. *Nature Educat* 1/1:100.

Qing T et al. (2020). Germline variant burden in cancer genes correlates with age at diagnosis and somatic mutation burden. *Nature Communicat* 11/1.

Ramazi S et al. (2020). Evaluation of post-translational modifications in histone proteins: A review on histone modification defects in developmental and neurological disorders. *J Biosci* 45/1.

Ravanbakhsh M et al (2023). Effect of Polycyclic Aromatic Hydrocarbons (PAHs) on respiratory diseases and the risk factors related to cancer. *Polycyclic Aromatic Compounds* 43/9.

Rekha Mol KR, Mohamed Hatha AA. (2023). Use of lectin-functionalized and lectin-targeted nanoparticles for multiple therapeutic applications. In: Thomas S et al., eds, *Applications of Multifunctional Nanomaterials*. Elsevier.

Saleem M et al. (2020). The BRCA1 and BRCA2 genes in early-onset breast cancer patients. *Adv Experim Med Biol* 1292/1–12.

Sandoval J, Esteller M. (2012). Cancer epigenomics: Beyond genomics. *Curr Opinion Genet Developm* 22/1:50–55.

Sankpal UT et al. (2012). Environmental factors in causing human cancers: Emphasis on tumorigenesis. *Tumor Biol* 33/5.

Shlien, A., & Malkin, D. (2009). Copy number variations and cancer. *Genome Med* 1/6.

Siegel RL et al. (2023). Cancer statistics, 2023. *CA* 73/1:7–48.

Skourti E, Dhillon P. (2022). Cancer epigenetics: Promises and pitfalls for cancer therapy. *FEBS J* 289/5.

Smith R et al. (2020). Silicon nanowires and their impact on cancer detection and monitoring. *ACS Applied Nano Mat* 3/9.

Soverini S et al. (2011). BCR-ABL kinase domain mutation analysis in chronic myeloid leukemia patients treated with tyrosine kinase inhibitors: Recommendations from an expert panel on behalf of European LeukemiaNet. *Blood* 118/5:1208–1215.

Stenson PD et al. (2020). The Human Gene Mutation Database (HGMD®): Optimizing its use in a clinical diagnostic or research setting. *Human Genet* 139/10:1197–1207.

Syeda ZA et al. (2020). Regulatory mechanism of microrna expression in cancer. *Int J Molec Sci* 21/5.

Taieb J, Gallois C. (2020). Adjuvant chemotherapy for stage iii colon cancer. *Cancers* 12/9.

Tajaldini M, et al. (2023). Strategy of targeting the tumor microenvironment via inhibition of fibroblast/fibrosis remodeling new era to cancer chemo-immunotherapy resistance. *Eur J Pharmacol* 957.

Taylor AM et al. (2018). Genomic and functional approaches to understanding cancer aneuploidy. *Cancer Cell* 33/4.

Van Bockstal MR et al. (2020). Somatic mutations and copy number variations in breast cancers with heterogeneous HER2 amplification. *Molec Oncol* 14/4:671–685.

Wang H et al. (2021). Characteristics of pre-metastatic niche: The landscape of molecular and cellular pathways. *Molec Biomed* 2/1.

Wang Q et al. (2023). Role of tumor microenvironment in cancer progression and therapeutic strategy. *Cancer Med* 12/10.

Wu C et al. (2021). Near-infrared-responsive functional nanomaterials: The first domino of combined tumor therapy. *Nano Today* 36.

Wu Y et al. (2022). A pH-sensitive supramolecular nanosystem with chlorin e6 and triptolide co-delivery for chemo-photodynamic combination therapy. *Asian J Pharmaceut Sci* 17/2.

Xu HZ et al. (2014). Hepatitis B virus-related hepatocellular carcinoma: Pathogenic mechanisms and novel therapeutic interventions. *Gastrointest Tumors* 1/3.

Yang H et al. (2021). Chronic inflammation and long-lasting changes in the gastric mucosa after Helicobacter pylori infection involved in gastric cancer. *Inflammation Res* 70:10–12.

You JS, Jones PA. (2012). Cancer genetics and epigenetics: Two sides of the same coin? *Cancer Cell* 22/1:9–20.

Zhang Y et al. (2020). Long noncoding RNA HCG11 inhibited growth and invasion in cervical cancer by sponging miR-942-5p and targeting GFI1. *Cancer Med* 9/19.

4

Inherited Cancer Syndromes
Recognition and Management

Muskan Verma and Parul Sharma

4.1 INTRODUCTION

The understanding of hereditary cancer syndromes plays a pivotal role in the early detection, treatment, and prevention of many types of cancers. This chapter provides a comprehensive overview of most hereditary cancer syndromes, focusing on the basic genetics and mechanism of inheritance of common inherited cancer syndromes (*e.g.,* Lynch syndrome, BRCA, and gastrointestinal stromal tumor). This chapter provides a better understanding of these diseases for clinicians to identify at-risk individuals, carry out individualized surveillance, and implement preventive interventions. To reduce the risk of cancer in future generations, understanding these syndromes is crucial for the patients and their families to make educated healthcare decisions. This chapter describes an outline of 20 hereditary syndromes, shedding a light on cancer as a major characteristic feature (Figure 4.1, Table 4.1).

4.2 LYNCH SYNDROME (HNPCC)

Lynch syndrome (hereditary non-polyposis colorectal cancer) is an inherited disorder that confers a 70–80% risk of developing colorectal cancer, which occurs at the age of 45–50 years in the United States (Davidson *et al*, 2021). Lynch syndrome (LS) is caused by mutations in DNA-MMR genes such as MLH1, MSH2, MSH6, PMS2, and EPCAM. These mutations cause genetic instability and

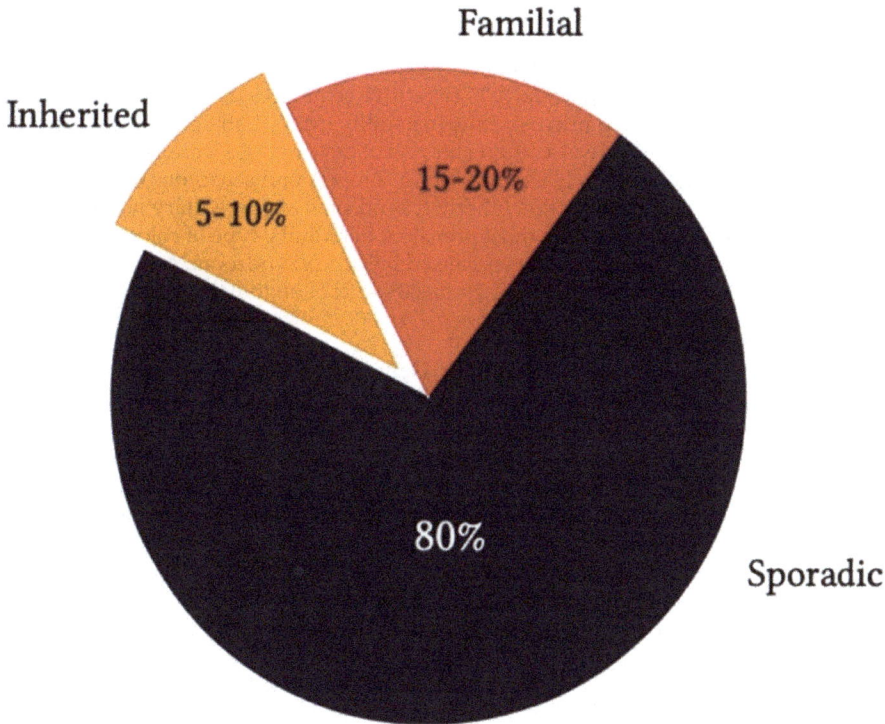

Figure 4.1 Cancer aetiology distribution by genetic contribution. The percentages of cancer cases according to genetic and familial factors are depicted in the pie chart. Five to ten percent of all cancer cases are caused by inherited cancer syndromes, which are defined by germline mutations in particular genes.

DOI: 10.1201/9781003542162-4

Table 4.1: **List of Hereditary Cancer Syndromes with their Gene Involved, Mode of Inheritance and Associated Cancer Risks**

HCS	Gene	Inheritance	Associated Cancers
Lynch syndrome	MLH1, MSH2, MSH6, PMS2, EPCAM	Autosomal dominant (AD)	Colorectal, endometrial, ovarian, gastric, and others.
Hereditary Breast and Ovarian Cancer Syndrome	BRCA1, BRCA2	AD	Breast, ovarian, prostate, pancreatic, and melanoma.
Li-Fraumeni syndrome	TP53	AD	Breast, sarcomas, brain tumors, leukemia, and adrenocortical carcinoma.
Familial Adenomatous Polyposis	APC	AD	Colorectal, duodenal, and thyroid.
Peutz-Jeghers syndrome	STK11 (LKB1)	AD	Colorectal, gastric, pancreatic, breast, and ovarian.
Cowden syndrome	PTEN	AD	Breast, thyroid, endometrial, and renal cell carcinoma.
Ataxia-Telangiectasia	ATM	Autosomal recessive (AR)	Lymphomas and leukemias.
Tuberous sclerosis complex	TSC1, TSC2	AD	Renal angiomyolipomas, subependymal giant cell astrocytoma, and cardiac rhabdomyomas.
Von Hippel–Lindau syndrome	VHL	AD	Renal cell carcinoma, pheochromocytoma, and hemangioblastomas.
MutYH-Associated polyposis	MUTYH	AR	Colorectal and duodenal cancer.

Source: Adapted from Gomy and Diz (2016).

the development of cancer by impairing the body's capacity to correct errors made during DNA replication (Peltomäki *et al*, 2023) particularly in repetitive sequences of DNA known as microsatellites through a phenomenon called microsatellite instability (MSI) (Latham *et al*, 2019). Individuals suffering from Lynch syndrome are also at greater risk of developing severe skin lesions, typically keratoacanthomas, epitheliomas, glioblastomas (brain tumors), and sebaceous carcinomas. While the majority of cancer cases caused by this inherited syndrome are hereditary non-polyposis colorectal cancer (HNPCC), which is the most prevalent hereditary type of colorectal cancer having an incidence of 10% in all cancer cases caused by Lynch syndrome. As affected patients have an 80% lifetime risk of colorectal cancer and a 60% risk of endometrial cancer, it is critical to identify them (Bhattacharya *et al*., 2024).

4.2.1 Basic Genetics

Lynch syndrome is caused by germline mutations in DNA mismatch repair (MMR) genes. Germline mutations in DNA mismatch repair (MMR) genes, such as MLH1, MSH2, MSH6, PMS2, and deletions in EPCAM (which silences MSH2), result in Lynch syndrome, a hereditary cancer predisposition syndrome. These genes are essential for fixing mistakes in DNA replication. Microsatellite instability (MSI) is caused by mutations that affect their function and accumulate replication errors, particularly in repetitive DNA sequences known as microsatellites (Cerretelli *et al*, 2020). Because Lynch syndrome is inherited in an autosomal dominant manner, a person who has the mutation has a 50% chance of passing it on to their children (Sharaf *et al*, 2013). The two-hit theory of cancer development is consistent with the inactivation of the second allele, which frequently occurs somatically. Vigilant screening and preventive measures are necessary due to this genetic defect, which dramatically raises the risk of several cancers, especially colorectal and endometrial (Morrow *et al*, 2024). Lynch syndrome is inherited in an autosomal dominant manner, which means that a single copy of a mismatch repair (MMR) gene mutation is enough to make a person more likely to develop cancer. A germline mutation in one allele of an MMR gene (MLH1, MSH2, MSH6, PMS2, or EPCAM) is inherited from one parent by the affected person. The two-hit theory of carcinogenesis states that the second allele usually experiences a somatic mutation or loss of function in impacted tissues (Tamura *et al*, 2019).

4.2.2 Diagnostic Approach

To be diagnosed with HNPCC, individuals must meet the Amsterdam II criteria that enable clinicians to identify families that are likely to have Lynch syndrome. The Amsterdam series of clinical criteria in which a family must satisfy the conditions of the *3-2-1* rule, where at least three family members must have a Lynch syndrome-associated cancer, the cancer must have at least two successive affected generations, and one of the cancers is diagnosed before the age of 50 in the patient's family (Vasen *et al*, 1999). The individuals who test positive for the mutation in any of the MMR genes MSH2, MLH1, MSH6, or PMS2 are also considered to have Lynch syndrome. This technique is known as microsatellite instability (MSI) testing, which is used to detect genomic instability in microsatellite regions of a DNA sequence (Leclerc *et al*, 2021). It is used to compare the DNA of a tumor sample with normal tissue from the same individual. The diagnosis of Lynch syndrome is dependent on two results of MSI testing: MSI-high (MSI-H) indicating high potential risk of LS and MSI-stable (MSS) suggesting no MMR deficiency. Other major factor considered for diagnosis of LS is Bethesda guidelines considered to be broader than the Amsterdam criteria are used to identify LS families by classifying colorectal cancer cases in a community by further molecular evaluation using IHC analysis (Rodriguez-Bigas *et al*, 1997). Immunohistochemistry (IHC) for MMR proteins uses tumor tissue from the individual's family to evaluate the existence of MMR proteins (MLH1, MSH2, MSH6 and PMS2) by staining the tumor tissue to determine the expression of MMR proteins. The loss of protein expression in IHC suggests a potential MMR gene mutation, while the presence of all proteins indicates normal MMR function, ruling out Lynch syndrome (Jenkins *et al*, 2007). In addition to this, several other diagnostic methods when used in combination for the diagnosis of LS are MLH1 Promoter Methylation testing, Genetic testing for germline mutations, BRAF mutation testing and Family history analysis ensures the accuracy of the diagnosis and helps the clinicians to enable personalized cancer surveillance and risk reduction strategies. Moreover, genetic counseling before and after the diagnosis plays a crucial role in individuals and their families to fight against this inherited syndrome (Weissman *et al*, 2011).

4.3 BRCA1 AND BRCA2 HEREDITARY BREAST AND OVARIAN CANCER SYNDROME

One of the most well-known hereditary cancer syndromes is BRCA1 and BRCA2 hereditary breast and ovarian cancer syndrome, which is defined by an elevated lifetime risk of breast, ovarian, and other cancers. These genes, which are found on chromosomes 17 and 13, respectively, are essential for homologous recombination-based DNA repair and genomic stability. BRCA1 or BRCA2 germline mutations affect how well they function, which increases the risk of developing cancer and causes cumulative DNA damage (Welcsh & King, 2001). Because of the autosomal dominant pattern of inheritance, these mutations can be inherited and passed on by both men and women. Finding people who have BRCA mutations is essential for risk-reduction plans, targeted cancer screening, and individualized treatment plans into place, which can greatly improve outcomes for impacted families (Petrucelli *et al*, 2022).

4.3.1 Basic Genetics

Germline mutations in the BRCA1 (chromosome 17q21) and BRCA2 (chromosome 13q12.3) genes result in BRCA1 and BRCA2 hereditary breast and ovarian cancer syndrome. Through the homologous recombination repair pathway, a crucial mechanism for preserving genomic stability, these genes encode proteins essential for DNA repair. Both gene mutations affect DNA repair, which increases the risk of developing cancers, especially ovarian and breast cancers, and causes genetic damage to accumulate (Gayther & Ponder, 1997). Regardless of gender, people with a mutation in one copy of the BRCA1 or BRCA2 gene have a 50% chance of passing the mutation on to their offspring because the syndrome follows autosomal dominant inheritance. Men are more likely to develop prostate, pancreatic, and breast cancers, while women are much more likely to develop ovarian and breast cancers, even though both sexes can inherit these mutations. Crucially, penetrance differs based on the type of mutation and family history, and genetic counseling is crucial for determining who is at risk and directing treatment and prevention choices (Serova *et al*, 1997).

4.3.2 Diagnostic Approach

Genetic testing, family history analyses, and clinical evaluations are all used in the diagnosis of BRCA1 and BRCA2 syndrome. Finding patterns of early-onset breast or ovarian cancer, multiple affected relatives, or male breast cancer, all of which may indicate a hereditary cancer risk— requires a thorough family history. In order to help patients, navigate testing and interpret results, genetic counseling is essential. Comprehensive sequencing to find mutations across BRCA1 and BRCA2, tests for large genomic rearrangements, and targeted mutation analysis for known familial variants are all examples of diagnostic genetic testing (Eccles *et al*, 2015). Therapeutic decisions, especially the use of PARP inhibitors, can be influenced by tumor testing, such as evaluating somatic BRCA mutations or loss of heterozygosity. The use of multigene panel testing is growing since it enables the simultaneous assessment of BRCA and other genes linked to cancer susceptibility (Tung & Garber, 2018). In patients without a strong family history, histopathological characteristics such as triple-negative breast cancer or high-grade serous ovarian cancer may lead to genetic testing. In populations with a high frequency of BRCA mutations, like Ashkenazi Jews, population-based screening is also beneficial (Roa *et al*, 1996). Personalized cancer prevention and treatment plans are becoming possible thanks to emerging technologies like liquid biopsies and polygenic risk scores, which are improving diagnostic precision and risk stratification (Figure 4.2).

4.3.3 Diagnostic Challenges and Approaches

There are several difficulties in diagnosing BRCA1 and BRCA2 mutations, but focused approaches have increased precision and accessibility. Finding variants of uncertain significance (VUS), in which the clinical significance of mutations is unknown, is a major problem. Computational

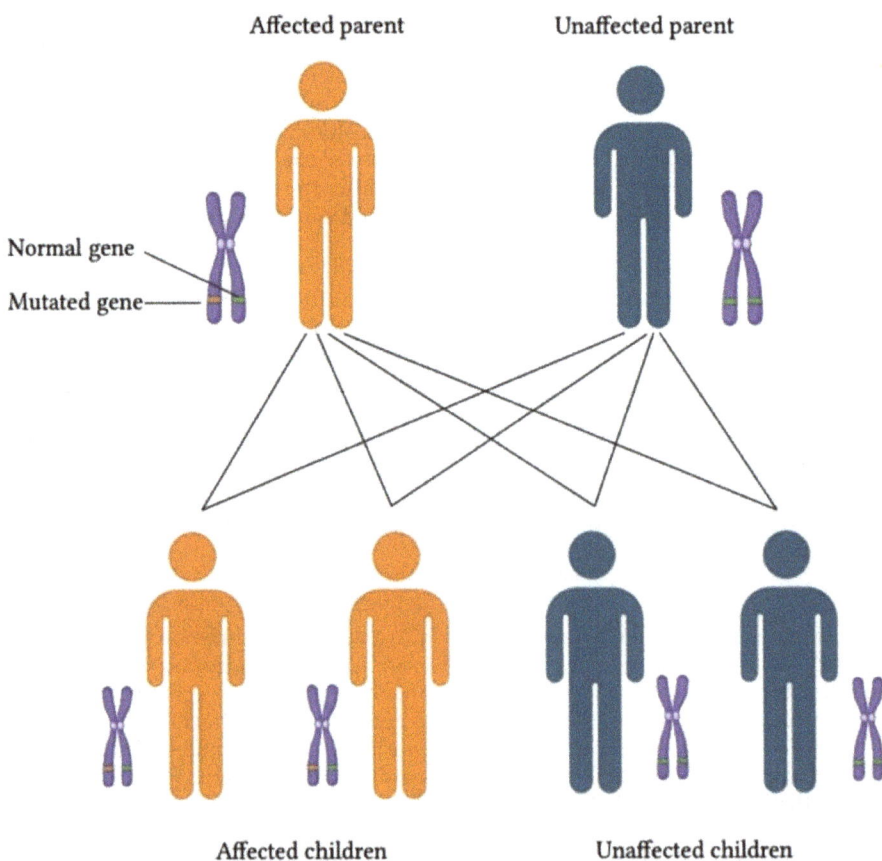

Figure 4.2 Autosomal dominance inheritance pattern. The transmission of genetic traits in autosomal inheritance patterns is depicted in this figure. A single copy of the mutated gene (shown by a shaded allele) is enough to cause the condition in autosomal dominant inheritance. Regardless of sex, an affected parent has a 50% chance of passing the mutation on to each child. For a person to have autosomal recessive inheritance, the condition must be mutated in both copies of the gene. There is a 25% chance of having an affected child, a 50% chance of having a carrier child, and a 25% chance of having an unaffected child if either of the carrier parents have one mutated allele. Because the genes are found on autosomes, or non-sex chromosomes, these inheritance patterns are the same for both males and females.

modeling, functional studies, and updates from genetic databases such as ClinVar can help with this (Arun *et al*, 2024). Missed diagnoses can also result from incomplete family histories, especially in those without clear inherited cancer patterns. This restriction can be addressed by extending the testing criteria and introducing population-based screening, particularly in high-risk populations such as Ashkenazi Jewish populations. Although technological advancements and expanded insurance coverage have lowered costs and improved availability, the high cost and restricted access to genetic testing in some areas continue to be obstacles. Large genomic rearrangements (LGRs) may be missed by conventional sequencing methods, but thorough mutation detection is ensured by combining methods like MLPA or advanced next-generation sequencing. While paired germline testing makes inheritance patterns clear, tumor-only testing may make it more difficult to distinguish between somatic and germline mutations (Feliubadaló *et al*, 2013). Positive test results can have psychological and ethical repercussions, including anxiety and family conflicts, which emphasize the value of genetic counseling in fostering emotional support and well-informed decision-making.

4.4 LI-FRAUMENI SYNDROME (LFS)

Mutations in the TP53 gene, which is essential for controlling the cell cycle and halting the development of tumors, result in Li-Fraumeni Syndrome (LFS), an uncommon hereditary cancer syndrome. The risk of getting many kinds of cancer, frequently at a young age, is greatly increased by this syndrome. Brain tumors, adrenocortical carcinoma, soft tissue sarcomas, osteosarcomas, and breast cancer are among the common cancers linked to LFS. Throughout their lives, people with LFS may get several primary cancers (Malkin, 1993). The syndrome can be brought on by a single copy of the mutated gene from either parent because it has an autosomal dominant inheritance pattern. Affected individuals need rigors surveillance and early intervention strategies to manage and lower cancer risks because of their high susceptibility to the disease (Kratz *et al*, 2017). The diagnosis of LFS requires genetic testing and counseling, and knowledge of the genetic mutation in impacted families can direct therapeutic and preventative strategies.

4.4.1 Basic Genetics

The TP53 gene, which codes for the p53 protein, is the primary source of mutations that cause Li-Fraumeni Syndrome (LFS). As it controls cell cycle progression, DNA repair, and the initiation of apoptosis (programed cell death) when DNA damage is irreparable, p53 is a crucial tumor suppressor that protects the genome. The principal role of p53 is to stop cells with damaged or mutated DNA from proliferating by either inducing apoptosis or arresting the cell cycle at the G1/S checkpoint. This prevents the accumulation of mutations that could lead to the development of cancer (Achatz *et al*, 2007).

The majority of TP53 mutations are point mutations, which can change the p53 protein's structure. These mutations frequently affect p53's capacity to interact with other proteins that control the cell cycle and apoptosis or to bind to DNA. These mutations can occasionally produce a protein that is unstable or truncated. Although the mutations can occur anywhere in the TP53 gene (Evans & Lozano, 1997), they frequently concentrate in specific areas, such as the DNA-binding domain, which is crucial for the tumor suppressor function of p53. TP53 mutations frequently cause a dominant negative effect, in which p53 function is lost due to one defective copy of the gene. This happens because of the mutant p53 protein's ability to combine with the normal protein to form inactive complexes that impair its functionality. The autosomal dominant inheritance pattern of Li-Fraumeni syndrome is caused by this mechanism (Schneider *et al*, 2024).

Even though LFS is inherited autosomally dominantly, the "two-hit" theory explains how cancer develops in LFS. Where, in the first hit a germline mutation occurs when a person inherits one TP53 mutated allele from either parent. Since the person still has one normal TP53 allele that still controls cellular processes, this is not enough to cause cancer on its own. Second hit dedicates to somatic cells, where the second mutation, or "hit," usually happens later in life. Random mutations, environmental influences, or other genetic changes could be the cause of this. The function of p53 is totally lost once the second mutation renders the remaining normal TP53 allele inactive. This results in unchecked cell division and the build-up of mutations that are responsible for the development of cancer (Srivastava *et al*, 1992).

4.4.2 Diagnostic Approach

In order to identify affected individuals and at-risk family members, Li-Fraumeni Syndrome (LFS) is diagnosed using a comprehensive approach that combines clinical evaluation, genetic testing, and family history assessment. Due to its rarity and wide range of related cancers, LFS requires a thorough assessment. A thorough family history is the first step in the clinical evaluation process, which focuses on indicators like multiple cancers in one person, early-onset cancers (before age 45), and cancers commonly linked to LFS, such as brain tumors, adrenocortical carcinoma, sarcomas, and breast cancer, that are clustered in relatives. Diagnostic frameworks such as the Chompret Criteria and Classic LFS Criteria help identify patients who need more research (Matzenbacher Bittar et al, 2021). Since germline TP53 mutations affect tumor suppression, genetic testing for them is essential. The diagnosis is confirmed by TP53 gene sequencing, and in cases that are unclear or to differentiate LFS from other syndromes, comprehensive cancer gene panels may be employed. Risk assessment and management are made easier when family members with known mutations undergo cascade testing (Sorrell et al, 2013). Additional evidence can be obtained through functional studies of tumor tissue and immunohistochemistry (IHC), especially by analysing the expression and activity of the p53 protein. Setting priority tests is aided by risk prediction tools like PREMM5, which calculate the probability of TP53 mutations based on cancer history. Prenatal testing and preimplantation genetic diagnosis (PGD) are reproductive options that help decrease the transmission of TP53 mutations in families with confirmed mutations (Mannucci et al, 2020). To differentiate LFS from other hereditary cancer syndromes, like those brought on by BRCA1/2 or PTEN mutations, differential diagnosis is crucial. Phenotypic variability, de novo mutations, and low-penetrance mutations are among the difficulties in diagnosing LFS, which all make clinical interpretation more difficult (Van Der Groep et al, 2011). Genetic counseling is essential for ensuring that families are aware of their options and risks. An integrated diagnostic approach is crucial because early diagnosis and focused surveillance can dramatically lower the risk of cancer.

4.5 FAMILIAL ADENOMATOUS POLYPOSIS (FAP)

Familial adenomatous polyposis (FAP) is a hereditary colorectal cancer syndrome characterized by the early onset of hundreds to thousands of adenomatous polyps in the colon and rectum. Without timely intervention, these polyps carry an almost inevitable risk of progressing to colorectal cancer, often by the age of 40 if untreated. FAP accounts for approximately 1% of all colorectal cancer cases and follows an autosomal dominant pattern of inheritance (Al-Sukhni et al., 2008). This syndrome is caused by germline mutations in the **APC gene** (adenomatous polyposis coli), a critical tumor suppressor gene that regulates cell growth and division. In addition to colorectal manifestations, FAP can involve extracolonic features, including polyps in the stomach and duodenum, as well as benign and malignant tumors in various tissues, such as the thyroid, liver, and central nervous system (Nieuwenhuis & Vasen, 2007). Along with colorectal symptoms, FAP can also cause benign and malignant tumors in the thyroid, liver, and central nervous system, as well as extracolonic features like stomach and duodenal polyps. To lower the risk of cancer and enhance patient outcomes, early diagnosis via genetic testing and endoscopic surveillance is essential. FAP is a prime example of how crucial it is to comprehend hereditary cancer syndromes to provide impacted individuals and their families with prompt interventions and genetic counseling (Figure 4.3).

4.5.1 Basic Genetics

A germline mutation in the APC gene, which is found on chromosome 5q21–q22, is the fundamental genetic cause of familial adenomatous polyposis (FAP). The Wnt signaling pathway, which is crucial for regulating cell growth, differentiation, and apoptosis, is regulated by the APC gene, which is a key tumor suppressor. The loss of the tumor-suppressive function of the APC gene due to mutations causes uncontrolled cell division and the development of adenomatous polyps in the intestinal epithelium. Given that the APC gene mutation in FAP is inherited autosomally dominantly, a high risk of developing the syndrome can be conferred by a single pathogenic variant from one parent (Segditsas & Tomlinson, 2006). While most FAP cases are inherited, de novo mutations, which arise spontaneously without a family history, account for about 20–25% of cases. The severity of FAP may vary depending on where the APC mutation is located in the gene. Mutations in the middle region of the gene, also referred to as the mutation cluster region (MCR), are associated with the classic FAP phenotype, which is characterized by hundreds to thousands of polyps. Mutations outside of this area may result in attenuated FAP (AFAP), a milder form of the disease with fewer polyps and a later onset of colorectal cancer (Tóth et al, 2024). Understanding the genetic basis is essential for accurate diagnosis, risk assessment, and the implementation of preventative measures like early screening and surgical interventions.

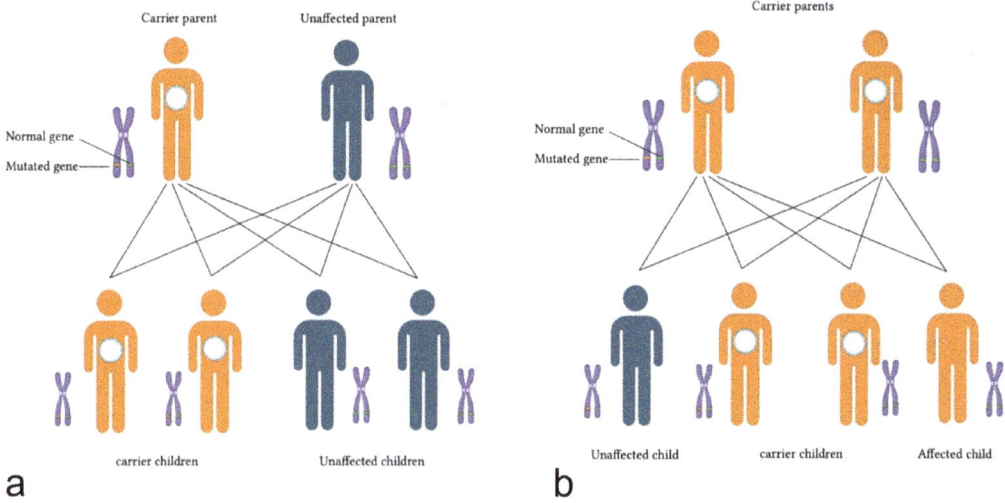

Figure 4.3 Autosomal recessive inheritance patterns. When a mutation in an autosomal gene (shown by a shaded allele) is carried by both parents, the inheritance pattern is shown in this figure. Two copies of the mutated gene are necessary for an individual to have the condition in autosomal recessive inheritance. The child has a 25% chance of inheriting two mutated alleles and being affected, a 50% chance of inheriting one mutated allele and being an unaffected carrier, and a 25% chance of inheriting two normal alleles and being totally unaffected for every pregnancy. Because the gene is found on an autosome, a non-sex chromosome, this inheritance pattern is equally present in males and females.

4.5.2 Diagnostic Approach

To be able to properly diagnose and treat familial adenomatous polyposis (FAP), a combination of clinical assessment, genetic testing, and endoscopic surveillance is used. A thorough personal and family history is the first step in the clinical evaluation process to spot important characteristics like a large number of adenomatous polyps, early-onset colorectal cancer, or related extracolonic manifestations like thyroid cancer and desmoid tumors. The diagnosis is confirmed by genetic testing for pathogenic mutations in the APC gene, which also makes it possible to use cascade testing to find family members who are at risk. Testing for MUTYH-associated polyposis (MAP) may be an option if APC mutations are not found. The main diagnostic method for identifying and measuring polyps is a colonoscopy, which is usually advised for people with a family history of FAP by the age of 10 or 12 (Aelvoet *et al*, 2022). Additionally, upper endoscopy is used to find duodenal and stomach polyps. Desmoid tumors and other extracolonic manifestations are assessed using imaging tests like MRIs and CT scans. To stop mutation transmission to subsequent generations, families with confirmed APC mutations may be offered reproductive options such as prenatal testing and preimplantation genetic diagnosis (PGD) (Kastrinos *et al*, 2007). To differentiate FAP from other polyposis syndromes, a differential diagnosis is essential, and thorough gene panel testing helps with this process. Periodic evaluations and routine endoscopic surveillance are crucial for at-risk individuals who do not exhibit symptoms. For people and families impacted by FAP, this multimodal strategy guarantees early detection, focused treatment, and genetic counseling to lower cancer risk and enhance outcomes.

4.5.3 Diagnostic Challenges

With regard to its clinical variability, genetic complexity, and overlap with other hereditary cancer syndromes, diagnosing familial adenomatous polyposis (FAP) is difficult. The phenotypic heterogeneity of FAP, which varies from the classic form with hundreds to thousands of polyps to attenuated FAP (AFAP), which has fewer polyps and colorectal cancer that develops later, is one of the main challenges. Particularly in AFAP cases where clinical suspicion may be lower, this variability can cause a delay in diagnosis.

The existence of de novo mutations, which make up 20–25% of FAP cases, presents another difficulty (Campos, 2014). It is challenging to identify at-risk individuals using family history alone because these mutations happen spontaneously without a family history. Furthermore, milder disease manifestations may arise from low-penetrance mutations in the APC gene, making diagnosis even more challenging. The complexity is increased by overlap with other hereditary syndromes, including Peutz-Jeghers syndrome, juvenile polyposis syndrome, and MUTYH-associated polyposis (MAP) (Funayama *et al*, 2024; Torrezan *et al*, 2013). In these situations, separating FAP from these disorders necessitates extensive gene panel testing, which isn't always practical or economical. Another diagnostic challenge is mosaicism, in which the mutation is found in only a portion of the person's cells. False-negative results could arise from traditional genetic testing techniques' inability to identify mosaic APC mutations. It can also be difficult to rely solely on endoscopic evaluation, especially in young children or people with incomplete penetrance, where polyp development may not be visible yet. Additionally, there is variation in how polyp count thresholds are interpreted, which may lead to the condition being incorrectly classified.

Furthermore, in environments with limited resources, access to genetic testing and counseling continues to be a major obstacle. Delays in diagnosis and treatment are made worse by patients' and healthcare professionals' lack of knowledge about FAP. Raising awareness, expanding access to genetic testing, and creating cutting-edge diagnostic tools are all necessary to address these issues and guarantee prompt identification and assistance for FAP-affected individuals and families.

4.6 PEUTZ-JEGHERS SYNDROME

The development of hamartomatous polyps in the gastrointestinal tract and characteristic mucocutaneous pigmentation are hallmarks of Peutz-Jeghers Syndrome (PJS), a rare hereditary cancer syndrome. Mutations in the tumor suppressor gene STK11 (LKB1), which is essential for controlling cell growth and metabolism, are the cause of this autosomal dominant disorder. PJS is linked to a higher lifetime risk of developing a number of cancers, such as breast cancer, gynecological cancers (ovarian and cervical), and gastrointestinal cancers (colorectal, gastric, and pancreatic) (Schumacher *et al*, 2005). PJS's defining characteristics, which include pigmented macules on the lips, mouth, and other mucosal surfaces, are important diagnostic markers and frequently manifest in childhood. Usually developing in adolescence or early adulthood, hamartomatous polyps can cause complications such as intussusception, gastrointestinal bleeding, and obstruction (Jiang *et al*, 2023). The syndrome emphasizes how crucial early detection and consistent monitoring are to controlling the elevated risk of cancer and averting complications.

The intersection of genetic mutations and cancer predisposition is highlighted by PJS, a well-known hereditary cancer syndrome. It also emphasizes the importance of genetic counseling, targeted surveillance, and individualized management strategies in reducing the risk of cancer for those who are affected and their families.

4.6.1 Basic Genetics

The STK11 (LKB1) gene, found on chromosome 19p13.3, is the site of germline mutations that cause Peutz-Jeghers Syndrome (PJS). A tumor suppressor protein called serine/threonine kinase, which is encoded by the STK11 gene, is essential for controlling cellular functions like cell growth, metabolism, and polarity. In addition to causing unchecked cell growth, loss of STK11 function puts people at risk for developing hamartomatous polyps and developing a number of malignancies. Since PJS is inherited autosomally dominantly, the syndrome can be brought on by a single pathogenic mutation in one copy of the STK11 gene. The likelihood that a person with PJS will pass the mutation on to their children is 50%. Although, the majority of cases are inherited from an affected parent, de novo mutations which happen on their own in people without a family history of the condition account for about 25 to 45% of cases. STK11 mutations frequently produce either a protein with reduced kinase activity or a shortened, non-functional protein. Tumorigenesis is encouraged by this loss of function, which upsets cellular homeostasis. Lack of functional STK11 causes cells to react improperly to metabolic stress, which increases the risk of malignant transformation and causes hamartomas to form. In order to identify at-risk individuals and effectively manage PJS, genetic testing, family history analysis, and appropriate counseling are essential. The genetic basis of PJS emphasizes the interaction between inherited mutations and cancer predisposition.

4.6.2 Diagnostic Approach

A combination of clinical assessment, genetic testing, and diagnostic imaging is used to diagnose Peutz-Jeghers Syndrome (PJS) to find characteristic traits and validate the condition. Clinically, gastrointestinal (GI) tract hamartomatous polyps and mucocutaneous pigmentation are hallmarks of PJS. A thorough medical and family history is frequently the first step in the diagnosis process. If characteristic features like pigmentation and GI polyps are seen, a clinical diagnosis may be made (Kopacova et al, 2009). The gold standard for confirming the diagnosis and enabling predictive testing for relatives who are at risk is genetic testing for pathogenic mutations in the STK11 (LKB1) gene. While imaging tests like MRI and CT scans help identify extracolonic polyps and screen for related cancers, endoscopic evaluations such as upper endoscopy, colonoscopy, and capsule endoscopy are crucial for identifying and characterizing polyps throughout the GI tract (Klimkowski et al, 2021). Polyps' hamartomatous nature is confirmed by histopathological examination. Given the increased risk of cancer, cancer surveillance protocols are essential, including routine endoscopic and imaging assessments specific to high-risk organs. To differentiate PJS from related syndromes like Cowden syndrome or juvenile polyposis, differential diagnosis is crucial. A systematic approach to early diagnosis enables prompt interventions, efficient surveillance, and better results for impacted individuals and their families.

4.7 COWDEN SYNDROME

Multiple non-cancerous, hamartomatous growths in different body tissues and organs are a hallmark of Cowden syndrome (CS), a rare genetic disorder. It belongs to a class of diseases called PTEN hamartoma tumor syndromes, which are brought on by germline mutations in the PTEN gene, which is an essential regulator of cell division and growth. The breast, thyroid, endometrial, and, less frequently, kidney and colon cancers are among the many cancers that people with Cowden syndrome are more likely to get (Hanssen & Fryns, 1995). Moreover, CS is linked to specific clinical characteristics like papillomatous lesions, trichilemmomas, macrocephaly, and other benign skin and mucous membrane tumors.

Cowden syndrome was first identified in the 1960s, but because of its link to cancer and other health issues, it is now understood to be a serious condition that needs to be identified early and managed carefully. The presentation of the syndrome varies; some people have mild symptoms, while others have a more severe course of the illness (Nelen, 2000). Improving outcomes and quality of life for individuals with Cowden syndrome requires genetic counseling, comprehensive surveillance, and customized risk management techniques.

4.7.1 Basic Genetics

Germline mutations in the PTEN gene, a tumor suppressor found on chromosome 10q23.31, are the main cause of Cowden syndrome. By blocking the PI3K/AKT/mTOR signalling pathway, the phosphatase and tensin homolog protein, which is encoded by the PTEN gene, is essential for controlling cell growth, proliferation, and survival. When PTEN is mutated, its tumor-suppressive function is lost, which causes unchecked cell division and a higher risk of developing benign and malignant tumors (Liaw et al, 1997). These mutations are inherited in an autosomal dominant fashion and can be point mutations, small insertions or deletions, or large genomic rearrangements. Genetic heterogeneity is reflected in the fact that about 80% of people with Cowden syndrome have a detectable PTEN mutation, with the remaining individuals possibly having mutations in related genes like KLLN, SDHB, SDHD, or PIK3CA. Knowing these genetic foundations has been crucial in creating risk assessment models, diagnostic instruments, and customized (Vida-Navas et al, 2024).

4.7.2 Diagnostic Approach

In an effort to confirm the diagnosis and control related risks, the diagnostic approach for Cowden syndrome combines clinical assessment, genetic testing, and surveillance techniques. Clinically, a thorough medical history, family history, and the presence of distinctive characteristics like papillomatous lesions, trichilemmomas, hamartomatous polyps in the gastrointestinal tract, and macrocephaly are used to diagnose Cowden syndrome. Frameworks for identifying people who might have the syndrome are provided by the NCCN Clinical Practice Guidelines and the International Cowden Consortium Criteria (Pilarski et al, 2013). The foundation of diagnosis is genetic testing, and the main method for confirming harmful mutations is PTEN gene sequencing.

To account for genetic heterogeneity, further testing for other related genes, such as KLLN, SDHB, SDHC, SDHD, or PIK3CA, may be carried out if PTEN mutations are not found. To find related cancers or precancerous lesions, imaging tests like thyroid ultrasounds, mammograms, endometrial biopsies, and colonoscopies are used (Takayama et al, 2023). To differentiate Cowden syndrome from other PTEN hamartoma tumor syndromes and hereditary cancer syndromes, differential diagnosis is necessary. Following a diagnosis, impacted individuals gain access to regular surveillance procedures and customized cancer risk management plans, which facilitate early cancer detection and intervention.

4.8 ATAXIA-TELANGIECTASIA (A-T)

Multiple body systems are impacted by the rare, autosomal recessive hereditary disorder known as ataxia telangiectasia (AT), which is characterized by progressive neurodegeneration, immune system dysfunction, and an increased risk of cancer. The ATM (ataxia-telangiectasia mutated) gene, which is essential for DNA repair, cell cycle control, and preserving genomic stability, is mutated in this condition. Clinically, AT manifests as a variety of symptoms, such as oculocutaneous telangiectasias (small, dilated blood vessels on the skin and eyes), early-onset ataxia brought on by cerebellar degeneration, and immunodeficiency-induced increased susceptibility to infections (Rothblum-Oviatt et al, 2016).

Along with these distinguishing characteristics, people with AT are more susceptible to ionizing radiation and have a higher lifetime risk of developing cancers, especially lymphoma and leukemia. Despite being a rare condition, AT has significant effects on those who are affected as well as their families because of its progressive nature and related complications (Crawford, 1998). Implementing supportive care, managing complications, and offering genetic counseling to families at risk all depend on early detection and diagnosis of AT.

4.8.1 Basic Genetics

ATM gene mutations on chromosome 11q22.3 cause ataxia telangiectasia (AT), an autosomal recessive disorder. By triggering repair pathways, controlling the cell cycle, and preserving genomic stability, the protein kinase encoded by the ATM gene is essential for the body's reaction to DNA damage, particularly double-strand breaks. Defective DNA repair and a build-up of genetic mutations are caused by mutations in the ATM gene, which cause a loss or marked decrease in ATM protein activity (Meyn, 1999). The progressive neurodegeneration, immunodeficiency, and elevated cancer risk seen in AT patients are all influenced by this genomic instability. Both copies of the ATM gene must have harmful mutations that are inherited from each parent for the disorder to appear. Although they are typically asymptomatic, heterozygous carriers of a single mutation may be marginally more susceptible to some cancers, including breast cancer (Hall et al, 2021). Accurate diagnosis, genetic counseling, and family risk assessment all depend on an understanding of the genetic basis and inheritance mechanism of AT.

4.8.2 Diagnostic Approach

Clinical criteria, genetic testing, and laboratory assessments are all used in the diagnosis of ataxia telangiectasia (AT). People who exhibit early-onset progressive cerebellar ataxia, oculocutaneous telangiectasias, recurrent infections, and symptoms like choreoathetosis or dysarthria are clinically suspected of having AT. The diagnosis is supported by laboratory results showing increased chromosomal breakage in lymphocytes exposed to ionizing radiation, low immunoglobulin levels (especially IgA, IgG, or IgE), and elevated serum alpha-fetoprotein (AFP) levels (Kilic et al, 2023; Pietrucha et al, 2007). Genetic testing to detect biallelic pathogenic mutations in the ATM gene establishes a definitive diagnosis. In cases that are unclear, complementary functional studies may be carried out, such as measuring ATM protein levels or kinase activity. Cerebellar atrophy may be seen on MRI imaging, and the diagnosis may be further supported by flow cytometry, which shows fewer T and B cells (Keklik et al, 2014). In addition to providing genetic counseling to families, early and accurate diagnosis is crucial for directing clinical management, which includes cancer surveillance, infection prevention, and supportive therapies.

4.9 TUBEROUS SCLEROSIS COMPLEX (TSC)

The development of benign tumors in the brain, skin, kidneys, lungs, and heart is a hallmark of the rare, multisystem genetic disease known as tuberous sclerosis complex (TSC). It results from changes in the TSC1 or TSC2 genes, which encode the proteins tuberin and hamartin, respectively. These proteins are important modulators of the mTOR signalling pathway, which regulates cell division and growth. Because of the condition's variable expressivity, even members of the same family may have very different symptoms and levels of severity. In addition to dermatological characteristics like hypomelanotic macules and facial angiofibroma, common manifestations include neurological symptoms like seizures, intellectual disability, and autism spectrum disorder (Henske *et al*, 2016). Additionally, TSC is linked to cardiac rhabdomyomas, pulmonary lymphangioleiomyomatosis (LAM), and renal angiomyolipomas. Even though TSC is a chronic illness, improvements in early detection and targeted treatments, such as mTOR inhibitors, have greatly enhanced treatment and quality of life for those who are impacted. Addressing the various clinical issues this complex disorder presents requires awareness and prompt action (Curatolo *et al*, 2018).

4.9.1 Basic Genetics

The genetic condition known as tuberous sclerosis complex (TSC) is brought on by harmful mutations in the TSC1 or TSC2 genes, which are found on chromosomes 9q34 and 16p13, respectively. The hamartin (TSC1) and tuberin (TSC2) that are encoded by these genes work together to block the mammalian target of rapamycin (mTOR) signalling pathway. Cell growth, proliferation, and metabolism are all regulated by this pathway. This inhibitory function is disrupted by mutations in either gene, which results in the mTOR pathway becoming hyperactivated, unchecked cell growth, and the development of benign tumors (hamartomas) in various organs. Because tuberin plays a crucial role in mTOR regulation, mutations in TSC2 are frequently linked to a more severe phenotype than those in TSC1 (Salussolia *et al*, 2019).

Since TSC is inherited in an autosomal dominant fashion, the condition can be brought on by a mutation in just one copy of the gene. Nonetheless, de novo mutations, which lack a previous family history, account for about 65–70% of cases. There is a 50% chance of passing the mutation on to children in familial cases (Salussolia *et al*., 2019). For the purposes of diagnosis, family counseling, and focused management techniques, it is crucial to comprehend the genetic foundation and inheritance pattern of TSC.

4.9.2 Diagnostic Approach

A combination of genetic testing, imaging studies, and clinical evaluation is used in the diagnosis of tuberous sclerosis complex (TSC). Major and minor features, such as hypomelanotic macules, facial angiofibroma, ungual fibromas, cortical tubers, and renal angiomyolipomas, are among the established criteria used in clinical diagnosis. When two or more major features, or one major feature and two or more minor features, are found, a diagnosis is considered definitive. Finding distinctive lesions like cortical tubers, subependymal nodules, or cardiac rhabdomyomas requires imaging tests like brain MRI, renal ultrasound, and echocardiography.

By detecting harmful mutations in the TSC1 or TSC2 genes, genetic testing is essential for confirming the diagnosis. It is especially beneficial for younger patients whose physical manifestations may not yet be evident or for cases with unclear clinical findings. Families with known mutations can also receive preimplantation genetic diagnosis (PGD) and prenatal genetic testing. Affected people's outcomes and quality of life are eventually improved by early and accurate diagnosis, which makes it possible to start surveillance and management plans on time. These strategies include monitoring for seizures, renal function, and possible complications.

4.10 VON HIPPEL–LINDAU SYNDROME (VHL)

The development of tumors and cysts in different body parts, such as brain, spinal cord, and retinal hemangioblastomas; renal cell carcinoma; pheochromocytomas; and pancreatic tumors, is a rare hereditary condition known as von Hippel-Lindau (VHL) syndrome. The VHL gene, which is essential for controlling how cells react to oxygen levels, is mutated in this condition. Tumor formation results from the disruption of normal cell growth control caused by this gene's alteration. Early adulthood is when VHL syndrome usually manifests, and even within families, symptoms can vary greatly in intensity (Lonser *et al*, 2003). Multidisciplinary care, genetic testing, and early detection are essential for efficient management and better results.

A single copy of the mutated gene is enough to confer risk because the condition is inherited in an autosomal dominant manner. About 1 in 36,000 people worldwide suffer from VHL syndrome, and symptoms usually start to appear in young adulthood. Early diagnosis and treatment of VHL syndrome are essential because of its multisystem involvement and potential for life-threatening complications (Nordstrom-O'Brien *et al*, 2010). Thorough surveillance procedures, such as routine imaging and biochemical testing, are used to identify and treat tumors early on, greatly enhancing the prognosis and quality of life for those who are impacted.

4.10.1 Basic Genetics

Germline mutations in the VHL gene, which is found on chromosome 3p25-26, are the cause of von Hippel-Lindau (VHL) syndrome. As a tumor suppressor, the VHL gene is essential for controlling how cells react to oxygen levels via the hypoxia-inducible factor (HIF) pathway. The VHL protein inhibits excessive angiogenesis and cell proliferation by targeting HIF for degradation under normal oxygen conditions. When the VHL gene is mutated, this regulatory function is lost, which causes angiogenesis, unchecked cell growth, and the formation of tumors and cysts in various organs (Chittiboina & Lonser, 2015). Since VHL syndrome is inherited in an autosomal dominant fashion, the disorder can be brought on by a single copy of the mutated gene. One faulty allele of the VHL gene is inherited by people with VHL syndrome from an affected parent, while the second allele is usually rendered inactive by somatic mutations in particular tissues, which results in the development of tumors. About 20% of cases are de novo mutations, which happen in people who have no family history (Nielsen *et al*, 2016). In order to identify carriers and provide early surveillance and management for at-risk individuals and their families, genetic testing is essential.

4.10.2 Diagnostic Approach

von Hippel-Lindau (VHL) syndrome is diagnosed using a multidisciplinary approach that includes genetic testing, imaging studies, clinical evaluation, and family history assessment. Given the autosomal dominant inheritance pattern of VHL, a thorough clinical evaluation concentrates on hallmark features like hemangioblastomas, renal cell carcinoma, pheochromocytomas, and pancreatic tumors, as well as any family history of these conditions. Imaging tests, such as brain and spinal cord MRIs, abdominal ultrasounds or CT scans, and retinal exams, are essential for detecting distinctive tumors and cysts (Maher *et al*, 1990). When pheochromocytomas are suspected, biochemical testing is done to find catecholamine levels. A conclusive diagnostic step that allows for early identification and predictive testing for family members who are at risk is genetic testing to confirm mutations in the VHL gene. Comprehensive genetic panels may be necessary for differential diagnosis of diseases such as multiple endocrine neoplasia type 2 or other hereditary cancer syndromes (Binderup, 2018). Following a diagnosis, patients are placed in ongoing surveillance programs to track the growth and spread of their tumors, guaranteeing prompt treatment and better results.

4.11 MUTYH-ASSOCIATED POLYPOSIS (MAP)

Mutations in the MUTYH gene result in the hereditary colorectal cancer syndrome known as MutYH-associated polyposis (MAP). People with this condition are more likely to develop multiple colorectal adenomas, which, if untreated, can eventually develop into colorectal cancer. Numerous polyps in the colon and rectum, which usually manifest in adulthood by the age of 50, are a characteristic of MAP (Nielsen *et al*, 2011). MAP is inherited in an autosomal recessive fashion, which means that people must inherit two mutated copies of the MUTYH gene one from each parent in contrast to other hereditary polyposis syndromes like familial adenomatous polyposis (FAP). Defects in the base excision repair pathway, which is essential for repairing DNA damage, result from this, which raises the risk of cancer and promotes the growth of polyps (Kashfi *et al*, 2013). In order to manage the condition and prevent colorectal cancer, early diagnosis and routine screening including colonoscopies are crucial.

4.11.1 Basic Genetics

Mutations in the MUTYH gene, which codes for an enzyme involved in the base excision repair (BER) pathway and is found on chromosome 1p34.1, result in MutYH-associated polyposis (MAP). Mutations in MUTYH hinder this pathway's capacity to repair oxidative DNA damage, which results in the accumulation of mutations in the genome and encourages the development of colorectal adenomas. An individual must inherit two mutated copies of the MUTYH gene, one from each parent, to develop MAP because the condition is inherited in an autosomal recessive manner (Cheadle & Sampson, 2007). Carriers are people who have one mutated allele; they typically don't exhibit any symptoms, but they can pass the mutation on to their children. MAP is distinct from other hereditary colorectal cancer syndromes, like familial adenomatous polyposis (FAP), which usually exhibits an autosomal dominant inheritance pattern, due to its autosomal recessive inheritance (Rashid *et al*, 2016).

4.11.2 Diagnostic Approach

MutYH-associated polyposis (MAP) is diagnosed by a combination of genetic testing, imaging, clinical evaluation, and family history assessment. Assessing the clinical presentation is the first step in diagnosing MAP. Multiple colorectal adenomas are frequently discovered during a colonoscopy. Adenomas can vary in number and are typically discovered in people by the age of 50. A family history of polyposis or colorectal cancer may raise suspicions of MAP. Since MAP is an autosomal recessive disorder, genetic testing for mutations in the MUTYH gene is essential for confirming the diagnosis (Sutcliffe *et al*, 2019). In order to find harmful mutations, genetic testing usually entails sequencing the MUTYH gene, with a focus on common mutations like Y179C and G396D. A person is diagnosed with MAP if they have two mutations in the MUTYH gene, one from each parent. When a single mutation is found, family members may undergo genetic testing to identify carriers and evaluate the likelihood of inheritance (Nielsen *et al*, 2009).

In MAP patients, colorectal polyps are detected and tracked using imaging tests, especially colonoscopies. Frequent colonoscopies are advised for the early detection of polyps because, by promptly removing adenomas, they can lower the risk of colorectal cancer progression. Genetic counseling is also crucial in informing families about the risks, inheritance pattern, and significance of early surveillance.

4.12 CHALLENGES TO CURRENT DIAGNOSTICS

Genetic conditions known as hereditary cancer syndromes are caused by inherited mutations in particular genes that predispose people to particular cancer types. These syndromes make up 5–10% of all cancers, which highlights how critical it is to identify and treat their distinct clinical and genetic traits. Comprehending hereditary cancer syndromes is essential for risk assessment, early detection, and customized treatment plans. Tumor formation results from mutations in DNA mismatch repair genes (e.g., MLH1, MSH2, MSH6, and PMS2), tumor suppressor genes (e.g., BRCA1, BRCA2, TP53, APC, PTEN, and STK11), and other cancer-related genes that interfere with normal cell growth control mechanisms. Every syndrome displays a distinct range of cancers (Stoffel & Chittenden, 2010). For instance, Lynch syndrome raises the risk of colorectal and endometrial cancers, Li-Fraumeni syndrome predisposes to a variety of early-onset cancers, and BRCA1/BRCA2 mutations are linked to hereditary breast and ovarian cancer. With a few exceptions, like MutYH-associated polyposis (autosomal recessive), these syndromes usually have autosomal dominant inheritance patterns. Since not all carriers of mutations develop cancer or display the hallmarks of the classic syndrome, variations in gene penetrance and expressivity can make clinical presentations more challenging. Genetic testing, tumor profiling, family history analysis, and clinical evaluation are all integrated into diagnostic methods. Instruments such as immunohistochemistry, microsatellite instability testing, and multigene panels aid in the confirmation of diagnoses and the differentiation of overlapping syndromes (Feliubadaló *et al*, 2019). Early diagnosis lowers cancer-related morbidity and mortality by enabling customized surveillance, such as breast imaging for carriers of BRCA mutations or colonoscopies for Lynch syndrome. Lack of knowledge, restricted access to genetic testing, and the psychological effects of a diagnosis on families are among the difficulties. Identification and management techniques have been enhanced by developments in risk prediction models, genomic technologies, and genetic counseling. Additional chances to reduce the risk of inherited cancer in subsequent generations are provided by reproductive options, such as preimplantation genetic diagnosis (Weitzel *et al*, 2011).

All things considered, hereditary cancer syndromes emphasize the interaction between oncology and genetics and the value of interdisciplinary cooperation in enhancing the prognosis of afflicted individuals and their families.

4.13 LIMITATIONS OF CURRENT DIAGNOSTIC CRITERIA

Despite being useful, the diagnostic criteria for hereditary cancer syndromes have significant drawbacks that affect how well they work. Numerous criteria, like the Amsterdam II guidelines for Lynch syndrome, may overlook cases with atypical presentations because they narrowly focus on particular cancers or clinical characteristics. There are problems with relying too much on family history, especially for people who don't know enough about their family's medical history. Li-Fraumeni syndrome and other syndromes with variable expressivity and incomplete penetrance make diagnosis even more difficult because carriers of the mutation might not show the typical symptoms. De novo mutations, which are prevalent in diseases such as Tuberous Sclerosis

Complex, frequently cause people without a family history to be disregarded by conventional standards (Samadder *et al*, 2021).

Furthermore, established guidelines may underrepresent rare syndromes like Birt-Hogg-Dubé or hereditary diffuse gastric cancer, which could delay diagnosis. Diagnostic complexity is increased by overlapping clinical features between syndromes, such as Lynch syndrome and BRCA1/BRCA2 mutations. Furthermore, the availability of sophisticated testing techniques and the quick growth of genetic knowledge frequently surpass current standards, rendering them obsolete. Disparities in diagnosis are made worse by technological and resource constraints, especially in environments with limited resources (Sessa *et al*, 2023). Updated, thorough criteria, increased access to genetic testing, and increased awareness among medical professionals are required to address these issues and guarantee prompt and precise diagnoses.

4.14 FUTURE PERSPECTIVES

With exciting developments aimed at enhancing diagnosis, treatment, and results for afflicted people and their families, the field of hereditary cancer syndromes is developing quickly. Enhancing diagnostic instruments, increasing genetic testing, improving risk assessment models, and creating targeted treatments should be the main goals of future initiatives. The incorporation of whole-genome sequencing (WGS) and next-generation sequencing (NGS) into standard clinical practice is one important avenue. These technologies are able to detect complex rearrangements, uncommon variants, and novel genetic mutations that are overlooked by conventional techniques. A more inclusive diagnostic framework can be provided by thorough multigene panel testing, which can also reveal less-studied syndromes. Polygenic risk scores (PRS), which take into consideration the combined effects of several genetic variations, are another area of emphasis for enhancing risk prediction models. Even those without a known pathogenic mutation or family history can receive personalized cancer risk assessments from these tools. In order to improve the predictive accuracy of hereditary cancer syndromes and analyse large datasets, researchers are also investigating the use of artificial intelligence and machine learning algorithms. The biological significance of unknown or novel variants could be clarified by developments in functional genomics and transcriptomics, which would close the gap between genetic results and clinical significance. Functional studies can provide vital information for patient care by assisting in determining whether variants of uncertain significance (VUS) impact cellular pathways, protein function, or gene expression.

Additionally, the range of therapeutic approaches for hereditary cancer syndromes is growing. Precision medicine is being made possible by targeted treatments like PARP inhibitors for carriers of BRCA1/BRCA2 mutations. Similar strategies will probably be investigated in the future for other hereditary syndromes, such as those involving TP53 mutations or mismatch repair (MMR). Furthermore, pathogenic mutations may be corrected by gene-editing technologies like CRISPR, providing a long-term curative option. More personalization will help surveillance programs and preventive measures. It is possible to maximize early detection and reduce needless procedures by customizing screening protocols according to each person's genetic risk, lifestyle choices, and environmental exposures. By making it possible to monitor circulating tumor DNA (ctDNA) and other biomarkers noninvasively, advances in liquid biopsy technologies have the potential to further transform early cancer detection.

REFERENCES

Achatz MIW et al. (2007) The TP53 mutation, R337H, is associated with Li-Fraumeni and Li-Fraumeni-like syndromes in Brazilian families. *Cancer Lett* 245:96–102.

Aelvoet AS et al. (2022) Management of familial adenomatous polyposis and MUTYH-associated polyposis; new insights. *Best Pract Res Clin Gastroenterol* 58:101793.

Al-Sukhni W et al. (2008) Hereditary colorectal cancer syndromes: familial adenomatous polyposis and lynch syndrome. *Surg Clin North Am* 88:819–844.

Arun B et al. (2024) BRCA-mutated breast cancer: the unmet need, challenges and therapeutic benefits of genetic testing. *Br J Cancer* 131:1400–1414.

Bhattacharya P et al. (2024) *Lynch Syndrome (Hereditary Nonpolyposis Colorectal Cancer)*. StatPearls Publishing Treasure Island (FL) StatPearls Publishing.

Binderup MLM (2018) von Hippel-Lindau disease: Diagnosis and factors influencing disease outcome. *Dan Med J* 65:B5461.

Campos FG (2014) Surgical treatment of familial adenomatous polyposis: dilemmas and current recommendations. *World J Gastroenterol* 20:16620.

Cerretelli G et al. (2020) Molecular pathology of Lynch syndrome. *J Pathol* 250:518–531.

Cheadle JP, Sampson JR (2007) MUTYH-associated polyposis—from defect in base excision repair to clinical genetic testing. *DNA Repair* 6:274–279.

Chittiboina P, Lonser RR (2015) von Hippel–Lindau disease. *Handb Clin Neurol* 132:139–156.

Crawford TO (1998) Ataxia telangiectasia. *Semin Pediatr Neurol* 5(4):287–294. WB Saunders.

Curatolo P et al. (2018) Management of epilepsy associated with tuberous sclerosis complex: updated clinical recommendations. *Eur J Paediat Neurol* 22:738–748.

Davidson KW et al. (2021) Screening for colorectal cancer: US Preventive Services Task Force recommendation statement. *JAMA* 325:1965–1977.

Eccles D et al. (2015) BRCA1 and BRCA2 genetic testing—pitfalls and recommendations for managing variants of uncertain clinical significance. *Ann Oncol* 26:2057–2065.

Evans SC, Lozano G (1997) The Li-Fraumeni syndrome: an inherited susceptibility to cancer. *Molec Med Today* 3:390–395.

Feliubadaló L et al. (2013) Next-generation sequencing meets genetic diagnostics: development of a comprehensive workflow for the analysis of BRCA1 and BRCA2 genes. *Eur J Hum Genet* 21:864–870.

Feliubadaló L et al. (2019) Opportunistic testing of BRCA1, BRCA2 and mismatch repair genes improves the yield of phenotype driven hereditary cancer gene panels. *Int J Cancer* 145:2682–2691.

Funayama Y et al. (2024) Advancements in endoscopic management of small-bowel polyps in Peutz–Jeghers syndrome and familial adenomatous polyposis. *Ther Adv Gastroenterol* 17:1–11.

Gayther SA, Ponder BA (1997) Mutations of the BRCA1 and BRCA2 genes and the possibilities for predictive testing. *Mol Med Today* 3:168–174.

Gomy I, Diz MDPE (2016) Hereditary cancer risk assessment: insights and perspectives for the Next-Generation Sequencing era. *Genet Molec Biol* 39:184–188.

Hall MJ et al. (2021) Germline pathogenic variants in the ataxia telangiectasia mutated (ATM) gene are associated with high and moderate risks for multiple cancers. *Cancer Prev Res* 14:433–440.

Hanssen A, Fryns J (1995) Cowden syndrome. *J Med Genet* 32:117–119.

Henske EP et al. (2016) Tuberous sclerosis complex. *Nature Rev Dis Prim* 2:1–18.

Jenkins MA et al. (2007) Pathology features in Bethesda guidelines predict colorectal cancer microsatellite instability: a population-based study. *Gastroenterol* 133:48–56.

Jiang L-X et al. (2023) Peutz-Jeghers syndrome without STK11 mutation may correlate with less severe clinical manifestations in Chinese patients. *World J Gastroenterol* 29:3302.

Kashfi SMH et al. (2013) MUTYH the base excision repair gene family member associated with colorectal cancer polyposis. *Gastroenterol Hepatol Bed Bench* 6:S1.

Kastrinos F et al. (2007) Attitudes toward prenatal genetic testing in patients with familial adenomatous polyposis. *ACG* 102:1284–1290.

Keklik M et al. (2014) Detection of acute lymphoblastic leukemia involvement in pleural fluid in an adult patient with ataxia telangiectasia by flow cytometry method. *Ind J Hematol Blood Transfus* 30:73–76.

Kilic M et al. (2023) Evaluation of clinical and laboratory features of patients with ataxia-telangiectasia. *Asthma Allergy Immunol* 21:287–294.

Klimkowski S et al. (2021) Peutz–Jeghers syndrome and the role of imaging: pathophysiology, diagnosis, and associated cancers. *Cancers* 13:5121.

Kopacova M et al. (2009) Peutz-Jeghers syndrome: diagnostic and therapeutic approach. *World J Gastroenterol* 15:5397.

Kratz CP et al. (2017) Cancer screening recommendations for individuals with Li-Fraumeni syndrome. *Clin Cancer Res* 23:e38–e45.

Latham A et al. (2019) Microsatellite instability is associated with the presence of Lynch syndrome pan-cancer. *J Clin Oncol* 37:286–295.

Leclerc J et al. (2021) Diagnosis of Lynch syndrome and strategies to distinguish Lynch-related tumors from sporadic MSI/dMMR tumors. *Cancers* 13:467.

Liaw D et al. (1997) Germline mutations of the PTEN gene in Cowden disease, an inherited breast and thyroid cancer syndrome. *Nature Genet* 16:64–67.

Lonser RR et al. (2003) von Hippel-Lindau disease. *Lancet* 361:2059–2067.

Maher E et al. (1990) Clinical features and natural history of von Hippel-Lindau disease. *QJM* 77:1151–1163.

Malkin D (1993) p53 and the Li-Fraumeni syndrome. *Cancer Genet Cytogenet* 66:83–92.

Mannucci A et al. (2020) Comparison of colorectal and endometrial microsatellite instability tumor analysis and Premm5 risk assessment for predicting pathogenic germline variants on multigene panel testing. *J Clin Oncol* 38:4086–4094.

Matzenbacher Bittar C et al. (2021) Clinical and molecular characterization of patients fulfilling Chompret criteria for Li-Fraumeni syndrome in Southern Brazil. *PLoS One* 16:e0251639.

Meyn MS (1999) Ataxia-telangiectasia, cancer and the pathobiology of the ATM gene. *Clin Genet* 55:289–304.

Morrow A et al. (2024) Bridging the gap between intuition and theory: a comparison of different approaches to implementation strategy development for improving lynch syndrome detection. *Publ Health Genom* 27:110-123.

Nelen MR (2000) A molecular genetic study on Cowden disease. Thesis, University Medical Centre, Utrecht.

Nielsen M et al. (2009) Analysis of MUTYH genotypes and colorectal phenotypes in patients with MUTYH-associated polyposis. *Gastroenterol* 136:471–476.

Nielsen M et al. (2011) MUTYH-associated polyposis (MAP). *Crit Rev Oncol Hematol* 79:1–16.

Nielsen SM et al. (2016) von Hippel-Lindau disease: genetics and role of genetic counseling in a multiple neoplasia syndrome. *J Clin Oncol* 34:2172–2181.

Nieuwenhuis M, Vasen H (2007) Correlations between mutation site in APC and phenotype of familial adenomatous polyposis (FAP): a review of the literature. *Crit Rev Oncol Hematol* 61:153–161.

Nordstrom-O'Brien M et al. (2010) Genetic analysis of von Hippel-Lindau disease. *Hum Mutat* 31:521–537.

Peltomäki P et al. (2023) Lynch syndrome genetics and clinical implications. *Gastroenterol* 164:783–799.

Petrucelli N et al. (2022) *BRCA1-and BRCA2-Associated Hereditary Breast and Ovarian Cancer.* Seattle, WA: University of Washington, Seattle; 1993, p. 998.

Pietrucha B et al. (2007) Clinical guidelines Ataxia-Telangiectasia: guidelines for diagnosis and comprehensive care. *Central Eur J Immunol* 32:234–238.

Pilarski R, et al. (2013) Cowden syndrome and the PTEN hamartoma tumor syndrome: systematic review and revised diagnostic criteria. *J Nat Cancer Instit* 105:1607–1616.

Rashid M et al. (2016) Adenoma development in familial adenomatous polyposis and MUTYH-associated polyposis: somatic landscape and driver genes. *J Pathol* 238:98–108.

Roa BB et al. (1996) Ashkenazi Jewish population frequencies for common mutations in BRCA1 and BRCA2. *Nature Genet* 14:185–187.

Rodriguez-Bigas MA et al. (1997) A National Cancer Institute workshop on hereditary nonpolyposis colorectal cancer syndrome: meeting highlights and Bethesda guidelines. *J Nat Cancer Instit* 89:1758–1762.

Rothblum-Oviatt C et al. (2016) Ataxia telangiectasia: a review. *Orphanet J Rare Dis* 11:1–21.

Salussolia CL et al. (2019) Genetic etiologies, diagnosis, and treatment of tuberous sclerosis complex. *Ann Rev Genom Hum Genet* 20:217–240.

Samadder NJ et al. (2021) Comparison of universal genetic testing vs guideline-directed targeted testing for patients with hereditary cancer syndrome. *JAMA Oncol* 7:230–237.

Schneider K et al. (1993–2025) Li-Fraumeni syndrome. In: Adam MP, Ardinger HH, Pagon RA, et al., editors. GeneReviews®. Seattle (WA): University of Washington.

Schumacher V et al. (2005) STK11 genotyping and cancer risk in Peutz-Jeghers syndrome. *J Med Genet* 42:428–435.

Segditsas S, Tomlinson I (2006) Colorectal cancer and genetic alterations in the Wnt pathway. *Oncogene* 25:7531–7537.

Serova OM et al. (1997) Mutations in BRCA1 and BRCA2 in breast cancer families: are there more breast cancer-susceptibility genes? *Am J Hum Genet* 60:486.

Sessa C et al. (2023) Risk reduction and screening of cancer in hereditary breast-ovarian cancer syndromes: ESMO Clinical Practice Guideline. *Ann Oncol* 34:33–47.

Sharaf RN et al. (2013) Uptake of genetic testing by relatives of lynch syndrome probands: a systematic review. *Clin Gastroenterol Hepatol* 11:1093–1100.

Sorrell AD et al. (2013) Tumor protein p53 (TP53) testing and Li-Fraumeni syndrome: current status of clinical applications and future directions. *Molec Diagnos Ther* 17:31–47.

Srivastava S et al. (1992) Detection of both mutant and wild-type p53 protein in normal skin fibroblasts and demonstration of a shared 'second hit'on p53 in diverse tumors from a cancer-prone family with Li-Fraumeni syndrome. *Oncogene* 7:987–991.

Stoffel EM, Chittenden A (2010) Genetic testing for hereditary colorectal cancer: challenges in identifying, counseling, and managing high-risk patients. *Gastroenterol* 139:1436–1441.e1431.

Sutcliffe EG et al. (2019) Multi-gene panel testing confirms phenotypic variability in MUTYH-associated polyposis. *Famil Cancer* 18:203–209.

Takayama T et al. (2023) Clinical guidelines for diagnosis and management of Cowden syndrome/PTEN hamartoma tumor syndrome in children and adults-secondary publication. *J Anus Rectum Colon* 7:284–300.

Tamura K et al. (2019) Genetic and genomic basis of the mismatch repair system involved in Lynch syndrome. *Int J Clin Oncol* 24:999–1011.

Torrezan GT et al. (2013) Mutational spectrum of the APC and MUTYH genes and genotype–phenotype correlations in Brazilian FAP, AFAP, and MAP patients. *Orphanet J Rare Dis* 8:1–12.

Tóth M et al. (2024) Integrated genotype–phenotype analysis of familial adenomatous polyposis-associated hepatocellular adenomas. *Virchows Archiv* 484:587–595.

Tung NM, Garber JE (2018) BRCA 1/2 testing: therapeutic implications for breast cancer management. *Br J Cancer* 119:141–152.

Van Der Groep P et al. (2011) Pathology of hereditary breast cancer. *Cellul Oncol* 34:71–88.

Vasen HF et al. (1999) New clinical criteria for hereditary nonpolyposis colorectal cancer (HNPCC, Lynch syndrome) proposed by the International Collaborative group on HNPCC. *Gastroenterol* 116:1453–1456.

Vida-Navas E et al. (2024) Constitutional mutation of PIK3CA: a variant of Cowden syndrome? *Genes* 15:1209.

Weissman SM et al. (2011) Genetic counseling considerations in the evaluation of families for Lynch syndrome—A review. *J Genet Counsel* 20:5–19.

Weitzel JN et al. (2011) Genetics, genomics, and cancer risk assessment: state of the art and future directions in the era of personalized medicine. *CA* 61:327–359.

Welcsh PL, King M-C (2001) BRCA1 and BRCA2 and the genetics of breast and ovarian cancer. *Hum Molec Genet* 10:705–713.

5

Molecular Diagnostic Tools in Cancer Detection

Aastha Dagar, Ashutosh Kumar Tiwari, Vivek Uttam, Manasranjan Parida, Kanupriya Medhi, Sia Daffara, Sanjana Bana, Sagarika Mukherjee, Raman Tikoria, and Aklank Jain

Abbreviation	Full Forms
AI	Artificial intelligence
AFP	Alfa fetoprotein
BDA	Blocker Displacement Amplification
BRCA	Breast cancer gene
CA125	Cancer antigen 125
CAD	Computer-aided diagnostic
μCAE	Capillary array electrophoresis
CBC	Complete blood count
CD	Cluster of differentiation
CEA	Carcinoembryonic antigen
CEUS	Contrast-enhanced ultrasound
CHRDL	Chordin like 2
CiRS	Circular RNA
CISH	Chromogenic insitu hybridization
CLSTN3	Calsyntenin 3
CNN	Convolutional neural networks
CRC	Colorectal cancer
CRISPR	Clustered regularly interspaced short palindromic repeats
CSF	Cerebrospinal fluid
CSF2RA	Colony stimulating factor 2 receptor subunit alpha
CT	Computed tomography
CTC	Circulating tumor cells
CTLA	Cytotoxic T-lymphocyte antigen
DCIS	Ductal carcinoma in-situ
DNA	Deoxyribonucleic acid
DIA	Digital image analysis
EFNB2	Ephrin-B2
EGFR	Epidermal growth factor receptor
ERBB	Erythroblastic oncogene B2
FDA	Food and drug administration
FDG	Fluorodeoxyglucose
FFPE	Formalin-fixed, paraffin-embedded
FISH	Fluorescence in-situ hybridization
FIT	Fecal immunochemical test
FITC	Fluorescein isothiocyanate
GPC	Glypican
GREM	Gremlin
hCG	Human chorionic gonadotropin
HER	Human epidermal growth factor receptor
HICs	High-income countries
HPV	Human papilloma virus
HSP	Heat shock protein
IL	Interleukin
KRAS	Kirsten rat sarcoma viral oncogene homolog

DOI: 10.1201/9781003542162-5

LDH	Lactate dehydrogenase
LG3BP	Galectin-3-Binding Protein
LM	Leptomeningeal metastases
LMICC	Low and middle-income countries
mPTGER4	Methylated Prostaglandin E Receptor 4
MRI	Magnetic resonance imaging
NGS	Next-generation sequencing
NLST	National lung screening trial
NMP22	Nuclear matrix protein 22
NRAS	Neuroblastoma RAS viral oncogene homolog
NLST	National lung screening trial
NSLCC	Non-small cell lung cancer
OSCC	Oral squamous cell carcinoma
PCA	Prostate cancer antigen
PCGEM	Prostate cancer gene expression
PCNSL	Primary central nervous system lymphoma
PCR	Polymerase chain reaction
PD	Programmed death
PDL1	Programmed death ligand 1
PET	Positron emission tomography
PENK	Proenkephalin
PIK3CA	Phosphatidylinositol-4,5-bisphosphate 3-kinase catalytic subunit alpha
PSA	Prostate-specific antigen
qPCR	Quantitative polymerase chain reaction
RNA	Ribonucleic acid
rtPCR	Real time polymerase chain reaction
SCLC	Small cell lung cancer
SGS	Sanger sequencing
SNV	Single-nucleotide variant
SPA	Sperm associated antigen
SPAG6	Sperm associated antigen 6
SPECT	Single-photon emission computed tomography
TNF-alpha	Tumor necrosis factor-alpha
VAF	Variant allele frequency
VEGFR2	Vascular endothelial growth factor receptor2
VC	Virtual colonoscopy
VOC	Volatile organic compounds
WHO	World Health Organization
WSI	Whole slide image

5.1 INTRODUCTION

The global burden of cancer is escalating, with both incidence and mortality rates rising rapidly. According to the Global Cancer Observatory by WHO, cancer incidence reached 19.9 million cases worldwide in 2022, with lung cancer being mainly reported in males and breast cancer in females (Bray et al. 2024). After lung cancer, incidences of cases reported were highest for prostate, colorectum, stomach, and liver cancer in males. In females, following breast cancer, incidence rates were observed to be highest for lung, colorectum, cervix uteri, and thyroid cancer respectively (Bray et al. 2024).

Cancer not only exhibits a higher incidence rate but also shows an elevated mortality rate, reporting approximately 9.7 million deaths worldwide. Lung and liver cancer reported the highest deaths in males, and when it comes to females, breast cancer and lung cancer were the leading causes of death. The rising incidence and mortality rates of cancer underscore the urgent need for improved detection and early diagnosis. With cancers increasingly contributing to global morbidity and mortality, early-stage identification becomes crucial in reducing cancer-related deaths (Sung et al. 2021).

Advancements in molecular diagnostic techniques have revolutionized the landscape of cancer detection, offering high precision in identifying malignancies at the molecular level both invasively and non-invasively. Molecular diagnostics comprise a range of methods, including polymerase chain reaction (PCR), fluorescence in situ hybridization (Schiffman, Fisher, and Gibbs 2015), and next-generation sequencing (NGS), which allow for the detection of epigenetic alterations, genetic mutations, and other biomarkers associated with cancer. Tissue biopsy involves the analysis of biofluids such as blood, urine, and saliva, allowing real-time, dynamic monitoring of tumor evolution (Ahmad et al. 2022). Computer-aided diagnostic (CAD) imaging techniques such as positron emission tomography (PET) scan, computed tomography (CT scan), magnetic resonance imaging (MRI), and X-ray serve the purpose of cancer diagnosis non-invasively by generating 2D or 3D images (Gillies and Schabath 2020). Endoscopic techniques are utilized to detect cancer in internal organs, such as colonoscopy, cystoscopy, bronchoscopy, etc. These technologies increase sensitivity and enable personalized approaches to treatment. Invasive techniques like biopsy and endoscopy involve penetrating the body through incisions, needles, or natural openings to examine or remove suspicious cells and often come with the risk of pain, discomfort, and complications. On the other hand, non-invasive techniques are typically used for initial screening and are less specific but involve no risk of infection or bleeding.

This chapter highlights the importance of molecular diagnostic techniques in early cancer detection, diagnosis, and management, underscoring their potential to transform oncological practice and improve survival rates.

5.2 BIOMARKERS IN CANCER DETECTION

A biological marker, also termed as a biomarker, is a measurable indicator of a biological state, condition, or process. Though challenging to identify, it can provide critical insights into significant clinical outcomes. They are applied in identifying, characterizing, and monitoring disease, including cancer (Das et al. 2023). A clear understanding of the intrinsic connection between a biomarker and its clinical outcomes is crucial for the precise evaluation of its importance (Das et al. 2023).

Cancer Biomarkers encompass a diverse range of biochemical entities, including proteins, nucleic acids, carbohydrates, cytogenetic and cytokinetic parameters, small metabolites, and any tumor cells released into body fluids (Wu and Qu 2015). These are used for screening, diagnosis, staging, or disease monitoring (Schiffman, Fisher, and Gibbs 2015). Detection of these biomarkers can be done both *in vivo* and *in vitro* by various techniques (Sarhadi and Armengol 2022). Various cancer biomarkers along with their detection methods are listed in Table 5.1. Sample collection for detection can be done invasively by intruding the body's physical barriers or non-invasively from body fluids like blood, urine, saliva, or stool (Sarhadi and Armengol 2022). We discuss the various types of biomarkers involved in cancer detection in the following section and illustrated in Figure 5.1.

5.2.1 Proteins

The proteome offers distinct insights into biology that extend beyond those provided by the genome and transcriptome (Das et al. 2023). Most cancer biomarkers approved by the FDA for clinical use are individual proteins found in serum, with Prostate-specific antigen (PSA) being the first (Das et al. 2023). Along with early detection, proteins hold significant potential as valuable biomarkers due to their role in disease staging and real-time patient monitoring (Das et al. 2023). Heat shock proteins like Hsp27, Hsp70, Hsp90, Methylated prostaglandin E2 receptor EP4 subtype (mPTGER4), and Hsp60 are implicated in a wide range of human cancers, including lung cancer (Mittal and Rajala 2020; Zhang Y 2020). Hsp27 expression is elevated in several types of cancers, including pancreatic cancer (Baylot et al. 2011). Alfa fetoprotein (AFP), Lactate dehydrogenase (LDH), and Human chorionic gonadotropin (hCG) are employed for staging testicular cancer. Likewise, Cluster of differentiation (CD)171, CD151, and Tetraspanin are associated with lung cancer, and CD44 and CD24 with breast cancer (Das et al. 2023; Camerlingo et al. 2014). Upregulated PSA levels suggest prostate cancer. Testicular and ovarian cancer show raised levels of Human chorionic gonadotropin (hCG) (Das et al. 2023) and several early preclinical studies have identified human epidermal growth factor receptor 2 (HER2) as a potential therapeutic target in ovarian cancer and its amplification in breast and gastric cancer (Shu et al. 2017). HER-2 mutations in non-small cell lung cancer (NSCLC) primarily occur in the kinase domain of the HER-2 gene (Xu and Wang 2020) while p53 changes in lung cancer are most common in the types of bronchial

Table 5.1: Various Cancer Biomarkers and their Detection

S.No.	Cancer	Nature of Biomarker	Biomarker	Detection Tools
1	Breast Cancer	Protein	HER2, CD44, CD24	Western Blotting, RT-PCR, NGS, Histopathology, qPCR, IHC
		Gene	BRCA1, BRCA2, P53	
		Carbohydrate	CEA	
		Non-Coding RNA	LINCC00152, MALAT1	
		Immune Check Point	PD-L1, PD-1	
2	Lung Cancer	Protein	Hsp27, Hsp70, Hsp90, Hsp60, CD171, CD151, Tetraspanin, HER2,	Western Blotting, RT-PCR, NGS, Histopathology, qpcr, IHC
		Gene	P53, mPTGER4	
		Carbohydrate	CEA, CA125, CEA15-3,	
		Non-Coding RNA	miRNA	
		Immune Check Point	PD-L1	
3	Prostate Cancer	Protein	PSA	Western Blotting, RT-PCR, NGS, Histopathology, qPCR, IHC
		Gene	TMPRSS2-ERG	
		Carbohydrate	CEA	
		Non-Coding RNA	PCA3, PCGEM,	
4	Ovarian Cancer	Protein	hCG, HER2	Western Blotting, RT-PCR, NGS, Histopathology, qPCR, IHC
		Gene	BRCA1, BRCA2, P53	
		Carbohydrate	CA125, CEA	
		Non-Coding RNA	AFAP1-AS1	
		Immune Check Point	CTLA4	
5	Colorectal Cancer	Protein	GREM1, CLSTN3, CSF2RA, CD86	Western Blotting, RT-PCR, NGS, Histopathology, qPCR, IHC
		Gene	KRAS, P53, BRAF, NRAS, PIK3CA	
		Carbohydrate	CEA, CA19-9, CA72-4,	
		Non-Coding RNA	FBXL19-AS1, BCYRN1	
6	Pancreatic Cancer	Protein	HSP27	Western Blotting, RT-PCR, NGS, Histopathology, qPCR, IHC
		Gene	GPC2, NCAPG2, KRT7	
		Carbohydrate	CA19-9, CEA, CA125, CA242	
		Non-Coding RNA	SNHG7, SNHG16	

cancer strongly linked to smoking, especially small cell lung cancer (SCLC) and squamous cell carcinomas (Campling and el-Deiry 2003). Genetically predicted levels of 13 proteins were linked to the risk of colorectal cancer (CRC). Increased levels of two proteins (GREM1 and CHRDL2) and reduced levels of 11 proteins were associated with a higher CRC risk. Among these, four proteins (GREM1, CLSTN3, CSF2RA, and CD86) were identified as having the strongest evidence (Sun et al. 2023).

5.2.2 Genetic Biomarkers

Mutations and genetic alterations serve as critical cancer biomarkers, offering valuable insights into the genetic changes underlying the development and progression of cancer. The KRAS gene is located at 12p12.1, indicative of colorectal cancer. KRAS mutations predominantly occur in codons 12 and 13, accounting for 95% of all the mutations (Dinu et al. 2014). The most common mutations in codon 12 are G12D and G12V, while G13D is the most frequent mutation in codon 13 (Dinu et al. 2014). Mutations in RAS, BRAF, PIK3CA, TP53, BCYRN1 are the genetic abnormalities found in metastatic colorectal cancer (mCRC) (Afrasanie et al. 2023; Yang et al. 2020). Similarly, BRCA1/BRCA2 mutations are related to breast or ovarian cancer. AFAP1-AS1 is seen to be overexpressed in both ovarian cancer and their cell lines when compared to their equivalents (Yang et al. 2016). The mutation of the p53 gene at the 17p13.1 locus is also the prevalent single genetic change found in sporadic human epithelial ovarian cancer (EOC) (Corney et al. 2008). The P53 gene is the most mutated in breast cancer, accounting for around 30% of all cases. Most p53 mutations occur within the DNA-binding domain and result from missense point mutations that impair its transcriptional function (Marvalim, Datta, and Lee 2023).

Biomarkers in Cancer Detection

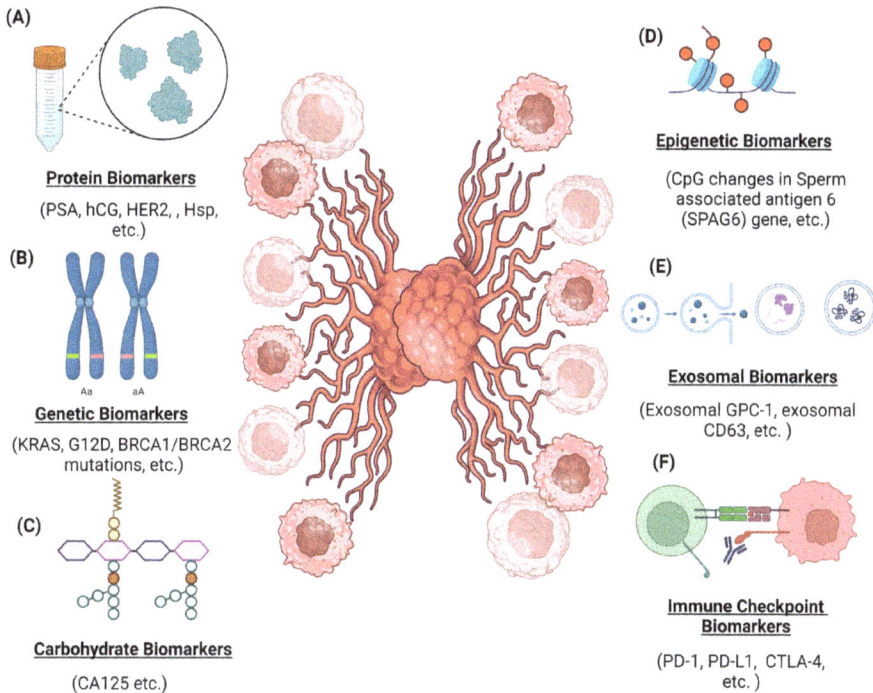

Figure 5.1 Biomarkers in cancer detection: (A) Protein, (B) Genetic, (C) Carbohydrate, (D) Epigenetic, (E) Exosome, (F) Immune checkpoint biomarkers.

DNA circulates in the blood of both healthy and sick individuals. Leon and colleagues, in 1977, determined the levels of cell-free DNA (cf-DNA) in cancerous patients (Pessoa, Heringer, and Ferrer 2020). Circulating tumor DNA (ct-DNA) has been extensively studied and utilized as a biomarker for screening of cancer (Pessoa, Heringer, and Ferrer 2020). Although detecting this early-stage biomarker remains a significant challenge, it demonstrates greater sensitivity than traditional blood-based biomarkers (Pessoa, Heringer, and Ferrer 2020).

CiRS-7 RNA is a circular, non-coding RNA that functions in gene regulation. Dysregulation of ciRS-7 has been associated with various human diseases and numerous types of cancer (Rahmati et al. 2021). Its overexpression has been shown to promote a malignant phenotype by enhancing cell proliferation, migration, and invasion, both in-vitro and in-vivo (Rahmati et al. 2021). Upregulation of miR-1269, a microRNA, promotes the formation and progression of gastric cancer (He et al. 2020). In the same way, the downregulation of miR-9 is associated with oral squamous cell carcinoma (OSCC) (He et al. 2020). Prostate cancer antigen3 (PCA3), a lncRNA transcribed from 9q21.22, is overexpressed in prostate cancer (Bhan, Soleimani, and Mandal 2017). This is the urinary biomarker for prostate cancer that offers good specificity and sensitivity as a minimally invasive test. When combined with PSA, the PCA3 test can help identify the need for a repeat biopsy in men who have had one or more negative prostate biopsies (Gunelli, Fragala, and Fiori 2021). PCGEM1 is the lncRNA Prostate cancer gene expression marker from locus 2q32, suppresses doxorubicin-induced apoptosis and contributes to chemoresistance by inhibiting PARB (poly-ADP-ribose polymerase) cleavage and delaying the activation of tumor suppressors p53 and p21 (Bhan, Soleimani, and Mandal 2017).

5.2.3 Carbohydrates

Carbohydrate Antigen, CA125, is among the most significant and commonly utilized biomarkers in clinical practice. The levels of CA153, CA125, and CEA in the blood were noticeably higher in the group with cancer (Li et al. 2022) (It's crucial role in the prognosis of ovarian cancer is well established (Zhang et al. 2021). Abnormal glycosylation of CA19-9 acts as an indicator for pancreatic cancer (Luo et al. 2021). Increased levels of Carcinoembryonic antigen (CEA), a glycoprotein involved with a high risk of gastric, colorectal, breast, ovarian, and lung cancer (Das et al. 2023). The combined measurement of CEA, CA19-9, and CA72-4 is very important for assessing the prognoses of colorectal cancer patients. This approach aids in predicting the outcomes for patients with stages I-III colorectal cancer (Wu, Mo, and Wu 2020). The serum levels of CA19-9, CEA, CA125, and CA242 is recorded higher in patients with pancreatic cancer (Gu et al. 2015; Chen et al. 2015).

5.2.4 Epigenetics

Epigenetic alterations serve as potent biomarkers for cancer due to their gene-specific frequency, stability, and detectability through minimally invasive methods. DNA methyltransferases, which add methyl groups to cytosine residues in DNA, are altered in cancerous cells (Das et al. 2023). CpG changes in the Sperm-associated antigen 6 (SPAG6) gene and hypermethylation's are linked to breast cancer. Genetic changes, like mutations in oncogenes and tumor suppressor genes, are not the only factors in breast cancer. Epigenetic changes, including the methylation of promoter CpG islands and modifications to histones, also play important roles in starting, promoting, and spreading the disease (Wu, Sarkissyan, and Vadgama 2015). Silencing of transcription factor RUNX3 seen in esophageal cancer and silencing of GATA-4 and GATA-5 in colorectal and gastric cancers are induced by promoter hypermethylation. Methylation levels of tumor suppressor genes **RASSF1A, RARβ2,** and **MINT13, MINT17** are associated with progression of breast cancer development. CpG islands in the GSTP1, APC, PTGS2, RASSF1A and MDR1 genes were found to be hypermethylated in over 85% of prostate cancers and cancer cell lines (Wu, Sarkissyan, and Vadgama 2015). Histone acetyltransferases (HATs) function by adding acetyl groups to lysine residues on histone tails, resulting in a more open chromatin structure. This conformational change increases DNA accessibility to transcription factors, thereby promoting active transcription. In small cell lung cancer (SCLC), mutations frequently occur in the CREBBP/EP300 family of HATs, which may disrupt this regulatory process. Chromatin remodeling and changes in structure play a crucial role in whether genes are turned on or off. Chromatin remodeling complexes help to pack and unpack DNA into chromatin. In non-small cell lung cancer (NSCLC) and small cell lung cancer (SCLC), mutations often impact parts of the SWI/SNF chromatin remodeling complex. Specifically, chromatin regulators like SMARCA4 (BRG1) and ARID1A are frequently mutated in lung adenocarcinoma (ADC) and are linked to the development of lung cancer (Chao and Pecot 2021).

5.2.5 Exosomes

Recent research has highlighted exosomes' significant potential as valuable diagnostic, prognostic, and therapeutic biomarkers (Hanjani et al. 2022). These membrane-bound, nanosized extracellular vesicles, which carry RNA, DNA, and proteins, are found in various body fluids (Hanjani et al. 2022). They play a pivotal role in cellular communication, thus contributing significantly to tumor progression and metastasis (Hanjani et al. 2022). The cargo within the exosomes has demonstrated considerable promise in early-stage detection of various types of cancer, offering high specificity and sensitivity (Hanjani et al. 2022). Glypican-1 (GPC-1) is markedly elevated in serum exosomes from patients with pancreatic cancer. Similarly, exosomal CD63 is found to be high in ovarian cancer (Yu et al. 2022).

5.2.6 Immune Checkpoint

Cancer cells have the ability to evade the immune system's detection and destruction by manipulating immune checkpoint pathways (Darvin et al. 2018). These pathways include key molecules such as Programmed Death-1 (PD-1), a receptor located on T-cell surfaces, and its ligand, Programmed Death-Ligand 1 (PD-L1), which is present on various cells, including those of tumors (Darvin et al. 2018). The binding of PD-L1 to PD-1 on T-cells sends an inhibitory signal that can lead to T cell apoptosis. Research has identified multiple forms of PD-1 and PD-L1 in the bloodstream of patients with cancer. By overexpressing PD-L1, cancer cells can effectively deactivate T-cells that are specifically targeting the tumor, thereby hindering their ability to attack the cancerous cells (Darvin et al. 2018). Immune checkpoint inhibitors, such as those that target PD-1, PD-L1, and CTLA-4 (Cytotoxic T-Lymphocyte antigen 4), work by blocking the interactions between these immune checkpoints and their ligands, which helps to restore the immune system's capacity to identify and combat cancer cells (Darvin et al. 2018).

5.3 CANCER DETECTION THROUGH IMAGING TECHNIQUES

Imaging techniques use energy waves to generate an image or scan of body tissues. These can be in the form of X-rays, sound waves, gamma rays, radioactive particles, or magnetic fields based on the technique used. These are also denoted as early detection or cancer screening tests as they provide an insight into cancer at early stages even when cancer has not spread throughout. Imaging techniques alone cannot be considered effective, but they are followed by other testing methods like a biopsy, endoscopy, cystoscopy, etc., if the scan shows tumor growth or traces of it. Several imaging techniques have been found effective in early-stage cancer detection, such as MRI, CT-scan, X-ray, PET scan ultrasound, etc. These imaging techniques are routinely used for cancer diagnosis, detecting cancer recurrence, and monitoring treatment efficacy (Gillies and Schabath 2020; Schiffman, Fisher, and Gibbs 2015). PET scans are generally considered more reliable and are frequently preferred because of their high sensitivity and accuracy as shown in Figure 5.2. They have the capability to identify abnormalities at the cellular level, often detecting issues before any structural changes become apparent on other imaging techniques.

5.3.1 X-Ray

Starting from the early use of X-ray films as detectors, medical X-ray imaging has evolved into a diverse array of specialized devices designed for various applications (Pfeiffer, Pfeiffer, and Rummeny 2020). The remarkable penetrating power of X-rays has established X-ray as a highly effective medical imaging technique for prognosis and screening of lung and breast cancer (Ou et al. 2021). It has emerged as the most widely accessible, typically fastest, and most cost-effective medical screening technique available today. Although CT scans are commonly employed to identify different types of cancer, X-rays continue to be the primary screening method for lung cancer (Bradley et al. 2021). It is a non-invasive technique that uses radiographic images to detect cancers originating in the lungs, bones, and other body parts. The primary applications of X-ray to detect lung cancer, bone cancer, and breast cancer are discussed below-

X-ray serves as a more favorable prognostic tool for early-stage lung cancer, increasing five-year survival rates reaching up to 70% for patients with small, localized tumors (Bradley et al. 2021). It is categorized into two main types based on biological behavior: non-small cell lung cancer (NSCLC) and small-cell lung cancer (SCLC), as their symptoms may result from endobronchial growth (tumors within the airways), intrathoracic extension (tumor spread within the chest), or distant metastases (spread to other parts of the body). Lung cancer typically does not show clear early symptoms, leading to diagnosis often at a more advanced stage (Hammerschmidt and Wirtz 2009).

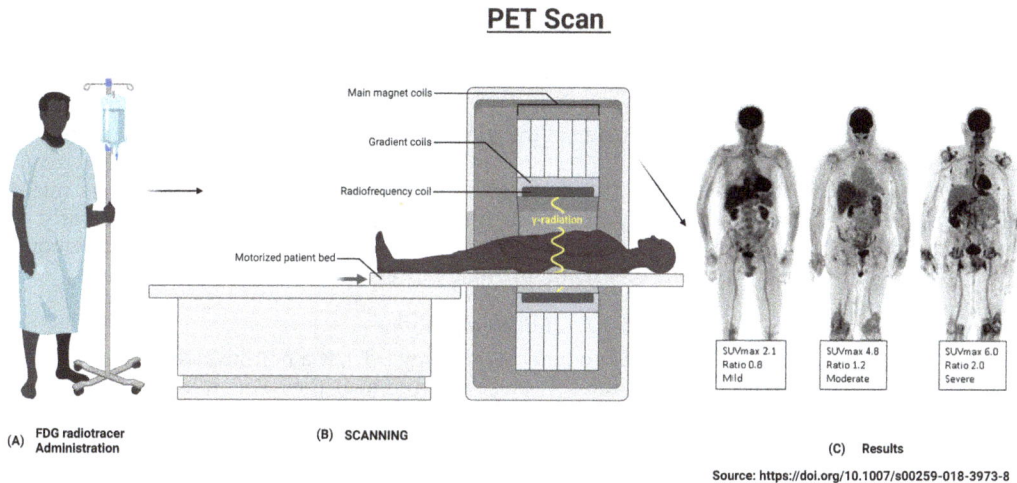

Source: https://doi.org/10.1007/s00259-018-3973-8

Figure 5.2 FDG-PET. Low (grade 1), intermediate (grade 2), and high (grade 3) LVV FDG uptake patterns including SUVmax values of the thoracic aorta in patients with GCA. The ratio is defined as the average SUVmax of the thoracic aorta divided by the liver region. The total vascular score (TVS) is the highest for the right-positioned patient. (From Slart RHJA et al. FDG-PET/CT(A) imaging in large vessel vasculitis and polymyalgia rheumatica: joint procedural recommendation of the EANM, SNMMI, and the PET Interest Group (PIG), and endorsed by the ASNC. Eur J Nucl Med Mol Imaging 2018;45:1250–1269, under Creative Commons Attribution.)

X-ray mammography is the most commonly used screening method proven to reduce breast cancer mortality rates worldwide (Heijblom et al. 2011). It is the diagnostic imaging technique used for screening early lesions that may be malignant, and it utilizes a low-energy X-ray beam, delivering a low dose of radiation, typically around 2–3 mGy, to the breast tissue. The goal is to screen and detect breast cancer at an early stage, where prompt treatment can reduce mortality rates by 15% to 30% (Pereira et al. 2021). However, this morphology-sensitive technique has several limitations. Breast cancers are often missed by mammograms, especially in women with dense breast tissue, where the low contrast between benign and malignant tissues reduces accuracy (Heijblom et al. 2011).

Plain radiography is the diagnostic test for bone cancer. Osteosarcoma is one of the most prevalent forms of bone cancer, predominantly impacting children and teenagers. This type of cancer usually develops in the metaphysis of long bones, especially in areas such as the distal femur, proximal tibia, and proximal humerus, and it frequently spreads to the lungs (Ferguson and Turner 2018). The sole reliance on X-rays for cancer therapy results in inadequate energy deposition from radiation, given that living tissues and organs exhibit low attenuation coefficients for X-rays. Consequently, this approach leads to unavoidable overexposure to radiation, which can inflict significant harm on healthy areas of the body (Chen et al. 2019b). Therefore, a CT scan is more effective in cancer detection than an X-ray, which is briefly discussed below.

5.3.2 Computed Tomography (CT-Scan)

CT-scan is a non-invasive detection technique discovered by Godfrey Hounsfield in 1979 (Benya 2008). As the most commonly used medical imaging technology, it is extensively employed for detecting lung lesions (Hirsch 2022). This tool provides high-density resolution, allowing it to distinguish even small density differences, such as those found in human soft tissues, which is a major advantage. However, with ongoing advancements in imaging technology and growing clinical demands, particularly with high-resolution CT, the volume of medical imaging data is increasing rapidly (Jiang et al. 2022b). It is designed to measure tumor volume and assess enhancement patterns following the injection of contrast agents. While CT plays a key role in guiding clinical decision-making and developing treatment plans, it provides limited information on specific immunologic pathways crucial for immunotherapy's effectiveness (Xiao and Pure 2021).

In 1989, the introduction of spiral or helical CT technology marked a significant advancement, as it enabled the simultaneous movement of both the gantry and the table, facilitating the acquisition of volumetric CT data. At the outset, these systems were equipped with a single X-ray source and a corresponding set of detectors within the gantry (Benya 2008). Low-dose spiral CT is far more effective than conventional chest radiographs at detecting lung cancer in its early stages. A meticulously structured protocol that includes follow-up CT scans to track the development of small nodules revealed that 86% of lung cancers identified in asymptomatic patients were classified as stage I. Additional research utilizing spiral CT has produced comparable results, although there are some differences in the percentage of individuals who received positive CT findings (Bastarrika et al. 2005).

Although CT is less effective than MRI at distinguishing between soft tissues and organs, micro CT excels with its high resolution (<50 μm) and fast imaging capabilities, which are particularly useful for detecting cancer lesions in the lungs and bones. This is crucial, as bones are a common metastatic site for major cancers like breast and prostate cancer (Serkova et al. 2021).

5.3.2.1 CT-Colonography

CT-colonography (CTC), often known as virtual colonoscopy (VC), is a non-invasive imaging technique employed to assess the large intestine, also referred to as the colon. It involves a modified CT scan performed after the patient has undergone bowel preparation and colonic distention. The resulting images are analyzed using advanced 2D and 3D display techniques. Since its debut in the mid-1990s, CTC has seen ongoing improvements in its technique and the sophisticated software used for image interpretation (Serkova et al. 2021). It is a minimally invasive colonoscopy that has been proven to be accurate, safe, and well-tolerated in the detection of advanced adenomas and cancer. Compared to colonoscopy's 95% sensitivity, CTC's average sensitivity for colorectal cancer (CRC) is 96%. Furthermore, CTC has a sensitivity of 83–93% for large polyps (≥10 millimeters) and 60–86% for intermediate polyps (6–9 millimeters). With a specificity of 95% to 97%, CTC is also very specific for lesions bigger than 9 millimeters (Sali, Grazzini, and Mascalchi 2017). CT-Colonography exhibits high specificity but varying sensitivity, and it is generally not as sensitive or specific as conventional colonoscopy. Despite this, it can be a valuable screening tool for populations at average risk of colorectal cancer (CRC) (Martin-Lopez et al. 2014).

5.3.2.2 Single-Photon Emission Computed Tomography (SPECT)

Single-photon emission computed tomography (SPECT) is used to determine the three-dimensional distribution of a radiopharmaceutical within the body by measuring the intensity of gamma rays emitted from the suspected tissue or organ (Coleman 1991). It is a type of medical imaging employed to detect biomarkers within tissues, aiding in diagnosing conditions such as strokes, fractures, infections, and cancers by providing detailed images of the body's internal structures (Coleman 1991). Camera-based SPECT systems provide an advantage as it capture data from multiple angles during a single rotation around the body, enabling the production of numerous contiguous images in both transverse and longitudinal sections. These three-dimensional images eliminate interference from overlapping structures, thus significantly enhancing image contrast compared to planar imaging which consequently, detect lesions (Coleman 1991). Apart from SPECT, PET imaging is more sensitive and advanced technique compared to SPECT (Sahin and Sanli 2023).

5.3.3 Magnetic Resonance Imaging (MRI)

Magnetic resonance technology is a non-invasive tool that has significantly influenced medical imaging (Tripathi, Rao, and Zeng 2017). Unlike x-ray methods, magnetic resonance imaging (MRI) does not rely on ionizing radiation; instead, it employs a powerful external magnetic field generated by a superconducting magnet, along with radiofrequency radiation, to produce cross-sectional images in any plane. The contrast between tissues is determined by various factors that are related to the magnetic properties of the material (Smith and McCarthy 1992), and this superior soft-tissue contract (Derks, van der Veldt, and Smits 2022) can be further enhanced with the use of exogenous paramagnetic contrast agents (Serkova et al. 2021; Stafford 2020).

MRI scans offer anatomical cross-sections that are more effective than pathological examinations for detecting invasion in medium to large blood vessels. Tumors with high-grade venous invasion can cause significant damage to normal vascular structures, often leaving little to no visible trace (Tripathi, Rao, and Zeng 2017). It is also commonly used to detect soft-tissue lesions, including liver and lung metastases. In addition to high-resolution anatomical imaging, physiological MRI techniques like diffusion-weighted imaging can quantify tumor cellular density and edema by assessing water molecules' restricted or enhanced diffusion (Serkova et al. 2021).

5.3.4 Positron Emission Tomography (PET Scan)

Positron emission tomography (PET) combined with computed tomography (Carvalho et al. 2025) is a valuable, non-invasive hybrid imaging technique that merges nuclear imaging with CT for various applications. It was developed by the Mallinckrodt Institute of Radiology in 1970 and significantly advances anatomic imagining in oncologic studies. It is the technology that subsequently distinguishes between benign and malignant tumors. It can detect both morphological changes and functional alterations by assessing tissue avidity for isotope uptake. The most commonly used isotope in these scans is fluorodeoxyglucose (FDG). However, other isotopes, such as florbetapir for amyloid detection and quantification, have also been introduced recently (Selva-O'Callaghan et al. 2019). FDG, a glucose analog, offers important functional insights by highlighting the increased glucose uptake and glycolysis in cancer cells. This allows it to detect metabolic abnormalities before any visible morphological changes appear as shown in Figure 5.2 (Almuhaideb, Papathanasiou, and Bomanji 2011).

FDG PET/CT is particularly sensitive and specific for certain cancers and is primarily used for staging and restaging, helping to guide patient management. It is also useful in distinguishing responders from non-responders to treatment, even before any measurable reduction in tumor size is observed (Almuhaideb, Papathanasiou, and Bomanji 2011). While the role of FDG PET/CT in assessing the primary tumor is somewhat limited, its sensitivity can be significantly improved when combined with contrast-enhanced head and neck CT, achieving a high sensitivity of 96%. A prevalent challenge associated with numerous PET agents is their tendency to be absorbed in non-malignant conditions, such as benign prostatic hyperplasia or prostatitis, which reduces their effectiveness for initial diagnostic purposes. Furthermore, many of these agents exhibit decreased sensitivity in the advanced stages of the disease, particularly when adenocarcinomas experience neuroendocrine trans-differentiation (Mena et al. 2021).

5.3.5 Ultrasound

Ultrasound imaging (also known as sonography or ultrasonography) is considered a highly sensitive tool, frequently used in routine clinical exams. It is the world's second most utilized imaging modality because it is widely accessible, robust, and safe (de Leon et al. 2018). In recent decades, ultrasound contrast agents have been used extensively in molecular cancer imaging to enhance tumor detection, characterization, and measurement. Several promising preclinical and clinical applications of ultrasound molecular cancer imaging are under investigation (Zhang et al. 2022). Ultrasonic diagnosis can produce tomographic images of various organs by detecting tissue changes and the morphological alterations associated with pathological anatomy. These images are consistent with the morphological manifestations, enabling accurate localization and qualitative diagnosis based on the tomographic image of the lesions (Wang and Yang 2021). Imaging with contrast-enhanced ultrasound (CEUS) is a useful diagnostic technique for preclinical and clinical settings. Microbubbles are the ultrasonic contrast agent most commonly utilized. In addition to them, new materials with a nanoscale are being studied. Using a site-specific ligand, the ultrasonic contrast agents are altered to target disease-associated molecular markers for molecular CEUS actively. The most often used markers for tumor imaging are those associated with neoangiogenesis, such as αvβ3 integrin and vascular endothelial growth factor receptor-2 (VEGFR2) (Baier, Rix, and Kiessling 2020).

5.3.6 Endoscopy-Based Cancer Detection

Several diagnostic methods are employed for cancer detection, each with distinct advantages and limitations. Endoscopy, a widely used diagnostic technique, involves the insertion of a long, flexible tube equipped with a light source and camera through a natural orifice such as the mouth or rectum. Various endoscopic procedures are used to detect cancers in different body parts (Ahmed et al. 2018). For instance, bronchoscopy examines the trachea, bronchi, and lungs for the presence of the tumor (Dumoulin 2018). Similarly, laparoscopy is employed to visualize the abdomen and pelvic cancer. Cystoscopy is used to examine bladder and urethra cancer (Amling 2001), and colonoscopy is considered as a valuable tool for early detection of colorectal cancer (Vleugels, van Lanschot, and Dekker 2016).

5.4 BIOFLUID-BASED CANCER DETECTION

Cancer, being the second leading cause of death globally, is one of the major threats to our society. Recently, personalized medicine has attracted significant attention as one of the most promising approaches in cancer therapy. Understanding the molecular landscapes of tumors is essential for guiding and improving treatment options in clinical practice (Marrugo-Ramirez, Mir, and Samitier 2018). Tissue biopsies are the standard methods for obtaining molecular information about tumors, necessary for identifying cancer types, gene and mutation expressions, and for screening purposes. However, this approach has several drawbacks, including the need for invasive surgical procedures that cause discomfort and pain and pose risks to patients. These procedures carry inherent clinical risks and potential surgical complications (Marrugo-Ramirez, Mir, and Samitier 2018). Additionally, some tumors are located in anatomical regions that are difficult or impossible to access for biopsy, and in some cases, extracting a biopsy may increase the risk of metastatic lesions. Moreover, monitoring tumor evolution at different stages of the disease is crucial for effective treatment, but repeated solid biopsies are impractical due to their highly invasive nature. The time required for sample analysis can delay the initiation of therapy, potentially compromising the prognosis. Typically, optic methods are used for monitoring, though they fail to provide comprehensive information about the tumors. Radiology is commonly employed, but excessive radiation exposure poses health risks to the patients. Non-radiation methods, such as MRI, provide limited information and are considered ineffective for detecting cancer at early stages. A promising alternative to traditional tissue biopsy is the examination of interactions between cancer cells and various cancer-associated biomolecules, including cells, nucleic acids, proteins, and microvesicles, as well as their surrounding environment (Kwong et al. 2021).

Liquid biopsy has emerged as a significant method for capturing tumor-related biomarkers from liquid samples, attracting considerable interest due to its minimally invasive nature, reduced reagent requirements, and user-friendly application. This technique primarily targets the analysis of circulating tumor cells (CTCs), circulating tumor nucleic acids (ctNAs), and tumor-derived extracellular vesicles (exosomes), which are released into the bloodstream, saliva, urine, cerebrospinal fluid (CSF), and other bodily fluids by tumors and their metastatic sites in cancer patients as demonstrated in Figure 5.3 (Kwong et al. 2021).

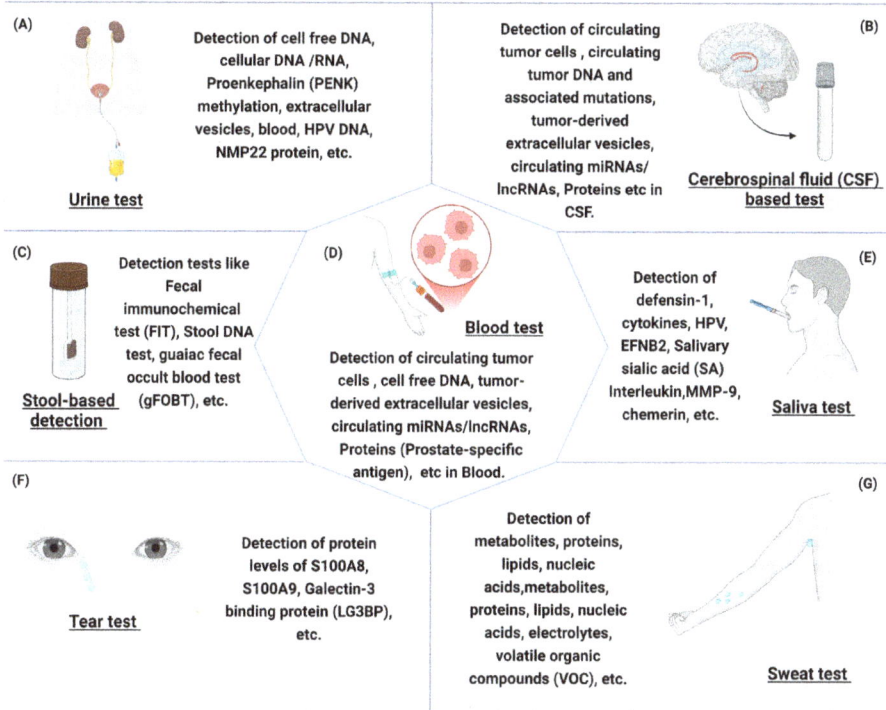

Figure 5.3 Biofluid-based cancer detection. (A) Urine, (B) Cerebrospinal fluid, (C) Stool, (D) Blood, (E) Saliva, (F) Tear, (G) Sweat test.

5.4.1 Urine Test

Urine is produced by blood filtration in the kidneys, where it removes unwanted substances from the blood to excrete them out of the body (Dunphy et al. 2021). Urine composition is an indirect reflection of plasma composition and kidney function, and it can serve as an essential tool for detecting various abnormalities in the body. The presence of specific biomarkers in the urine samples indicates a specific type of cancer (Dunphy et al. 2021).

Urine analysis can serve as a detection source for bladder cancer, kidney cancer, and cancer of the uterus or urethra (Wood et al. 2013). Urine proteins are less susceptible to proteolysis and have less complexity than plasma proteins, which makes it easy to identify differences in urine proteomics in healthy and cancerous patients (Kalantari et al. 2015). Alterations in body metabolism and pathophysiology can also be detected via volatile organic compounds (VOCs) found in urine. Butyrolactone and 2-methoxy-5-methylphenol are among the VOCs found in the urine of bladder cancer patients.

Urine testing is done for various analytes like cfDNA, cellular DNA/RNA, extracellular vesicles, and proteins. The presence of blood in the urine (hematuria) can be a sign of early-stage bladder cancer (Oh et al. 2023). Colorectal cancer screening for the presence of certain metabolites is indicative of cancer polyps and tumors in the colon and rectum. Proenkephalin (PENK) methylation, a type of DNA methylation, also acts as a diagnostic marker for various cancer types, including bladder cancer (Oh et al. 2023).

NMP22 (Nuclear Matrix Protein 22) protein is released from disintegrating cells whose increased levels in urine serve as a marker for bladder cancer (Sarhadi and Armengol 2022). Meta-analysis of urine and HPV DNA serves the diagnostic purpose for cervical cancer (Yin et al. 2017). Although urine cytology is widely used for cancer detection, it has certain limitations. Urine tests, being a non-invasive, easy-to-collect sample detection technique, has limited sensitivity (Jeong and Ku 2022). If any abnormalities are found in urine composition, a biopsy is performed as a confirmatory test.

5.4.2 Cerebrospinal Fluid Based Detection

Biopsy-based diagnosis of central nervous system malignancies comes with certain challenges and risks. Imaging techniques are less specific and sensitive in detecting these cancers. The introduction of liquid biopsy has enabled molecular testing in cancer patients to incorporate the analysis of biofluids from readily accessible compartments (Dunphy et al. 2021). Liquid biopsy of CSF obtained by lumbar puncture or from the ventricular access device provides a convenient approach to cancer detection by analyzing genetic alterations from circulating tumor DNA (ctDNA) (Hickman, Miller, and Arcila 2023). ctDNA secreted from viable tumor cells or released from apoptotic or necrotic cells with the CNS parenchyma may enter the CSF, or CSF can collect ctDNA through direct contact with the tumor (Hickman, Miller, and Arcila 2023). Cerebrospinal fluid also contains other biomarkers derived from brain tumor cells like miRNA, proteins, and EVs. ctDNA-associated gene mutations in IDH1, TP53, EGFR, ERBB2, and FGFR2 derived from CSF serve as biomarkers for glioblastoma patients (Hickman, Miller, and Arcila 2023). Primary central nervous system lymphoma (PCNSL) is detected by CSF-derived MYD88 mutation. Brain metastasis originating from primary lung cancer correlates to EGFR and KRAS mutations in ctDNA derived from CSF. Similarly, TP53 and AKT2 mutations in CSF-derived ctDNA denote brain metastasis from primary bladder cancer.

5.4.3 Stool Test

Both colorectal polyps and cancers have the potential to cause bleeding, and stool-based tests are designed to detect trace amounts of blood in feces that are not visibly apparent. Stool DNA tests are carried out in asymptomatic patients with colon cancer (Dickinson et al. 2015). The stool DNA test detects any DNA changes and/or the presence of a small amount of blood shed from polyps into the stool. These polyps can be removed surgically before they become cancerous (Dickinson et al. 2015).

Notably, the presence of blood in the stool can also indicate non-malignant conditions such as hemorrhoids. If any sort of abnormality is detected through stool tests, a colonoscopy is performed as a confirmatory test for colorectal cancer. Three stool tests have been confirmed by the U.S. Food and Drug Administration (FDA) for diagnosis of colorectal cancer-Guaiac based fecal occult blood test and Fecal immunochemical test (Crosby et al. 2022), to specifically target and detect heme presence in stool samples (Gomez-Molina et al. 2024). The FIT test employs the use of specific antibodies to serve the purpose. Multitarget stool DNA test detects both hemoglobin and specific DNA biomarkers associated with colorectal neoplasms (Dickinson et al. 2015). Stool test helps detect cancer in its early stages, even before the appearance of symptoms, thus enhancing the survival chances of patient by providing them with appropriate treatment (Gomez-Molina et al. 2024). Although stool-based cancer screening is a non-invasive, painless diagnostic approach, it comes with certain limitations. Stool-based cancer detection tests are less sensitive and often show false positive results. Additional tests like colonoscopy are required after stool DNA test (Carvalho et al. 2025).

5.4.4 Blood Test

Blood composition provides insight into various physiologic and pathologic states, such as cancer and other disease (Dunphy et al. 2021). CTCs, cfDNA, cfRNA, miRNA, proteins, and other macromolecules derived from cancerous cells can be detected in blood. Blood serves as a rich source of cancerous biomarkers (Dunphy et al. 2021). CTCs are circulating tumor cells shed from the tumor into the bloodstream that may behave as an indicator of early steps of cancer metastasis. These are transported via the bloodstream to different regions of the body, where they may leak out, multiply, and form metastatic lesions (Lawrence et al. 2023).

Prostate-specific antigen (PSA) is a protein produced by the cells of the prostate gland and found in the bloodstream, with elevated levels serving as an indicator of prostate cancer (Das et al. 2023). Carcinoembryonic antigen (CEA) is an antigen present in developing fetus and absent in the blood of healthy adults. The presence of CEA in the blood is indicative of several forms of cancer, including cancer in the rectum, pancreas, colon, or ovary (Hao, Zhang, and Zhang 2019). Cancer antigen 125 (CA125) associated with ovarian cancer can be measured through blood tests (Margoni, Gargalionis, and Papavassiliou 2024). The elevated Blood levels of CA 27.29 are indicative of breast cancer (Rack et al. 2016); similarly, CA19-9 is associated with cancer of the pancreas (Zhu et al. 2024).

CBC (Complete Blood Count) test measures the levels of various blood cells in blood. Abnormalities in the count of white blood cells (WBC) may suggest the presence of leukemia (a type of blood cancer), lymphoma (cancer of the lymphatic system), or multiple myeloma (a cancer that impacts plasma cells in the bone marrow). Blood tests are conducted to detect circulating tumor cells (CTCs), circulating tumor nucleic acids, or tumor-derived extracellular vesicles (exosomes) (Lozar et al. 2019). The presence of cell-free DNA in blood is indicative of apoptosis in actively proliferating / tumor cells. Blood testing is a non-invasive, risk-free, painless, non-surgical cancer diagnostic approach without any side effects or the risk of infection (Das et al. 2023).

5.4.5 Saliva test

Saliva is a complex biofluid that constitutes proteins, peptides, electrolytes, gingival crevicular fluid, serum transudate, leukocytes, epithelial cells, and microorganisms, along with various inorganic and organic salts secreted from salivary glands (Zhou and Liu 2023). It consists of omics molecular biomarkers similar to that found in blood and urine, which can serve as indicators for various types of cancer, including oral, lung, pancreatic, breast, and gastric cancers (Zhou and Liu 2023; Birknerova et al. 2022; Mishra et al. 2016).

Saliva testing is the least-invasive, safest, noncoagulated biofluid used in the clinical diagnosis of cancer. Saliva directly interacts with oral cancer lesions, increasing saliva's specificity and sensitivity as a screening tool. Over 100 salivary biomarkers have been identified, including defensin-1, cytokines (IL-8,1b, TNF-alpha) (Khurshid et al. 2018; Kaczor-Urbanowicz et al. 2019).

Enhanced levels of Salivary sialic acid (SA) also serve as potential biomarkers for breast cancer and oral cancer. Human papillomavirus (HPV) was one of the earliest-developed salivary biomarkers used for the screening of cervical cancer. Expression of gene EFNB2 is useful for prognostic evaluation in patients with Oral squamous cell carcinoma (OSCC). Increased levels of post-inflammatory cytokines, Interleukin 6 (IL-6), and IL-8 associated with OSCC are biomarkers of oral malignant and premalignant lesions. MMP-9 and chemerin salivary biomarkers are used to screen oral cancers with high sensitivity and accuracy. Salivary biomarkers serve the purpose of early-stage detection of head and neck carcinoma and oral squamous cell carcinoma) (Nguyen et al. 2020; Mishra et al. 2016; Khijmatgar et al. 2024).

5.4.6 Tear Analysis

High protein concentration, ease of collection, and relatively low complexity of tear fluid compared to blood make it an ideal candidate for diagnostic purposes (Daily et al. 2022). Furthermore, the accessibility of low molecular weight proteins in tear fluid enhances its potential for the identification of critical cancer biomarkers (Daily et al. 2022).

Raised levels of S100A8 and S100A9, a family of calcium-binding proteins, were detected in tear samples of patients with breast cancer. These proteins, with high sequence and folding similarity, are involved in differentiation, migration, invasion, and inflammation(Daily et al. 2022). A heavily glycosylated protein, Galectin-3 binding protein (LG3BP) expressed in various body fluids and cancerous cells, serves as binding sites for proteins known to be involved in metastasis. Elevated levels of LG3BP reduce the overall survival chances of breast cancer patients (Daily et al. 2022).

5.4.7 Sweat Analysis

Non-invasive methods are widely used for screening and diagnosing several types of cancers, and sweat analysis is one of these approaches. Numerous biomarkers like metabolites, proteins, lipids, nucleic acids, and electrolytes in sweat reflect various physiological changes. The presence of specific volatile organic compounds (VOC) in the sweat samples is a possible biomarker for specific cancer screening like that for breast cancer and lung cancer. Metabolically high, active cancerous cells release these VOC that are absent in non-cancerous patients (Leemans et al. 2023). Earlier, lung cancer detection approaches based on X-ray and sputum cytology had a high chance of false positive results associated with other health issues (Calderon-Santiago et al. 2015). Sweat being less complex in composition, has the diagnostic advantage of not being interfered by other pathological conditions.

5.5 HISTOPATHOLOGY-BASED DETECTION

The study of disease indicators through microscopic analysis of a biopsy or surgical specimen is known as histopathology. A histopathologist examines tissues that may be abnormal or carcinogenic providing early diagnosis and effective treatment plans. A detailed microscopic examination is more widely called a biopsy since it can identify malignant cells. The pap smear test used for screening cervical cancer involves scraping off cellular material from the cervix's squamocolumnar junction with a brush or spatula, which is then smeared onto a glass slide and examined under the microscope, the cells are fixed, stained, and visually inspected for any alterations in the cells.

Personalized cancer therapy relies heavily on precise biomarker evaluation, making accurate diagnosis critical for effective treatment plans. The emergence of digital image analysis (Hanjani et al. 2022) algorithms presents significant potential to enhance the efficiency and accuracy of histomorphological assessments, offering improved precision in evaluating cancerous tissues (Acs, Rantalainen, and Hartman 2020).

5.5.1 AI Tools Used in Cancer Detection

The integration of artificial intelligence (AI)-based tools into clinical practice represents a significant advancement in the digitalization of medical imaging. Computer-aided detection (CADe) tools have been commercially available for pulmonary nodule detection since the 2000s. Data collected from the National Lung Screening Trial (NLST) has supported the creation of many computer-aided diagnostic (CADx) tools aimed at improving lung cancer diagnosis using chest computed tomography (Carvalho et al. 2025). convolutional neural networks (CNNs) are the most common type of deep learning algorithms for image analysis (Chassagnon et al. 2023).

The GALEN algorithm is one of the several AI platforms that are currently available for evaluating the histology of breast core biopsies. In order to identify a variety of breast diseases, such as invasive and in situ carcinomas, precursors such as typical hyperplasia, and benign disorders, GALEN can analyze whole slide images (WSIs) from core needle biopsies. GALEN has demonstrated high accuracy, achieving an area under the curve (Gomez-Molina et al. 2024) of 0.99 for detecting invasive carcinoma (specificity and sensitivity of 93.6% and 95.5%, respectively) and 0.98 for ductal carcinoma in situ (DCIS). GALEN was developed using a deep learning ensemble of Convolutional Neural Networks (CNNs) trained on over 2 million labeled image patches from 2,153 H&E-stained slides. This artificial intelligence technique helps pathologists detect breast cancers more precisely and has the potential to prevent non-aggressive DCIS from requiring needless therapies, such as surgery or radiotherapy. Standard H&E slides provide quicker diagnosis, more affordable care, and improved risk management for both over and under-treatment (Liu et al. 2023) (Sandbank et al. 2022).

Looking ahead, prevention rather than treatment may emerge as the most impactful application of artificial intelligence (AI) in cancer care. Seminal research has already identified a comprehensive portfolio of cancer risk factors, and technological advancements now allow for the collection of extensive data at the individual patient level. Beyond genetic testing and electronic health records (Khehra, Padda, and Swift 2024), sensors embedded in smartphones and wearable devices gather vast quantities of data points for each patient. By integrating these data, AI can enhance diagnostic precision by analyzing physiological and environmental parameters, paving the way for more personalised and proactive cancer prevention strategies (Bhinder et al. 2021).

5.6 OTHER TECHNIQUES FOR CANCER DETECTION

A broad range of biochemical entities lies under cancer biomarkers, such as protein, sugar, small metabolites, nucleic acids, cytokinetic parameters, and even the body fluid containing the entire tumor. These biomarkers are used in risk assessment, diagnosis, prognosis, even in determining the efficacy of the treatment. The cancer biomarker field aims to develop detection and monitoring strategies that are reliable, cost-effective, and powerful for cancer risk indicators and tumor classification so that the patient with cancer can get the most appropriate treatment and doctors can monitor the progression and regression, as well as recurrence of the disease. This field has made significant progress in the past few decades. Detection methods that recognize intracellular biomarkers on the cancer cell surface have been discovered by the use of tools like polymerase chain reaction, colorimetric assay, fluorescence method, electrophoresis, next-generation sequencing and Flow cytometry-based assays, etc.

5.6.1 Polymerase Chain Reaction (PCR)

The polymerase chain reaction (PCR) is a laboratory technique for nucleic acid amplification that involves denaturing and renaturing small fragments of deoxyribonucleic acid (DNA) or ribonucleic acid (RNA) sequences with the help of the DNA polymerase I enzyme, specifically Taq DNA, isolated from Thermus aquaticus. Introduced in 1985 by Mullis and his team, for which they were awarded the Nobel Prize, PCR has become an essential tool in biomolecular sciences due to its remarkable capability to amplify and detect DNA components (Khehra, Padda, and Swift 2024).

Real-time qPCR is widely applied in various fields and is a fundamental molecular and genomic research technique. It is commonly used for gene quantification and expression analysis through relative and absolute quantification. Relative quantification compares gene expression between different samples, while absolute quantification relies on a standard curve with known template concentrations to measure gene expression (Harshitha and Arunraj 2021). These advancements in real-time RT-PCR technology have led to substantial progress in cancer diagnostics by delivering precise, quantitative data on gene expression in an automated, rapid, versatile, and cost-effective manner. Recently, real-time RT-PCR has been employed to diagnose circulating tumor cells (CTCs) in persons with metastatic breast cancer's peripheral blood and lymph nodes by identifying the differential expression of marker genes through multigene RT-PCR assays (Park et al. 2017).

5.6.2 Fluorescence in Situ Hybridization

Fluorescence in situ hybridization, which was created in the 1980s and uses fluorescent probes to precisely pinpoint particular DNA targets, is still a common therapeutic tool (Ordulu and Nardi 2022). This technique has bridged the gap between molecular genetics and traditional cytogenetics (Ordulu and Nardi 2022) as it is the principal method for evaluating a broad range of genetic abnormalities, including rearrangements resulting from translocations, insertions, inversions, deletions, and amplifications (Kato 2023; Chrzanowska, Kowalewski, and Lewandowska 2020; Ahmad et al. 2022). Chromogenic in situ hybridization, or CISH, is occasionally used in oncology and molecular pathology as well. The underlying idea of both techniques is annealing to the target region, followed by evaluation, detection, and spatial localization. The primary labeling difference between the two is that FISH uses fluorescent tags, each with its own detection method, whereas CISH uses biotin or digoxigenin (Chrzanowska, Kowalewski, and Lewandowska 2020).

This tool helps spot irregularities in different types of cancer, like multiple myeloma, pulmonary adenocarcinoma, prostate cancer, and breast carcinoma, among others. It is often used to check for changes in the ROS1 gene, which is found in about 1–2% of non-small cell lung cancer (NSCLC) cases. It works by using a dual-color break-apart probe to detect any ROS1 rearrangements (Ahmad et al. 2022).

5.6.3 Sanger Sequencing

The gold standard for detecting DNA mutations has been Sanger sequencing (SGS). Sanger and his team came up with the first DNA sequencing technique that used modified nucleotides to stop DNA polymerase from extending the chain (Sabour, Sabour, and Ghorbian 2017).

Sanger sequencing (SGS) of PCR-amplified products remains the most commonly employed method for detecting KRAS mutations in colorectal cancer in routine clinical practice (Malapelle et al. 2012). BDA (Blocker Displacement Amplification) is a technique that selectively amplifies DNA sequences by using blocker oligonucleotides. BDA along with Sanger sequencing is involved in the detection of low variant allele frequency (VAF) mutations of EFGR in ctDNA from plasma samples of lung cancer patients (Jiang et al. 2022a). This sequencing method remains the ideal standard for nucleic acid-based tests, particularly in cases involving low-quality single-nucleotide variants (SNVs) or small deletions and insertions of up to 10bp. Sanger sequencing can be used to screen BRCA1 c.68_69del, BRCA2 c.5946del, and BRCA1 c5266dup mutations in DNA extracted from pap smears in females (Lee et al. 2016).

Sanger sequencing combined with BDA technology has been employed in various applications, including the detection of low-level PIK3CA mutations in melanoma tumor sections, estimation of variant allele frequency (VAF) for low-level mosaic mutations in families with alveolar capillary dysplasia, and identification of BRAF mutations at VAFs as low as 0.2% in formalin-fixed, paraffin-embedded (FFPE) lymph node tissue samples from metastatic melanoma patients. Furthermore, BDA has been utilized in multiplex PCR and integrated with amplicon sequencing to enhance the detection of low-level variants in next-generation sequencing (NGS) workflows (Yan et al. 2021).

SGS has limitations, including limited sensitivity and the inability to investigate multiple targets simultaneously. Additionally, because somatic cancers are heterogeneous and frequently mixed with normal tissue, it can be challenging to detect somatic cancer mutations using SGS without performing microdissections (Sabour, Sabour, and Ghorbian 2017).

5.6.4 Next-Generation Sequencing

Next-generation sequencing (NGS), also known as massively parallel sequencing, was developed over the last ten years to allow for the concurrent sequencing of hundreds of thousands of DNA fragments without the need for prior sequence information. This cutting-edge technology marks a substantial advancement over conventional sequencing techniques, which typically permit the sequencing of only one or a few short DNA fragments that have been previously amplified using Polymerase Chain Reaction (PCR) in a single tube. Traditional sequencing was limited to specific DNA regions and samples due to its high cost and labor-intensive process (Kamps et al. 2017). Since the advent of Sanger sequencing, next-generation sequencing (NGS) technologies have advanced considerably, offering greater data output, improved efficiencies, and broader applications (Hu et al. 2021). NGS methods provide a significantly higher molecular detail at a relatively low cost, enabling comprehensive analysis of both normal human and cancer genomes. Additionally, NGS allows for the study of mutational signatures across different cancers, which can be linked to potential causes, such as exposure to genotoxic agents or defects in DNA repair mechanisms (Ning et al. 2014).

NGS has become important in cancer genomics research and has recently been integrated into clinical oncology to enhance personalized cancer treatment. NGS is used to identify novel diagnostic and rare cancer mutations, detect translocations, inversions, insertions, deletions, and copy number variants, and identify familial cancer mutation carriers. Additionally, NGS provides the molecular basis for selecting appropriate targeted therapies and making therapeutic and prognostic decisions (Sabour, Sabour, and Ghorbian 2017; Choi and Ro 2023). Tumor mutation profiling through NGS has become a standard practice for many patients with advanced cancer, either at the outset for selecting first-line treatments or later in the course of the disease (Schmid et al. 2022).

Cancer is a disease that can be caused by genetic alterations. In particular, single-nucleotide variants, which appear as germline or somatic point mutations, are crucial in driving cellular proliferation and cancer development across various human cancer types. Next-generation sequencing (NGS) technologies allow for the simultaneous sequencing of thousands of DNA molecules, offering high speed and throughput. These technologies can generate both quantitative and qualitative sequence data, comparable to the scale of the Human Genome Project, in just two weeks. Next-generation sequencing (NGS) has been integrated into clinical oncology to enhance personalized cancer treatment. NGS is used to identify novel diagnostic markers and rare cancer mutations, detect translocations, inversions, insertions, deletions, and copy number variants, as well as identify carriers of familial cancer mutations. Additionally, NGS provides a molecular basis for selecting appropriate targeted therapies and improving prognostic assessments (Sabour, Sabour, and Ghorbian 2017). When broad NGS testing is conducted, discussing the results at a molecular tumor board is essential to maximize the potential benefits for the patient. This is particularly important when alterations are found for which there are no approved targeted therapies, ensuring that the cost of molecular testing translates into meaningful clinical outcomes (Schmid et al. 2022).

5.6.5 Flow Cytometry

Cells can be characterized or sorted based on their fluorescent or light-scattering properties. Various fluorescent reagents are employed in this process, including fluorescently labeled antibodies, nucleic acid-binding dyes, viability dyes, ion indicator dyes, and fluorescent proteins (McKinnon 2018). Flow cytometry provides high sensitivity and specificity, allowing for the precise distinction of cancer cell populations (Georvasili et al. 2022). Its use in cancer diagnosis is expanding rapidly, and it is now routinely employed to help classify leukemia's and lymphomas (Mishra 2023). This tool plays a crucial role in diagnosing and monitoring hematologic neoplasms. It enables the identification, quantification, and detailed characterization of hematopoietic cells in both peripheral blood and bone marrow (Saft 2023). There are multiple applications of flow cytometry in detecting tumor-related abnormalities in patients. These include identifying unusual cell distributions in various tissues, analyzing DNA content, assessing cell proliferation rates, detecting abnormal expression of surface receptors, and identifying tumor antigens. Different flow cytometry techniques can be applied to characterize these anomalies effectively (Mishra 2023).

Flow cytometry has also been valuable in analyzing tumor dissemination in cerebrospinal fluid (CSF). Leptomeningeal metastases (LM), also called meningeal carcinomatosis, involve the spread of tumor cells into the CSF and leptomeninges. Despite treatment, approximately 5–10% of cancer patients with solid tumors will develop LM (D'Amato Figueiredo et al. 2022). In patients with invasive breast cancer and DNA ploidy can be determined in the early stages of carcinogenesis. Chromosomal instability, which is linked to aneuploidy (an abnormal number of chromosomes), is directly associated with cancer progression and poor prognosis. The main advantage of Intraoperative flow cytometry is that it offers the potential to provide real-time information on DNA ploidy, aiding in the assessment of tumor characteristics during surgery (D'Amato Figueiredo et al. 2022).

5.6.6 CRISPR-Based Diagnostic

Clustered regularly interspaced short palindromic repeats and CRISPR-associated proteins together were expected to be an adaptive immunological management identified in most of the bacteria and archaea, cross better-called defence against the invasion of foreign nucleic acids(Rahimi et al. 2024; Gong et al. 2021). This genome editing technology has been categorized as an efficient genetic tool up until 2020 (de la Fuente-Nunez and Lu 2017). CRISPR is steadily becoming more popular for tasks like gene expression screening, site-directed mutagenesis, and functional gene studies. It is a powerful genome editing tool that offers many benefits, such as high precision, strong sensitivity, and excellent efficiency (Cheng et al. 2020).This technique is used increasingly in the experimental contexts enlisted for the treatment of cancers. CRISPR -Cas9 is under preliminary evaluation as an anti-tumor agent applicable to judicious therapy (Chen et al. 2019a).

This method can be used for the early detection and screening of cancer-associated mutations by capturing circulating tumor DNA (ctDNA) or circulating tumor cells (CTCs) from blood samples obtained through liquid biopsies. This non-invasive method allows the detection of cancer at an early stage and gives information on tumor dynamics over time, which can be important for insights into disease progression and potential resistance to therapy. The merger of CRISPR/Cas with biosensors converting biological replies into electrical signals can pose a great improvement to specificity with respect to several cancer-associated genetic sequences, helping in the identification of mutations in oncogenes such as KRAS and EGFR, along with tumor suppressor genes like TP53 (Di Carlo and Sorrentino 2024).

The epidermal growth factor receptor (EGFR) functions as a transmembrane receptor tyrosine kinase and is crucial in stimulating the growth and expansion of cancerous cells. As such, identifying EGFR mutations in circulating tumor DNA (ctDNA) obtained from body fluids—including blood plasma—offers significant promise for guiding clinical decisions regarding targeted therapies aimed at EGFR. Tsou et al. (2020) presented a technique that leverages the collateral cleavage ability of Cas12a on non-specific single-stranded DNA (ssDNA) reporters, which facilitates straightforward fluorescent readings for sensitive detection of EGFR point mutations within plasma-derived ctDNA (Rahimi et al. 2024).

Emerging CRISPR/Cas13-based technologies represent a noteworthy advancement in the early diagnosis of colorectal cancer (CRC) through monitoring circulating exosomal microRNAs (CEx-miRNAs) (Duran-Vinet et al. 2021). Strategies focusing on cell-free cancer-derived extracellular vesicles, particularly CEx-miRNAs present in circulation, have grown increasingly vital for both monitoring and diagnosing CRC at an early stage(Hibner, Kimsa-Furdzik, and Francuz 2018). The profiling of CEx-miRNAs is primarily conducted using reverse transcription-quantitative polymerase chain reaction (RT-qPCR), a method recognized for its high sensitivity and specificity concerning microRNA expression levels (Min et al. 2019). Furthermore, platforms based on CRISPR/Cas13 hold considerable potential as next-generation tools not only for early diagnosis but also for prognostic evaluations related to colorectal cancer—and their features may make them valuable candidates for similar applications across various other cancers(Duran-Vinet et al. 2021).

In ovarian cancer (OC), FCGR1A expression has been found to correlate positively with higher grades and stages of tumors. This factor plays a role in the metastasis of ovarian cancer cells; specifically, its involvement in promoting abdominal metastases appears linked to regulating epithelial-mesenchymal transition (EMT) through LSP1 signaling pathways. Thus, assessing FCGR1A levels could serve as a promising biomarker for predicting concealed abdominal metastases among patients experiencing recurrent ovarian cancer. Using tests for wound healing, Transwell invasion, and CCK-8, the functions of FCGR1A and LSP1 in ovarian cancer (OC) cell migration, invasion, and proliferation were evaluated. (Qi et al. 2024).

A central aspiration behind CRISPR/Cas-based diagnostics in breast cancer is to reduce the need for invasive procedures like tissue biopsies, which are vital to understand if the tissue abnormalities detected via mammography are cancerous. There are situations also when a biopsy fails to obtain cancerous tissue if the needle is not directed into a cancer tissue. Repeat biopsies could be expensive and even excruciating for cancer patients. Thus, CRISPR/Cas9 is envisaged as an extremely sensitive and minimally invasive tool that could assist in breast cancer diagnosis (Mintz et al. 2018). CRISPR/Cas11-based diagnostics can easily be coupled with microfluidic chip technologies to enhance the whole diagnostic process' sensitivity, speed, and portability through accurate manipulation and analysis of small volumes of fluid (Moltzahn et al. 2011).

Very notable advances have been achieved in developing microfluidic-based capillary array electrophoresis (µCAE) chips for oncogene parallel sequencing. For example, a spatial temperature gradient µCAE chip has been introduced for the detection of KRAS mutations in tissue biopsy specimens taken from colorectal cancer patients (Xu et al. 2010). The sensitivity of these microfluidic platforms can be enhanced by integrating SHERLOCK and CUT-PCR techniques, which amplify the signal of target RNA or DNA. Hence, combining CRISPR/Cas systems with microfluidic chips is likely to produce a robust lab-on-a-chip system for quick and accurate breast cancer diagnosis (Mintz et al. 2018).

5.7 CHALLENGES/LIMITATIONS

Most current tests for the diagnosis of cancer, like the computerized tomography scan, magnetic resonance imaging MRI scan, and positron emission tomography (PET) scan, are expensive, take considerable time, and lack sensitivity and resolution to detect ultrasmall tumor cells during the earlier stage of the disease (Hussain et al. 2022). Thus, there is an urgent need for a quick, inexpensive, and early cancer diagnosis and monitoring procedure besides being highly sensitive, specific, and wide-ranging to justify all the obstacles it currently faces (Sun and Chen 2024).

The lack of sensitivity and specificity of CRC screening tests, coupled with factors such as compliance on the part of the patient, issues of inequity in society, and primary barriers to accessing health services, create a complex situation that continues to impede the full realization by CRC screening. The attendant challenges of a modern screening techniques where factors such as interval cancers, overdiagnosis, missed lesions, and low sensitivity to serrated lesions beset the maximization of outcomes with their use are representative of the broader challenges encountered in achieving maximum benefit from screening due to the depressingly low sensitivity and specificity of other modalities (Tonini and Zanni 2024).

At present, there are great challenges to the diagnosis and treatment of pancreatic carcinoma (PC). The lack of noticeable symptoms in the early stages of the disease and its property of not necessarily showing certain clinical manifestations or reliable tumor markers make it a tough proposition. In fact, the imaging features of this cancer have been reported to be nonspecific. It could be stated that its pathogenesis and progression involve complex dynamics and that the same is a heterogeneous and a complex malignant tumor becalmed by a chronic genomic instability as is prominent in the progress of cancer. Gene rearrangements, however, show a considerable interpatient variability in their kinds and frequencies among the many forms of these rearrangements, within the first half forming during the very early phase of tumor development. Such variability makes diagnosis and treatment that much more difficult (Yang et al. 2023).

Late diagnoses of breast cancer is common in low and middle-income countries. In contrast, according to the available evidence, nearly 70% of patients diagnosed with breast cancer in high-income countries (Hickman, Miller, and Arcila 2023) do so at stage I or stage II, while in LMIC less than half of the patients with breast cancer are diagnosed at these early stages. The early detection of breast cancer may include two distinct approaches: early diagnosis of symptomatic patients and screening of asymptomatic persons. Both strategies vary in their costs, required infrastructures, and prerequisites for successful implementation. Thus, their efficiency will vary according to specific local needs and available resources (Barrios 2022).

The need for effective treatment to gynecological cancers, especially ovarian cancer, the most lethal gynecological malignancy, is an urgent clinical challenge. The insidious and nonspecific nature of ovarian cancer symptoms, however, is the major cause of the detrimental delay of diagnosis, resulting in such high late-stage diagnosis prevalence (Zhang et al. 2021). The complexities entailed in diagnosing and treating ovarian cancer have intensified the search for screening methodologies for early detection in asymptomatic individuals; however, evidence in randomized controlled trials has not shown that the use of follitropin-α propylamine and transvaginal ultrasound (TVS) reduces ovarian cancer mortality in asymptomatic populations (Hurwitz, Pinsky, and Trabert 2021).

The urgency is heightened further by the challenge posed by late-stage recurrent and drug-resistant forms of the disease that accentuate the need for a new generation of treatment paradigms (Li et al. 2024).This not only facilitates a more effective treatment but also improves the patients' quality of life and their chances of getting treatment for some other types of cancers

(Connal et al. 2023; Adashek, Janku, and Kurzrock 2021). The combination of tumor-derived signals with non-tumor-derived information will lead to better early-stage cancer detection based on the complementary information they can offer about the disease (Connal et al. 2023).It is widely accepted that early cancer diagnosis may lessen its costs by substituting extensive treatment with surgery, prolonged hospital stay, and continued care. On the other hand, due to high-level management for disease occurrence over such a long time duration, a later diagnosis leads to high costs (Nataren, Yamada, and Prow 2023).

5.8 CONCLUSION AND FUTURE ASPECT

Detecting cancer in its early stages results in more effective treatment and significantly higher survival rates. Nevertheless, nearly 50% of cancers are still identified at an advanced stage (Crosby et al. 2022). The survival rate for cancer patients remains low, primarily due to late-stage diagnosis and the poor prognosis of the disease (Jayanthi, Das, and Saxena 2017). Medical costs for medications, home care, clinical visits, and hospital treatment rise substantially as cancer progresses to more advanced stages (Connal et al. 2023). Conventional techniques, such as ultrasound, MRI, and biopsy, are inadequate for detecting cancer in its early stages, as they rely on the tumor's phenotypic characteristics. Cancer is a multistage condition, with its initiation and progression linked to a complex range of genetic or epigenetic changes that disrupt cellular signaling, leading to tumor development and malignancy (Jayanthi, Das, and Saxena 2017).

The cancer burden in low- and middle-income countries (LMICs) places additional strain on already fragile healthcare systems and struggling economies. Furthermore, this burden is often underrepresented due to the absence of reliable cancer registries and reporting systems. In contrast, cancer survival rates have steadily improved in high-income countries (HICs) thanks to earlier diagnoses and more advanced treatments (Connal et al. 2023). Enhancing early cancer detection could significantly boost survival rates. While recent breakthroughs in early detection have already saved lives, continued innovation and development of new detection methods remain essential. The field is advancing rapidly due to improvements in biological knowledge and the accelerating pace of technological progress (Crosby et al. 2022).

ACKNOWLEDGMENT

Prof. Aklank Jain, Department of Zoology, is thankful to the Central University of Punjab, DST-FIST, and the DST-PURSE Scheme.

REFERENCES

Acs B et al. 2020. Artificial intelligence as the next step towards precision pathology. *J Intern Med* 288(1):62–81.

Adashek JJ et al. 2021. Signed in blood: circulating tumor DNA in cancer diagnosis, treatment and screening. *Cancers (Basel)* 13(14).

Afrasanie VA et al. 2023. Clinical, pathological and molecular insights on KRAS, NRAS, BRAF, PIK3CA and TP53 mutations in metastatic colorectal cancer patients from Northeastern Romania. *Int J Mol Sci* 24(16).

Ahmad E et al. 2022. Molecular approaches in cancer. *Clin Chim Acta* 537:60–73.

Ahmed S et al. 2018. Molecular endoscopic imaging in cancer. *Dig Endosc* 30(6):719–729.

Almuhaideb A et al. 2011. 18F-FDG PET/CT imaging in oncology. *Ann Saudi Med* 31(1):3–13.

Amling CL 2001. Diagnosis and management of superficial bladder cancer. *Curr Probl Cancer* 25(4):219–278.

Baier J et al. 2020. Ultrasound imaging. *Recent Results Cancer Res* 216:509–531.

Barrios CH 2022. Global challenges in breast cancer detection and treatment. *Breast* 62(Suppl 1):S3–S6.

Bastarrika G et al. 2005. Early lung cancer detection using spiral computed tomography and positron emission tomography. *Am J Respir Crit Care Med* 171(12):1378–1383.

Baylot V et al. 2011. OGX-427 inhibits tumor progression and enhances gemcitabine chemotherapy in pancreatic cancer. *Cell Death Dis* 2(10):e221.

Benya EC 2008. Advances in computed tomography. *Pediatr Ann* 37(6):428–31.

Bhan A et al. 2017. Long noncoding RNA and cancer: a new paradigm. *Cancer Res* 77(15):3965–3981.

Bhinder B et al. 2021. Artificial intelligence in cancer research and precision medicine. *Cancer Discov* 11(4):900–915.

Birknerova N et al. 2022. Circulating cell-free DNA-based methylation pattern in saliva for early diagnosis of head and neck cancer. *Cancers* 14(19).

Bradley SH et al. 2021. Chest X-ray sensitivity and lung cancer outcomes: a retrospective observational study. *Br J Gen Pract* 71(712):e862–e868.

Bray F et al. 2024. Global cancer statistics 2022: GLOBOCAN estimates of incidence and mortality worldwide for 36 cancers in 185 countries. *CA* 74(3):229–263.

Calderon-Santiago M et al. 2015. Human sweat metabolomics for lung cancer screening. *Anal Bioanal Chem* 407(18):5381–5392.

Camerlingo R et al. 2014. The role of CD44+/CD24-/low biomarker for screening, diagnosis and monitoring of breast cancer. *Oncol Rep* 31(3):1127–1132.

Campling BG, el-Deiry WS. 2003. Clinical implications of p53 mutations in lung cancer. *Methods Mol Med* 75:53–77.

Carvalho B et al. 2025. Stool-based testing for post-polypectomy colorectal cancer surveillance safely reduces colonoscopies: the molecular stool testing for colorectal cancer surveillance study. *Gastroenterol* 168(1):121–135.e16.

Chao YL, Pecot CV 2021. Targeting epigenetics in lung cancer. *Cold Spring Harb Perspect Med* 11(6).

Chassagnon G et al. 2023. Artificial intelligence in lung cancer: current applications and perspectives. *Jpn J Radiol* 41(3):235–244.

Chen M et al. 2019a. CRISPR-Cas9 for cancer therapy: opportunities and challenges. *Cancer Lett* 447:48–55.

Chen X et al. 2019b. X-ray-activated nanosystems for theranostic applications. *Chem Soc Rev* 48(11):3073–3101.

Chen Y et al. 2015. Serum CA242, CA199, CA125, CEA, and TSGF are biomarkers for the efficacy and prognosis of cryoablation in pancreatic cancer patients. *Cell Biochem Biophys* 71(3):1287–91.

Cheng X et al. 2020. CRISPR/Cas9 for cancer treatment: technology, clinical applications and challenges. *Brief Funct Genomics* 19(3):209–214.

Choi JH, Ro JY 2023. The recent advances in molecular diagnosis of soft tissue tumors. *Int J Mol Sci* 24(6).

Chrzanowska NM et al. 2020. Use of Fluorescence In Situ Hybridization (FISH) in diagnosis and tailored therapies in solid tumors. *Molecules* 25(8).

Coleman RE 1991. Single photon emission computed tomography and positron emission tomography in cancer imaging. *Cancer* 67(4 Suppl):1261–1270.

Connal S et al. 2023. Liquid biopsies: the future of cancer early detection. *J Transl Med* 21(1):118.

Corney DC et al. 2008. Role of p53 and Rb in ovarian cancer. *Adv Exp Med Biol* 622:99–117.

Crosby D et al. 2022. Early detection of cancer. *Science* 375(6586):eaay9040.

D'Amato Figueiredo MV et al. 2022. Advances in intraoperative flow cytometry. *Int J Mol Sci* 23(21).

Daily A et al. 2022. Using tears as a non-invasive source for early detection of breast cancer. *PLoS One* 17(4):e0267676.

Darvin P et al. 2018. Immune checkpoint inhibitors: recent progress and potential biomarkers. *Exp Mol Med* 50(12):1–11.

Das S et al. 2023. Biomarkers in cancer detection, diagnosis, and prognosis. *Sensors (Basel)* 24(1).

de la Fuente-Nunez C, Lu TK 2017. CRISPR-Cas9 technology: applications in genome engineering, development of sequence-specific antimicrobials, and future prospects. *Integr Biol (Camb)* 9(2):109–122.

de Leon A et al. 2018. Ultrasound contrast agents and delivery systems in cancer detection and therapy. *Adv Cancer Res* 139:57–84.

Derks S et al. 2022. Brain metastases: the role of clinical imaging. *Br J Radiol* 95(1130):20210944.

Di Carlo E, Sorrentino C 2024. State of the art CRISPR-based strategies for cancer diagnostics and treatment. *Biomark Res* 12(1):156.

Dickinson BT et al. 2015. Molecular markers for colorectal cancer screening. *Gut* 64 9):1485–1494.

Dinu D et al. 2014. Prognostic significance of KRAS gene mutations in colorectal cancer--preliminary study. *J Med Life* 7(4):581–587.

Dumoulin E 2018. Recent advances in bronchoscopy. *F1000Res* 7.

Dunphy K et al. 2021. Clinical proteomics of biofluids in haematological malignancies. *Int J Mol Sci* 22(15).

Duran-Vinet B et al. 2021. CRISPR/Cas13-based platforms for a potential next-generation diagnosis of colorectal cancer through exosomes micro-RNA detection: a review. *Cancers* 13(18).

Ferguson JL, Turner SP 2018. Bone cancer: diagnosis and treatment principles. *Am Fam Physician* 98(4):205–213.

Georvasili VK et al. 2022. Detection of cancer cells and tumor margins during colorectal cancer surgery by intraoperative flow cytometry. *Int J Surg* 104:106717.

Gillies RJ, Schabath MB 2020. Radiomics improves cancer screening and early detection. *Cancer Epidemiol Biomarkers Prev* 29(12):2556-2567.

Gomez-Molina R et al. 2024. Utility of stool-based tests for colorectal cancer detection: a comprehensive review. *Healthcare* 12(16).

Gong S et al. 2021. CRISPR/Cas-based in vitro diagnostic platforms for cancer biomarker detection. *Anal Chem* 93(35):11899–11909.

Gu YL et al. 2015. Applicative value of serum CA19-9, CEA, CA125 and CA242 in diagnosis and prognosis for patients with pancreatic cancer treated by concurrent chemoradiotherapy. *Asian Pac J Cancer Prev* 16(15):6569–6573.

Gunelli R et al. 2021. PCA3 in prostate cancer. *Methods Mol Biol* 2292:105–113.

Hammerschmidt S, Wirtz H. 2009. Lung cancer: current diagnosis and treatment. *Dtsch Arztebl Int* 106(49):809–18; quiz 819–20.

Hanjani NA et al. 2022. Emerging role of exosomes as biomarkers in cancer treatment and diagnosis. *Crit Rev Oncol Hematol* 169:103565.

Hao C et al. 2019. Serum CEA levels in 49 different types of cancer and noncancer diseases. *Prog Mol Biol Transl Sci* 162:213–227.

Harshitha R, Arunraj DR. 2021. Real-time quantitative PCR: a tool for absolute and relative quantification. *Biochem Mol Biol Educ* 49(5):800–812.

He B et al. 2020. miRNA-based biomarkers, therapies, and resistance in Cancer. *Int J Biol Sci* 16(14):2628–2647.

Heijblom M et al. 2011. Imaging tumor vascularization for detection and diagnosis of breast cancer. *Technol Cancer Res Treat* 10(6):607–623.

Hibner G et al. 2018. Relevance of microRNAs as potential diagnostic and prognostic markers in colorectal cancer. *Int J Mol Sci* 19(10).

Hickman RA et al. 2023. Cerebrospinal fluid: a unique source of circulating tumor DNA with broad clinical applications. *Transl Oncol* 33:101688.

Hirsch B 2022. Lung cancer screening using low-dose computed tomography. *Radiol Technol* 93(3):303CT–321CT.

Hu,T et al. 2021. Next-generation sequencing technologies: An overview. *Hum Immunol* 82(11):801–811.

Hurwitz LM et al. 2021. General population screening for ovarian cancer. *Lancet* 397(10290):2128–2130.

Hussain SI et al. 2022. Modern diagnostic imaging technique applications and risk factors in the medical field: a review. *Biomed Res Int* 2022:5164970.

Jayanthi V et al. 2017. Recent advances in biosensor development for the detection of cancer biomarkers. *Biosens Bioelectron* 91:15–23.

Jeong SH, Ku JH. 2022. Urinary markers for bladder cancer diagnosis and monitoring. *Front Cell Dev Biol* 10:892067.

Jiang H et al. 2022a. Validation of a highly sensitive Sanger sequencing in detecting EGFR mutations from circulating tumor DNA in patients with lung cancers. *Clin Chim Acta* 536:98–103.

Jiang W et al. 2022b. Application of deep learning in lung cancer imaging diagnosis. *J Healthc Eng* 2022:6107940.

Kaczor-Urbanowicz KE et al. 2019. Clinical validity of saliva and novel technology for cancer detection. *Biochim Biophys Acta Rev Cancer* 1872(1):49–59.

Kalantari S et al. 2015. Human urine proteomics: analytical techniques and clinical applications in renal diseases. *Int J Proteomics* 2015:782798.

Kamps R et al. 2017. Next–generation sequencing in oncology: genetic diagnosis, risk prediction and cancer classification. *Int J Mol Sci* 18(2).

Kato TA 2023. FISH with whole chromosome painting probes. *Methods Mol Biol* 2519:99–104.

Khehra N et al. 2024. *Polymerase Chain Reaction (PCR)*. Treasure Island, FL: StatPearls.

Khijmatgar S et al. 2024. Salivary biomarkers for early detection of oral squamous cell carcinoma (OSCC) and head/neck squamous cell carcinoma (HNSCC): a systematic review and network meta-analysis. *Jpn Dent Sci Rev* 60:32–39.

Khurshid Z et al. 2018. Role of salivary biomarkers in oral cancer detection. *Adv Clin Chem* 86:23–70.

Kwong GA et al. 2021. Synthetic biomarkers: a twenty-first century path to early cancer detection. *Nat Rev Cancer* 21(10):655–668.

Lawrence R et al. 2023. Circulating tumour cells for early detection of clinically relevant cancer. *Nat Rev Clin Oncol* 20(7):487–500.

Lee SH et al. 2016. Sanger sequencing for BRCA1 c.68_69del, BRCA1 c.5266dup and BRCA2 c.5946del mutation screen on pap smear cytology samples. *Int J Mol Sci* 17(2):229.

Leemans M et al. 2023. Screening of breast cancer from sweat samples analyzed by 2-dimensional gas chromatography-mass spectrometry: a preliminary study. *Cancers* 15(11).

Li G et al. 2022. Serum markers CA125, CA153, and CEA along with inflammatory cytokines in the early detection of lung cancer in high-risk populations. *Biomed Res Int* 2022:1394042.

Li Y et al. 2024. Advancements in ovarian cancer immunodiagnostics and therapeutics via phage display technology. *Front Immunol* 15:1402862.

Liu Y et al. 2023. Applications of artificial intelligence in breast pathology. *Arch Pathol Lab Med* 147(9):1003–1013.

Lozar T et al. 2019. The biology and clinical potential of circulating tumor cells. *Radiol Oncol* 53(2):131–147.

Luo G. et al. 2021. Roles of CA19-9 in pancreatic cancer: biomarker, predictor and promoter. *Biochim Biophys Acta Rev Cancer* 1875(2):188409.

Malapelle U et al. 2012. Sanger sequencing in routine KRAS testing: a review of 1720 cases from a pathologist's perspective. *J Clin Pathol* 65(10):940–944.

Margoni A et al. 2024. CA-125:CA72-4 ratio - towards a promising cost-effective tool in ovarian cancer diagnosis and monitoring of post-menopausal women under hormone treatment. *J Ovarian Res* 17(1):164.

Marrugo-Ramirez J et al. 2018. Blood-based cancer biomarkers in liquid biopsy: a promising non-invasive alternative to tissue biopsy. *Int J Mol Sci* 19(10).

Martin-Lopez JE et al 2014. Comparison of the accuracy of CT colonography and colonoscopy in the diagnosis of colorectal cancer. *Colorectal Dis* 16(3):O82–O89.

Marvalim C et al. 2023. Role of p53 in breast cancer progression: an insight into p53 targeted therapy. *Theranostics* 13(4):1421–1442.

McKinnon KM 2018. Flow cytometry: an overview. *Curr Protoc Immunol* 120:5 1 11.

Mena E et al. 2021. Novel PET imaging methods for prostate cancer. *World J Urol* 39 3):687–699.

Min L et al. 2019. Evaluation of circulating small extracellular vesicles derived miRNAs as biomarkers of early colon cancer: a comparison with plasma total miRNAs. *J Extracell Vesicles* 8(1):1643670.

Mintz RL et al. 2018. CRISPR technology for breast cancer: diagnostics, modeling, and therapy. *Adv Biosyst* 2(11).

Mishra HK 2023. Clinical applications of flow cytometry in cancer immunotherapies: from diagnosis to treatments. *Methods Mol Biol* 2593:93–112.

Mishra S et al. 2016. Recent advances in salivary cancer diagnostics enabled by biosensors and bioelectronics. *Biosens Bioelectron* 81:181–197.

Mittal S, Rajala MS. 2020. Heat shock proteins as biomarkers of lung cancer. *Cancer Biol Ther* 21(6):477–485.

Moltzahn F et al. 2011. Microfluidic-based multiplex qRT-PCR identifies diagnostic and prognostic microRNA signatures in the sera of prostate cancer patients. *Cancer Res* 71(2):550–560.

Nataren N et al. 2023. Molecular skin cancer diagnosis: promise and limitations. *J Mol Diagn* 25(1):17–35.

Nguyen TTH et al. 2020. Salivary biomarkers in oral squamous cell carcinoma. *J Korean Assoc Oral Maxillofac Surg* 46(5):301–312.

Ning B et al. 2014. Toxicogenomics and cancer susceptibility: advances with next-generation sequencing. *J Environ Sci Health C Environ Carcinog Ecotoxicol Rev* 32(2):121–158.

Oh TJ et al. 2023. Evaluation of sensitive urine DNA-Based PENK methylation test for detecting bladder cancer in patients with hematuria. *J Mol Diagn* 25(9):646–654.

Ordulu Z, Nardi V. 2022. Molecular detection of oncogenic gene rearrangements. *Clin Lab Med* 42(3):435–449.

Ou X et al. 2021. Recent development in X-Ray imaging technology: future and challenges. *Research (Wash D C)* 2021:9892152.

Park HS et al. 2017. Detection of circulating tumor cells in breast cancer patients using cytokeratin-19 real-time RT-PCR. *Yonsei Med J* 58(1):19–26.

Pereira L et al. 2021. Biological effects induced by doses of mammographic screening. *Phys Med* 87:90–98.

Pessoa LS et al. 2020. ctDNA as a cancer biomarker: a broad overview. *Crit Rev Oncol Hematol* 155:103109.

Pfeiffer D et al. 2020. Advanced X-ray imaging technology. *Recent Results Cancer Res* 216:3–30.

Qi Y et al. 2024. CRISPR/Cas9-based genome-wide screening for metastasis ability identifies FCGR1A regulating the metastatic process of ovarian cancer by targeting LSP1. *J Cancer Res Clin Oncol* 150(6):306.

Rack B et al. 2016. CA27.29 is a tumour marker for risk evaluation and therapy monitoring in primary breast cancer patients. *Tumour Biol* 37(10):13769–13775.

Rahimi S et al. 2024. CRISPR-Cas target recognition for sensing viral and cancer biomarkers. *Nucleic Acids Res* 52(17):10040–10067.

Rahmati Y et al. 2021. CiRS-7/CDR1as; an oncogenic circular RNA as a potential cancer biomarker. *Pathol Res Pract* 227:153639.

Sabour L et al. 2017. Clinical applications of next-generation sequencing in cancer diagnosis. *Pathol Oncol Res* 23(2):225–234.

Saft L 2023. The role of flow cytometry in the classification of myeloid disorders. *Pathologie* 44(Suppl 3):164–175.

Sahin MC, Sanli S 2023. Vitamin-based radiopharmaceuticals for tumor imaging. *Med Oncol* 40(6):165.

Sali L et al. 2017. CT colonography: role in FOBT-based screening programs for colorectal cancer. *Clin J Gastroenterol* 10(4):312–319.

Sandbank J et al. 2022. Validation and real-world clinical application of an artificial intelligence algorithm for breast cancer detection in biopsies. *NPJ Breast Cancer* 8(1):129.

Sarhadi VK, Armengol G. 2022. Molecular biomarkers in cancer. *Biomolecules* 12(8).

Schiffman JD et al. 2015. Early detection of cancer: past, present, and future. *Am Soc Clin Oncol Educ Book*:57–65.

Schmid S et al. 2022. How to read a next-generation sequencing report-what oncologists need to know. *ESMO Open* 7(5):100570.

Selva-O'Callaghan A et al. 2019. PET scan: nuclear medicine imaging in myositis. *Curr Rheumatol Rep* 21(11):64.

Serkova NJ et al. 2021. Preclinical applications of multi-platform imaging in animal models of cancer. *Cancer Res* 81(5):1189–1200.

Shu T et al. 2017. Down-regulation of HECTD3 by HER2 inhibition makes serous ovarian cancer cells sensitive to platinum treatment. *Cancer Lett* 411:65–73.

Smith RC, McCarthy S. 1992. Physics of magnetic resonance. *J Reprod Med* 37(1):19–26.

Stafford RJ 2020. The physics of magnetic resonance imaging safety. *Magn Reson Imaging Clin N Am* 28 4):517–536.

Sun J et al. 2023. Identification of novel protein biomarkers and drug targets for colorectal cancer by integrating human plasma proteome with genome. *Genome Med* 15(1):75.

Sun S, Chen J. 2024. Recent advances in hydrogel-based biosensors for cancer detection. *ACS Appl Mater Interfaces* 16(36):46988–47002.

Sung H et al. 2021. Global Cancer Statistics 2020: GLOBOCAN Estimates of Incidence and Mortality Worldwide for 36 Cancers in 185 Countries. *CA Cancer J Clin* 71(3):209–249.

Tonini V, Zanni M 2024. Why is early detection of colon cancer still not possible in 2023? *World J Gastroenterol* 30(3):211–224.

Tsou JH, Leng Q, Jiang F. 2020. A CRISPR test for rapidly and sensitively detecting circulating EGFR mutations. *Diagnostics* 10(2):114.

Tripathi P et al. 2017. Clinical value of MRI-detected extramural venous invasion in rectal cancer. *J Dig Dis* 18(1):2–12.

Vleugels JL et al. 2016. Colorectal cancer screening by colonoscopy: putting it into perspective. *Dig Endosc* 28(3):250–9.

Wang X, Yang M 2021. The application of ultrasound image in cancer diagnosis. *J Healthc Eng* 2021:8619251.

Wood SL et al. 2013. Proteomic studies of urinary biomarkers for prostate, bladder and kidney cancers. *Nat Rev Urol* 10(4):206–18.

Wu L, Qu X 2015. Cancer biomarker detection: recent achievements and challenges. *Chem Soc Rev* 44(10):2963–97.

Wu T et al. 2020. Prognostic values of CEA, CA19-9, and CA72-4 in patients with stages I-III colorectal cancer. *Int J Clin Exp Pathol* 13(7):1608–1614.

Wu Y et al. 2015. Epigenetics in breast and prostate cancer. *Methods Mol Biol* 1238:425–66.

Xiao Z, Pure E. 2021. Imaging of T-cell Responses in the Context of Cancer Immunotherapy. *Cancer Immunol Res* 9(5):490-502.

Xu F, Wang Y 2020. [Current management and future prospect of HER-2 mutant non-small cell lung cancer]. *Zhonghua Zhong Liu Za Zhi* 42(10):829–837.

Xu ZR et al. 2010. A miniaturized spatial temperature gradient capillary electrophoresis system with radiative heating and automated sample introduction for DNA mutation detection. *Electrophoresis* 31(18):3137–43.

Yan YH et al. 2021. Confirming putative variants at </= 5% allele frequency using allele enrichment and Sanger sequencing. *Sci Rep* 11(1):11640.

Yang H et al. 2023. Progress on diagnostic and prognostic markers of pancreatic cancer. *Oncol Res* 31(2):83–99.

Yang L et al. 2020. Long non-coding RNA BCYRN1 exerts an oncogenic role in colorectal cancer by regulating the miR-204-3p/KRAS axis. *Cancer Cell Int* 20:453.

Yang SL et al. 2016. Expression and functional role of long non-coding RNA AFAP1-AS1 in ovarian cancer. *Eur Rev Med Pharmacol Sci* 20(24):5107–5112.

Yin B et al. 2017. Association between human papillomavirus and prostate cancer: a meta-analysis. *Oncol Lett* 14(2):1855–1865.

Yu D et al. 2022. Exosomes as a new frontier of cancer liquid biopsy. *Mol Cancer* 21 (1):56.

Zhang G et al. 2022. Ultrasound molecular imaging and its applications in cancer diagnosis and therapy. *ACS Sens* 7(10):2857–2864.

Zhang M et al. 2021. Roles of CA125 in diagnosis, prediction, and oncogenesis of ovarian cancer. *Biochim Biophys Acta Rev Cancer* 1875(2):188503.

Zhang Y 2020. Methylated PTGER4 is better than CA125, CEA, Cyfra211 and NSE as a therapeutic response assessment marker in stage IV lung cancer. *Oncol Lett* 19(4):3229–3238.

Zhou Y, Liu Z. 2023. Saliva biomarkers in oral disease. *Clin Chim Acta* 548:117503.

Zhu X et al. 2024. Pancreatic cancer: an exocrine tumor with endocrine characteristics. *Ann Surg* 280(6):e17–e25.

6

Cytogenetic Diagnostic Testing in Cancer

Sweety Mehra, Priyanka Bhardwaj, Madhu Sharma, Muskan Budhwar,
Anupriya Rana, and Mani Chopra

6.1 INTRODUCTION

Cancer cytogenetics constitutes a pivotal convergence of genetics and oncology, concentrating on the examination of cancer-linked chromosomal anomalies (Ribeiro et al., 2019; Balciuniene et al., 2024). The discovery of the Philadelphia chromosome in chronic myeloid leukemia (CML) signaled the start of a new era in cancer genetics (Koretzky, 2007). Cytogenetic testing for cancer diagnosis includes various methodologies, such as conventional karyotyping, molecular cytogenetic techniques like fluorescence in situ hybridization (FISH), and advanced genomic sequencing technologies (Gonzales et al., 2016; Ozkan and Lacerda, 2020). These methods offer critical insights into the structural and numerical chromosomal modifications that define various cancer types, facilitating diagnosis, prognosis, and treatment strategies (Kou et al., 2020). The incorporation of cytogenetic testing into clinical practice has been revolutionary, enabling the identification of specific genetic markers that can guide targeted therapies and personalized treatment approaches. Identification of specific chromosomal rearrangements can inform the choice of suitable therapeutic agents, enhancing patient outcomes. Nonetheless, despite these advancements, obstacles persist in the extensive adoption of cytogenetic testing owing to factors such as expense, accessibility, and the intricacy of result interpretation (Findley et al., 2023). This chapter seeks to examine the present state of cancer cytogenetics testing, outlining its methodologies, clinical ramifications through case studies, and the obstacles encountered in its execution. Additionally, it will address prospective avenues for research and practice in this swiftly advancing domain, emphasizing the continual necessity for enhanced incorporation of cytogenetic discoveries into standard oncology treatment. This work aims to highlight the crucial importance of cancer cytogenetics in improving diagnostic precision and refining treatment strategies in oncology by integrating recent advancements and addressing current deficiencies.

6.2 CANCER CYTOGENETICS

Cancer cells frequently exhibit changes in their chromosomes, including structural abnormalities, numeric abnormalities (such as aneuploidy), and gene mutations (Fröhling and Döhner, 2008). These alterations may contribute to carcinogenesis (the development of cancer) by activating oncogenes (genes that promote cell growth) or inactivating tumor suppressor genes (genes that inhibit unchecked cell proliferation such as TP53 (p53) or RB). One significant type of structural abnormality is translocations, rearrangements where parts of one chromosome are transferred to another chromosome, frequently resulting in fusion genes that drive cancer (Panagopoulos and Heim, 2022). A well-known example is the Philadelphia chromosome (t(9;22)), which is associated with Chronic Myelogenous Leukemia (CML). This translocation fuses the BCR gene on chromosome 22 with the ABL gene on chromosome 9, producing a constitutively active tyrosine kinase that promotes uncontrolled cell division (Sampaio et al., 2021). Another example is Burkitt Lymphoma (t(8;14)), where the MYC oncogene on chromosome 8 fuses with the immunoglobulin heavy chain gene on chromosome 14, leading to MYC overexpression and rapid cell growth (Yan et al., 2007).

There are other known structural alterations such as inversions, deletion, and duplications. Inversion, where a segment of a chromosome is reversed end to end, also contributes to cancer; for instance, inv(16) in acute myelomonocytic leukemia (AMML) results in the fusion of the CBFβ and MYH11 genes (Bain and Béné, 2019). Deletions involve the loss of sections of chromosomes, which can lead to the loss of tumor suppressor genes or other critical genetic material. These chromosomal deletions result in the removal of intergenic regions located between two adjacent genes, facilitating the formation of fusion genes by bringing together two genes that are transcribed in the same direction. An example of a significant gene fusion in prostate cancer is the TMPRSS2–ERG fusion, which occurs through an intron deletion between the TMPRSS2 gene and the ERG gene located on chromosome 21q22.2-3 (Taniue and Akimitsu, 2021). The TMPRSS2 gene encodes a prostate-specific androgen-regulated protein, while ERG is a member of the ETS family of transcription factors, known for its oncogenic potential. The TMPRSS2-ERG fusion has been associated

DOI: 10.1201/9781003542162-6

with a higher tumor stage, an increased risk of disease progression, and a greater likelihood of bone metastasis. This fusion not only alters normal gene regulation but also enhances the aggressiveness of prostate cancer, making it a critical factor in the disease's pathology. Duplications occur when segments of chromosomes are duplicated, leading to overexpression of certain genes, including oncogenes; for example, HER2 gene (located on chromosome 17) amplification in breast cancer results in overexpression of the HER2 receptor, promoting tumor growth (Iqbal and Iqbal, 2014).

Numerical abnormalities, known as aneuploidy, refer to gains or losses of entire chromosomes and are prevalent in many cancers. Aneuploidy can manifest as trisomy (three copies of a chromosome), such as trisomy 21, which is associated with an increased risk of leukemia (Baruchel et al., 2023). Monosomy involves the loss of one copy of a chromosome; monosomy 7 is often observed in acute myelogenous leukemia (AML) (Eldfors et al., 2024). Polyploidy, characterized by having more than two sets of chromosomes, is less common but may occur in some tumors. Chromosomal instability is another feature seen in certain cancers like colorectal and lung cancer, where cells exhibit multiple abnormal chromosome numbers. Overall, these chromosomal abnormalities play critical roles in cancer development by disrupting normal cellular functions and contributing to tumorigenesis through various mechanisms.

In addition to chromosomal abnormalities, gene mutations are critical in cancer development, as they can activate oncogenes or inactivate tumor suppressor genes, both of which lead to unregulated cell growth. Oncogene mutations, often referred to as gain-of-function mutations, result in the activation of genes that drive cancer. Notable examples include mutations in the RAS family, which are prevalent in various cancers such as pancreatic, colorectal, and lung cancers. These mutations lead to the constitutive activation of the RAS protein, a key regulator of cell signaling pathways that promote cell proliferation and survival (Molina and Adjei, 2006). Another significant oncogene is c-MYC; amplification or mutations in the MYC promoter region are associated with Burkitt lymphoma (t(8;14)) (Yan et al., 2007), small cell lung cancer, and breast cancer. HER2 (ERBB2) amplification in breast cancer results in overexpression of the HER2 receptor protein, which promotes increased cell proliferation and is targeted by therapies like trastuzumab (Herceptin). Additionally, mutations in the epidermal growth factor receptor (EGFR) are common in non-small cell lung cancer (NSCLC).

On the other hand, tumor suppressor gene mutations are classified as loss-of-function mutations that allow cells to escape normal growth regulation. The TP53 gene is the most commonly mutated gene across human cancers; its mutations lead to a loss of a critical tumor suppressor that normally induces apoptosis in cells with damaged DNA. This mutation is prevalent in various cancers including lung, colon, breast, and ovarian cancer (Chen et al., 2022). Similarly, mutations in the RB1 gene result in the loss of the retinoblastoma protein, which regulates the cell cycle and is associated with retinoblastoma as well as other cancers like osteosarcoma and small cell lung cancer. BRCA1 and BRCA2 mutations impair DNA repair mechanisms and predispose individuals to breast and ovarian cancers due to accumulated DNA damage (Mylavarapu et al., 2018). APC mutations are frequently observed in colorectal cancer and lead to activation of the Wnt signaling pathway that regulates cell growth and division. Lastly, PTEN mutations affect cell cycle regulation and are linked to various cancers including endometrial, breast, and prostate cancers (Bassi et al., 2021). Overall, these genetic alterations play crucial roles in cancer biology by disrupting normal cellular functions and contributing to tumorigenesis through various mechanisms.

Moreover, epigenetic dysregulation, including DNA methylation defects and abnormal post-translational modification processes, is commonly associated with all cancer types. These alterations have reversible effects on gene silencing and activation through epigenetic enzymes and related proteins. Abnormal DNA methylation of tumor suppressor genes can silence their expression, leading to loss of function. DNA methylation regulates gene expression, with hyper- and hypomethylation processes being independent in cancer genomes and tumor progression. Hypermethylated CpG islands in tumors are often located in promoter regions, linked to various carcinogenesis, including breast, liver, prostate, and small-cell bladder cancer (Yu et al., 2024).

Histone modifications also play a crucial role in regulating chromatin structure and gene expression. Changes such as acetylation and methylation of histones can either promote or repress gene activity by altering the accessibility of DNA to transcriptional machinery. In cancer cells, there is often a loss of acetylation marks due to increased activity of histone deacetylases (HDACs), which has been linked to unregulated gene expression and tumor progression. For example, upregulation of HDAC3 leads to colon cancer (Kanwal and Gupta, 2011).

Cancer cytogenetics reveals a wide array of chromosomal abnormalities and mutations that drive cancer development and progression. These changes can be structural or numerical, affecting key genes involved in cell regulation, growth, and survival. Identifying these genetic changes is essential for diagnosis, prognosis, and the development of targeted treatments.

6.3 CYTOGENETICS DIAGNOSTIC TESTING (CDT) IN CANCER

Modern oncology relies heavily on cytogenetic diagnostic testing (CDT), which examines chromosomal abnormalities that can reveal the type and presence of cancers. CDT in cancer involves conventional, molecular, and advanced sequencing techniques.

6.3.1 Conventional Cytogenetics in Cancer Diagnosis

Conventional cytogenetics is important in diagnosing and prognosing various cancers as it provides vital insights into chromosomal abnormalities that are often linked with cancer development (Ribeiro et al., 2019). Karyotyping and chromosome banding techniques allow the detection of quantitative and structural chromosomal alterations, which are crucial for classifying multiple kinds of cancer, particularly haematological malignancies such as leukemia and lymphoma (Wan, 2014).

a) Band-specific karyotyping and its role in cancer diagnosis

Karyotyping is an analytical method that delivers essential details regarding chromosomal number and structure by analyzing an individual's entire chromosome set (Levy and Wapner, 2018). Cell samples are obtained from bone marrow, blood, or amniotic fluid and subsequently cultured to encourage cell division. Colchicine arrests the cells in the metaphase stage when the chromosomes are compact. The cells are then processed hypotonically to expand the nuclei, further fixed and then stained with Giemsa. After the chromosomes' distinctive banding patterns are revealed by staining, they are photographed and arranged into a karyotype, a graphical representation that groups chromosomes into pairs according to size and shape (Zhao et al., 2001).

It has proven crucial in identifying particular genetic changes connected to various cancers. For example, karyotyping can identify the Philadelphia chromosome, a hallmark of chronic myeloid leukemia (CML) that is linked to a poor prognosis if treatment is not received (Kang et al., 2016). Furthermore, karyotyping is used to help with diagnosis and treatment choices in lymphomas like Burkitt lymphoma by identifying the t(8;14) translocation involving the MYC gene. Additionally, it is used to diagnose solid tumors and acute lymphoblastic leukemia (ALL), where chromosomal alterations in terms of number and structure can reveal the course of the disease or the effectiveness of treatment. Karyotyping is a vital tool in oncology because it allows for the visualization of these chromosomal changes, which improves diagnostic precision and helps guide treatment plans specific to the genetic makeup of the cancer (Wan, 2017).

b) Limitations of karyotyping

Despite being a vital method in cytogenetics for identifying chromosomal abnormalities, karyotyping has several significant drawbacks. Its incapacity to identify minute chromosomal changes, like tiny deletions or duplications, is a major disadvantage because of its resolution limit of roughly 5-10 megabases. This implies that minor genetic alterations that may have important clinical ramifications might go unrecognized. Moreover, karyotyping depends on identifying cells in the metaphase stage, which requires cell division and may make it difficult to collect sufficient samples for analysis. Testing for specific tissue types or conditions, such as solid tumors or samples with low mitotic indices, may become more challenging due to the requirement for actively dividing cells (Bridge, 2008).

6.3.2 Molecular Cancer Cytogenetics Testing

Molecular cytogenetics testing combines cytogenetic analysis and molecular biology to identify chromosomal abnormalities and holds a significant role in the diagnosis and treatment of cancer (Nowakowska and Bocian, 2004). This field relies heavily on key techniques like comparative genomic hybridization (CGH) and fluorescence in situ hybridization (FISH).

6.3.2.1 Comparative Genomic Hybridization (CGH)

Comparative genomic hybridization (CGH) is a molecular technique that evaluates the cancer-associated chromosomal copy number variations with a comprehensive picture of chromosomal gains and losses in the genome (Houldsworth and Chaganti, 1994). CGH is a reasonably quick screening method that can identify particular chromosomal areas involved in the development or progression of tumors (Weiss et al., 2003). In contrast to conventional karyotyping, CGH offers a whole genome view with greater resolution and has the potential to identify submicroscopic alterations that are essential for comprehending tumor biology. This technology helps to customize more effective, targeted therapies based on the precise genetic changes within a tumor and has proven efficient in identifying genetic alterations in a variety of cancers, including lung, prostate, and breast cancers (Krzyszczyk et al., 2018).

a) Process of the CGH

The procedure involves the isolation of genomic DNA from normal and tumor cells. Different fluorescent dyes are used to label these samples; normally, Cy3 is used for normal DNA (green) and Cy5 is used for tumor DNA (red). Further, the tagged DNAs are combined and hybridized to produce typical human metaphase chromosomes. The two DNA samples compete with one another to bind to their respective chromosomal loci during hybridization. A greater ratio of green to red denotes a gain in the tumor DNA, whereas a lower ratio implies a loss. The resulting fluorescence intensity ratios are then measured (Weiss et al., 1999). Specialized software like CGHPRO, CGH-Explorer, and CGH-Fusion facilitates this analysis by processing the fluorescence data to produce a thorough profile of chromosomal gains and losses throughout the genome, which helps to clarify the genetic changes linked to cancer (Lingjaerde et al., 2005). In this way, a comparative genomic analysis can be performed, which could be beneficial in evaluating the exact chromosomal alterations.

b) Limitations of CGH

Several restrictions may affect the efficiency of comparative genomic hybridization (CGH) in cancer research and diagnosis. Its relatively low resolution, which usually detects alterations at a scale of 5–10 megabases (Mb), offers a serious limitation as it may overlook smaller genomic alterations that could have clinical significance (Lichter et al., 2000). Furthermore, for CGH to be accurately analyzed, the sample must contain at least 50% aberrant cells, which presents difficulties in heterogeneous tumors where the percentage of cancerous cells may be lower. Additionally, CGH mainly detects quantitative changes like gains or losses in DNA and ignores balanced chromosomal rearrangements like translocations, which are also significant in cancer (Dong et al., 2018). Moreover, complex statistical methods for CGH analysis can cause noise and non-Gaussian distributions to overestimate or underestimate genomic alterations, presenting difficulties in interpreting results and questioning the validity of detected aberrations. Lastly, the selection of reference DNA may affect the precision of CGH results, adding variability if the reference does not accurately reflect typical genomic content (Redon and Carter, 2009). These drawbacks highlight the need for better techniques, like array CGH, which has better detection capabilities and higher resolution but still has problems with clinical application and data interpretation.

6.3.2.2 Fluorescence in Situ Hybridization (FISH)

The molecular cytogenetic method known as fluorescence in situ hybridization (FISH) is frequently used in cancer diagnosis to identify and localize particular genetic abnormalities within cells (Shakoori, 2017). Fluorescently labeled DNA probes attach to specific chromosomal sequences and detect cancer-associated gene alterations like inversions, deletions, duplications, and translocations under a fluorescent microscope (Cui et al., 2016).

a) Process of FISH

Several crucial steps are involved in the fluorescence in situ hybridization (FISH) process to identify specific genetic abnormalities linked to cancer. Firstly, a biological sample (either blood or tissue) is collected from the patient. The samples are processed in the lab, and particular fluorescently labeled DNA probes are made to attach to specific gene sequences on the relevant chromosomes. After that, the sample is exposed to these probes, which enable them to hybridize with complementary DNA (cDNA) sequences. Following hybridization, the samples are visualized under a fluorescence microscope to determine the presence and location of genetic changes based on the fluorescence produced (O'Connor, 2008).

b) Limitations

Although fluorescence in situ hybridization (FISH) is a useful method for diagnosing cancer, several loopholes may limit its applicability. One major drawback is that FISH is a targeted biotechnique, which means that only a certain number of probes can be analyzed in one go, usually only two or three colors, which restricts the technique from analyzing a large amount of genetic information (So et al., 2008). Furthermore, cell culture is necessary for metaphase FISH to synchronize cells at the metaphase stage, which is a time-consuming and labor-intensive procedure (Doležel et al., 2021). Moreover, FISH lacks the ability to detect important positional uniparental disomy or atypical rearrangements regarding chromosomal abnormalities, which could present difficulties in the diagnosis (Lindstrand et al., 2019). Additionally, manual counting of fluorescence signals can introduce variability; thus, the technique requires skilled analysts to interpret the results accurately. Lastly, this technique is not cost-effective and may not be widely used in clinical practice compared to other techniques like immunohistochemistry (IHC). These drawbacks emphasize the necessity of using complementary methods and exercising caution when applying FISH to cancer diagnosis.

6.3.3 Sequencing in Cancer Cytogenetics

Sequencing techniques have transformed cancer cytogenetics, offering unparalleled insights into the genetic and chromosomal modifications that distinguish various cancers. These advancements allowed researchers to detect mutations, structural variations, and epigenetic alterations contributing to cancer development, progression, and metastasis. The incorporation of next-generation sequencing (NGS) technologies, alongside other molecular methodologies, has markedly improved the understanding of cancer biology and enabled the formulation of personalized treatment approaches (LeBlanc and Marra, 2015).

6.3.3.1 Next Generation Sequencing (NGS)

NGS has become a key technology in cancer genomics owing to its rapid and economical analysis of large fluxes of genetic data. NGS enables the simultaneous sequencing of several genes or even entire genomes, in contrast to conventional sequencing techniques like Sanger sequencing, which can only evaluate one gene at a time (Qin, 2019). Finding new mutations and comprehending the intricate genetic makeup of tumors are two applications that greatly benefit from this high-throughput capability. Whole-genome sequencing (WGS), for example, can detect structural variations throughout the entire genome, copy number variations (CNVs), insertions/deletions (indels), and single nucleotide variants (SNVs). This comprehensive approach has been useful in characterizing cancers such as breast cancer, where specific gene mutations in BRCA1 and BRCA2 have been linked to hereditary breast and ovarian cancer syndromes (Zhang et al., 2023).

a) Process of NGS

Next-generation sequencing (NGS) encompasses several essential steps for analyzing the genetic nature of tumors. The procedure begins with the acquisition of biological tumor samples, which may be procured via surgical resection, biopsy, or liquid biopsy for circulating tumor DNA (Lin et al., 2021). Following sample collection, high-quality DNA or RNA is extracted, which frequently necessitates techniques such as laser capture microdissection to separate pure tumor cells from normal tissue. After extraction, the next phase is library preparation, during which nucleic acids are fragmented and specific adapters are ligated to both termini of the fragments, facilitating subsequent amplification and sequencing. The prepared library is subsequently loaded onto a next-generation sequencing (NGS) platform, such as those created by Illumina or Thermo Fisher Scientific, where extensive parallel sequencing takes place, producing substantial data rapidly. The data is analyzed with bioinformatics tools to align sequenced reads to a reference genome and identify genetic variants, such as single nucleotide variants (SNVs), insertions/deletions (indels), and structural variants in cancer. The findings can facilitate clinical decision-making by detecting relevant mutations that may be conveyed to targeted treatments.

b) Limitations

Next-generation sequencing (NGS) has various limitations that may impact clinical applicability in identifying a particular cancer. A significant challenge is the heterogeneity of tumor samples, as solid tumors frequently comprise a mixture of malignant and normal cells, which can dilute the concentration of tumor-derived DNA and impede the identification of low-frequency mutations. Moreover, preservation techniques such as formalin fixation can compromise sample quality, resulting in DNA degradation. Also, data interpretation is difficult due to the large amount of information generated, making it difficult to distinguish clinically relevant mutations from benign variants, especially since many mutations still need to be recognized. Next-generation sequencing may overlook specific genomic alterations, including structural variants and gene fusions unless specially engineered to detect them. Ultimately, regulatory obstacles hinder the clinical implementation of NGS results, as numerous targeted therapies are tissue-specific, thereby restricting their applicability based on detected mutations. These challenges highlight the necessity for meticulous evaluation when integrating NGS into clinical practice (Cheng et al., 2023).

6.3.3.2 Cancer Personalized Profiling by Deep Sequencing (CAPP-Seq)

Cancer personalized profiling by deep sequencing (CAPP-Seq) is a next-generation sequencing (NGS) technique aimed at measuring circulating tumor DNA (ctDNA) in cancer patients (Noguchi et al., 2020). CAPP-Seq facilitates the identification and surveillance of genetic modifications linked to multiple cancers via a quick blood test, offering a non-invasive substitute for conventional tumor biopsies (Newman et al., 2014).

CAPP-Seq is distinguished by its exceptional sensitivity, being able to detect one mutant DNA molecule among 10,000 normal DNA molecules and identifying multiple classes of genomic alterations, including single nucleotide variants (SNVs), insertions/deletions (indels), copy number variations (CNVs), and rearrangements (Kurtz et al., 2021). This allows clinicians to monitor tumor progression over time by examining circulating tumor DNA (ctDNA) from various blood samples collected at different treatment phases. The method has been effectively utilized across multiple cancer types, such as lung cancer, lymphoma, and gynecological cancers, illustrating its efficacy in monitoring treatment responses and identifying resistance mutations.

a) Process of CAPP-Seq

Cancer personalized profiling by deep sequencing (CAPP-Seq) is an advanced technique that facilitates non-invasive observation of tumor dynamics. The procedure starts with extracting ctDNA from a blood sample and then designing a "selector" that uses freely accessible sequencing data to target recurrent mutations associated with specific cancer types. The regions of interest in the ctDNA are bound by biotinylated DNA oligonucleotides, which make up this selector. Selector probes enrich the ctDNA library by attaching to these target regions during hybridization capture, which enables selective amplification (Newman et al., 2014). Next-generation sequencing (NGS) is then performed on the enriched ctDNA to detect and measure the mutations. With some sensitivities, this method enables the detection of extremely low levels of ctDNA. Clinicians can effectively monitor tumor evolution and treatment response by applying CAPP-Seq at multiple time points. Without requiring invasive biopsies, the incorporation of sophisticated bioinformatics tools facilitates the analysis of the sequencing data and offers insights into the genetic makeup of tumors.

b) Limitations

The clinical utility of CAPP-Seq is impacted by several limitations. One of the main issues is the sensitivity of detecting circulating tumor DNA (ctDNA), which can be reduced at low ctDNA levels, especially below a threshold of about 0.01% fractional abundance (Dang and Park, 2022). This restriction makes it more difficult to identify any remaining disease and track the tumor's dynamics while undergoing treatment, particularly when stable tumor growth may cause a decrease in ctDNA release. Furthermore, the method is vulnerable to errors that arise during the polymerase chain reaction (PCR) amplification or sequencing procedures, sample cross-contamination, and possible allelic bias introduced by the reaction reagents. Even though these mistakes are usually small, they can still affect how accurately mutations are detected. Additionally, some genomic changes, like gene fusions, may be difficult for CAPP-Seq to detect, which could result in an underestimation of tumor burden. Lastly, CAPP-Seq measures the amount of ctDNA present but does not reveal the anatomical location or histological features of the tumor, which restricts its ability to evaluate the total tumor burden without the use of additional imaging techniques. These drawbacks emphasize the need for cautious thought when integrating CAPP-Seq into clinical practice and emphasize its function as an additional diagnostic tool to be used in conjunction with other approaches.

6.4 CLINICAL IMPLICATIONS

Cytogenetic testing has emerged as an invaluable tool in oncology, profoundly influencing cancer diagnostics and therapeutic approaches. Despite some limitations, like the need for new tissue samples and the difficulties in deciphering intricate genetic information, developments in cytogenetic techniques are transforming the way cancer is treated (Table 6.1). The advancement of technologies such as fluorescence in situ hybridization (FISH) and next-generation sequencing (NGS)

Table 6.1: Summary of Case Studies Using Cytogenetic Testing in Analyzing Cancer-Related Alterations

S. No.	Cytogenetics Testing	Cancer Type	Findings of the Study	References
1.	Karyotyping	Breast cancer	Three breast cancer cell lines, T-47D, MDA-MB-361, and ZR-75-1.	Morris et al., 1997
		Human mammary sarcoma	Chromosome 1 is actively involved in the rearrangements Chromosome 2 and 7q were over-represented on the per-cell level, the 7q	Chen and Seman, 1981
2.	CGH	Breast cancer	Chromosomal alterations in 15 cancer lines **Chromosomal gain** in 1q, 8q, 20q, 7, 11q13, 17q, 9q, and 16p **Chromosomal losses** were most common at 8p, 11q14→qter, 18q, and Xq	Blegen et al., 2003
		Non-small cell lung cancer	5p, 3q, 8q, 11q, 2q, 12p and 12q to be commonly over-represented and regions on 9p, 3p, 6q, 17p, 22q, 8p, 10p, 10q and 19p to be commonly under-represented.	Berrieman et al., 2004
3.	FISH	Non-small cell lung cancer	Chromosome 12 alterations	Speicher et al., 2000
			• Numerous complex chromosomal rearrangements. • Translocations between chromosomes 5 and 14, 5 and 11 and 1 and 6 were observed in three of the six samples, with a further 14 translocations being observed in two samples each. • Loss of the Y chromosome and gains of chromosomes 20 and 5p were also frequent. • Chromosomes 4, 5, 8, 11, 12 and 19 were most frequently involved in interchromosomal translocations.	Berrieman et al., 2004
4.	NGS	Multiple primary tumors (gastric cancer and breast cancer, GIST gastrointestinal stromal tissue)	Detection of hereditary and germline mutations	Wu et al., 2022
		Lung cancer	Mutational status of EGFR, KRAS, BRAF and PIK3 CA	Jing et al., 2018
		Metastatic breast cancer and successive pulmonary lesions	Somatic mutations in PiK3CA and TP53 genes.	Choi et al., 2023
		Lung and colon carcinoma	Mutation hotspots of 48 genes. mutations in the KRAS and EGFR genes	Chevrier et al., 2014
		Multiple Primary Lung Cancer and intrapulmonary metastasis	Mutation KRAS	Ezer et al., 2021

has significantly improved the capacity to identify chromosomal abnormalities with remarkable accuracy. The application of these methodologies enables the precise identification of distinct genetic modifications, including translocations and mutations, while permitting an extensive examination of the tumor genome. This, in turn, uncovers vital information regarding tumor biology and its progression.

6.5 CHALLENGES AND FUTURE DIRECTIONS

Cancer cytogenetics testing encounters numerous challenges that can influence the accuracy, reliability, and clinical utility. Below are several primary challenges:

a) Heterogeneity in tumors

A major obstacle to cytogenetic testing is tumor heterogeneity, especially when looking for molecular predictive biomarkers for the diagnosis and treatment of cancer. Diverse genetic profiles within a single tumor complicate karyotype analyses, resulting in inconsistent outcomes that impede effective treatment planning. Intra-tumoral heterogeneity results from multiple mechanisms, such as genomic instability, epigenetic changes, and varying microenvironmental factors, leading to a diverse array of genetically distinct cell populations within a single tumor mass. The complexity may hinder the identification of specific chromosomal abnormalities essential for precise diagnosis and prognosis. Moreover, some genetic changes may be present in one area of the tumor but undetectable or mutated in another. Therefore, establishing a reliable biomarker profile that accurately depicts the nature of a tumor can be challenging. This variability complicates the discovery of effective therapeutic avenues and increases the likelihood of treatment resistance, as different subclonal populations may respond differently to therapies. Addressing tumor heterogeneity is essential for optimizing cytogenetic testing strategies and enhancing outcomes in precision oncology.

b) Evidence-based clinical practices

Advanced cytogenetic technologies like array Comparative Genomic Hybridization (aCGH) and Next-Generation Sequencing (NGS) hold great potential and could improve our understanding of cancer biology, but their adoption into routine clinical practice has been sluggish. A contributing factor in this disparity is the difficulty in interpreting the wide variety of genetic alterations detected by these techniques. Moreover, numerous identified biomarkers lack robust validation studies demonstrating their utility in improving patient outcomes or guiding treatment decisions. Clinicians may encounter difficulties in integrating these biomarkers into standard practice due to the lack of clear evidence regarding their influence on prognosis or therapy selection.

c) Sample viability challenges

Sample viability-related concerns pose a substantial obstacle in utilization of karyotyping for cancer diagnosis, chiefly because the technique relies on metaphase-stage cells. Conventional karyotyping requires the in-vitro cultivation of viable cells that must divide to attain the metaphase stage appropriate for chromosomal examination. However, obtaining a sufficient number of viable cells is often difficult, particularly in certain tumor types or when sample processing is delayed. Studies demonstrated that samples processed after 24 hours post-collection showed a considerably increased rate of culture failure, with cellular viability declining significantly over time. Insufficient cellularity, defined by a deficiency of nucleated cells, may lead to incomplete or inconclusive karyotypic results, hindering precise diagnosis and effective treatment strategies.

d) Cost-effectiveness of techniques

The expense and availability of advanced cytogenetic testing methods present considerable obstacles to their extensive adoption in clinical contexts. These sophisticated methodologies can be excessively costly, potentially limiting their accessibility to specialized centers possessing the requisite technology and expertise. Consequently, patients in low-income or rural regions may experience delays in diagnosis and treatment owing to insufficient access to these essential tests. It is imperative to tackle these challenges through policy reforms, augmented funding for healthcare infrastructure, and enhanced communication regarding costs to improve the incorporation of cytogenetic testing into standard clinical practice.

6.6 CONCLUDING REMARKS

Cytogenetic diagnostic testing (CDT) is essential in modern oncology, as it improves our knowledge of cancer biology and drives specific therapy approaches. As techniques progress, especially next-generation sequencing (NGS), detecting chromosomal abnormalities and their effects on tumor behavior becomes more precise. This advancement facilitates the identification of particular genetic markers linked to different cancers and promotes the creation of targeted therapies. Integrating cytogenetic testing into standard clinical practice is expected to enhance patient outcomes by facilitating more personalized and effective treatment strategies, signifying a notable advancement towards precision medicine in oncology.

REFERENCES

Bain B J, Béné MC (2019). Morphological and immunophenotypic clues to the WHO categories of acute myeloid leukaemia. *Acta Haematol* 141(4):232–244.

Balciuniene J et al. (2024). Cancer cytogenetics in a genomics world: wedding the old with the new. *Blood Rev* 66:101209.

Baruchel A et al. (2023). Down syndrome and leukemia: from basic mechanisms to clinical advances. *Haematol* 108(10):2570–2581.

Bassi C et al. (2021). The PTEN and ATM axis controls the G1/S cell cycle checkpoint and tumorigenesis in HER2-positive breast cancer. *Cell Death Different* 28(11):3036–3051.

Berrieman HK et al. (2004). Chromosomal analysis of non-small-cell lung cancer by multicolour fluorescent in situ hybridisation. *Br J Cancer* 90(4):900–905.

Blegen H et al. (2003). DNA amplifications and aneuploidy, high proliferative activity and impaired cell cycle control characterize breast carcinomas with poor prognosis. *Anal Cell Pathol* 25(3):103–114.

Bridge JA (2008). Advantages and limitations of cytogenetic, molecular cytogenetic, and molecular diagnostic testing in mesenchymal neoplasms. *J Orthopaed Sci* 13(3):273–282.

Chen TR, Seman G (1981). Karyotype analysis of a human mammary sarcoma explant in vitro. *Breast Cancer Res Treat* 1(3):203–208.

Chen X et al. (2022). Mutant p53 in cancer: from molecular mechanism to therapeutic modulation. *Cell Death Dis* 13(11).

Cheng C et al. (2023). Methods to improve the accuracy of next-generation sequencing. *Front Bioengineer Biotechnol* 11:982111.

Chevrier S et al. (2014). Next-generation sequencing analysis of lung and colon carcinomas reveals a variety of genetic alterations. *Int J Oncol* 45(3):1167–1174.

Choi JH et al. (2023). Prognostic significance of TP53 and PIK3CA mutations analyzed by next-generation sequencing in breast cancer. *Med* 102(38):e35267.

Cui C et al. (2016). Cell-based genetic diagnostic and research applications. *Front Cell Development Biol* 4:89.

Dang DK, Park BH (2022). Circulating tumor DNA: current challenges for clinical utility. *J Clin Investigat* 132(12):e154941.

Doležel J et al. (2021). Chromosome analysis and sorting. *Cytometry A* 99(4):328–342.

Dong Z et al. (2018). Identification of balanced chromosomal rearrangements previously unknown among participants in the 1000 Genomes Project: implications for interpretation of structural variation in genomes and the future of clinical cytogenetics. *Geneti Med* 20(7):697–707.

Eldfors S et al. (2024). Monosomy 7/del(7q) cause sensitivity to inhibitors of nicotinamide phosphoribosyltransferase in acute myeloid leukemia. *Blood Adv* 8(7):1621–1633.

Ezer N et al (2021). Integrating NGS-derived mutational profiling in the diagnosis of multiple lung adenocarcinomas. *Cancer Treat Res Communicat* 29:100484.

Findley TO et al. (2023). Challenges in the clinical understanding of genetic testing in birth defects and pediatric diseases. *Transl Pediatr* 12(5):1028–1040.

Fröhling S, Döhner H (2008). Chromosomal abnormalities in cancer. *New Engl J Med 359*(7):722–734.

Gonzales PR et al. (2016). Overview of clinical cytogenetics. *Curr Proto Hum Genet 89*:8.1.1–8.1.13.

Houldsworth J, Chaganti RS (1994). Comparative genomic hybridization: an overview. *Am J Pathol 145*(6):1253–1260.

Iqbal N, Iqbal N (2014). Human Epidermal Growth Factor Receptor 2 (HER2) in cancers: overexpression and therapeutic implications. *Molec Biol Int 2014*:1–9.

Jing C et al. (2018). Next-generation sequencing-based detection of EGFR, KRAS, BRAF, NRAS, PIK3CA, Her-2 and TP53 mutations in patients with non-small cell lung cancer. *Mol Med Rep 18*(2):2191–2197. doi: 10.3892/mmr.2018.9210. Epub 2018 Jun 22. PMID: 29956783; PMCID: PMC6072231.

Kang ZJ et al. (2016). The Philadelphia chromosome in leukemogenesis. *Chinese J Cancer 35*:48.

Kanwal R, Gupta S (2011). Epigenetic modifications in cancer. *Clin Genet 81*(4),:303–311.

Koretzky GA (2007). The legacy of the Philadelphia chromosome. *J Clin Investigat 117*(8):2030–2032.

Kou F et al (2020). Chromosome abnormalities: new insights into their clinical significance in cancer. *Molec Ther Oncolyt 17*:562–570.

Krzyszczyk P et al. (2018). The growing role of precision and personalized medicine for cancer treatment. *Technol 6*(3–4):79–100.

Kurtz DM et al. (2021). Enhanced detection of minimal residual disease by targeted sequencing of phased variants in circulating tumor DNA. *Nature Biotechnol 39*(12):1537–1547.

LeBlanc VG, Marra MA (2015). Next-generation sequencing approaches in cancer: where have they brought us and where will they take us?. *Cancers 7*(3):925–1958.

Levy B, Wapner R (2018). Prenatal diagnosis by chromosomal microarray analysis. *Fertil Steril 109*(2):201– 212.

Lichter P et al (2000). Comparative genomic hybridization: uses and limitations. *Sem Hematol 37*(4):348–357.

Lin C et al. (2021). Liquid biopsy, ctDNA diagnosis through NGS. *Life 11*(9):890.

Lindstrand A et al. (2019). From cytogenetics to cytogenomics: whole-genome sequencing as a first-line test comprehensively captures the diverse spectrum of disease-causing genetic variation underlying intellectual disability. *Genome Medi 11*(1):68.

Lingjaerde OC et al. (2005). CGH-Explorer: a program for analysis of array-CGH data. *Bioinformat 21*(6):821–822.

Molina JR, Adjei AA (2006). The RAS/RAF/MAPK pathway. *J Thorac Oncol 1*(1):7–9.

Morris JS et al. (1997). Cytogenetic analysis of three breast carcinoma cell lines using reverse chromosome painting. *Genes Chrom Cancer 20*(2):120–139.

Mylavarapu S et al. (2018). Role of BRCA mutations in the modulation of response to platinum therapy. *Front Oncol 8*.

Newman AM et al. (2014). An ultrasensitive method for quantitating circulating tumor DNA with broad patient coverage. *Nature Med 20*(5):548–554.

Noguchi T et al. (2020). Changes in the gene mutation profiles of circulating tumor DNA detected using CAPP-Seq in neoadjuvant chemotherapy-treated advanced ovarian cancer. *Oncol Letters* 19(4):2713–2720.

Nowakowska B, Bocian E (2004). Cytogenetyka molekularna -- techniki badawcze i ich zastosowanie w diagnostyce klinicznej [Molecular cytogenetic techniques and their application in clinical diagnosis]. *Medycyna wieku rozwojowego* 8(1):7–24.

O'Connor C (2008). Karyotyping for chromosomal abnormalities. *Nature Educat* 1(1):27.

Ozkan E, Lacerda MP (2020). *Genetics, Cytogenetic Testing and Conventional Karyotype*. StatPearls.

Panagopoulos I, Heim S (2022). Neoplasia-associated chromosome translocations resulting in gene truncation. *Cancer Genom Proteom* 19(6):647–672.

Qin D (2019). Next-generation sequencing and its clinical application. *Cancer Biol Medi* 16(1):4–10.

Redon R, Carter NP (2009). Comparative genomic hybridization: microarray design and data interpretation. *Meth Molec Biol* 529:37–49.

Ribeiro IP et al. (2019). Cytogenetics and cytogenomics evaluation in cancer. *Int J Molec Sci* 20(19):4711.

Sampaio MM et al. (2021). Chronic myeloid leukemia-from the Philadelphia chromosome to specific target drugs: a literature review. *World J Clin Oncol* 12(2):69–94.

Shakoori AR (2017). Fluorescence In Situ Hybridization (FISH) and its applications. *Chromosome Structure and Aberrations*, 343–367.

So CC et al. (2008). A dual colour dual fusion fluorescence in situ hybridisation study on the genesis of complex variant translocations in chronic myelogenous leukaemia. *Oncol Rep* 19(5):1181–1184.

Speicher MR et al. (2000). Analysis of chromosomal alterations in non-small cell lung cancer by multiplex-FISH, comparative genomic hybridization, and multicolor bar coding. *Lab Investigat* 80(7):1031–1041.

Taniue K, Akimitsu N (2021). Fusion genes and RNAs in cancer development. *Non-Coding RNA* 7(1):10.

Wan TS (2014). Cancer cytogenetics: methodology revisited. *Ann Lab Med* 34(6):413–425.

Wan TS (2017). Cancer cytogenetics: an Introduction. *Meth Molec Biol* 1541:1–10.

Weiss MM et al. (1999). Comparative genomic hybridisation. *Molec Pathol* 52(5):243–251.

Weiss MM et al. (2003). Comparative genomic hybridisation as a supportive tool in diagnostic pathology. *J Clin Pathol* 56(7):522–527.

Wu T et al. (2022). Case report: next-generation sequencing-based detection in a patient with three synchronous primary tumors. *Front Oncol* 12:910264.

Yan Y et al (2007). In a model of immunoglobulin heavy-chain (IGH)/MYC translocation, the Igh 3′ regulatory region induces MYC expression at the immature stage of B cell development. *Genes Chromosomes Cancer* 46(10):950–959.

Yu X et al. (2024). Cancer epigenetics: from laboratory studies and clinical trials to precision medicine. *Cell Death Disc* 10(1).

Zhao L et al. (2001). Spectral karyotyping study of chromosome abnormalities in human leukemia. Cancer Genet Cytogenet 127(2):143–7. doi: 10.1016/s0165-4608(00)00438-6. Erratum in: *Cancer Genet Cytogenet* 2001 Nov;131(1):94–5. PMID: 11425454.

Zhang Y et al. (2023). Detection of clinically important BRCA gene mutations in ovarian cancer patients using next generation sequencing analysis. *Am J Cancer Res 13*(10):5005–5020.

7

Genomic Profiling

A Paradigm Shift in Precision Oncology

Arshiya Sood, Gangandeep Singh, Dipansh Katoch, Lata Kumari, and Neelam Thakur

ABBREVIATIONS

Acronym	Full Form
Array CGH	Array comparative genomic hybridization
CNVs	Copy number variations
CML	Chronic myeloid leukemia
CGP	Comprehensive genome profiling
CGH	Comparative genomic hybridization
ctDNA	Circulating tumor DNA
DNA	Deoxy ribonucleic acid
FISH	Fluorescence in situ hybridization
MSI	Microsatellite instability
mNSCLC	Metastatic non-small cell lung cancer
LSV	Large structural variants
PCR	Polymerase chain reaction
NGS	Next-generation sequencing
HGP	Human Genome Project
SNVs	Single nucleotide variants
RT-PCR	Reverse transcriptase -polymerase chain reaction
TMB	Tumor mutational burden
TGP	Tumor genomic profiling
TSG	Tumor suppressor gene
VUS	Variants of uncertain significance

7.1 INTRODUCTION

Genomic profiling provides the genetic information associated with an individual person or cell type, as well as how their genes interact with one another and with the environment. The genetic modifications that have occurred allow for more effective treatment techniques that are specific to the genetic profile pertaining to each patient (Pankiw, Brezden-Masley, and Charames 2024). This method examines a wide array of genomic features, including structural variants, single nucleotide variants (SNVs), gene fusions, insertions and deletions, and copy number variations (CNVs), offering a thorough overview of the genomic landscape. Currently, genomic profiling is integral to genetic counseling, cancer diagnosis, molecular characterization, and serves as a biomarker for prognosis and therapy response (Mathew et al. 2022).

The scope of genomic profiling extends beyond merely identifying mutations; it encompasses the assessment of microsatellite instability (MSI) tumors and mutational burden (TMB), both of which can influence treatment strategies and predict responses to therapies, especially immunotherapies. By comparing tumor DNA to normal germline DNA, genomic profiling can also uncover inherited mutations that may indicate a predisposition to certain cancers, thus offering insights into hereditary cancer risks (Mathew et al. 2022; Garofalo et al. 2016). New possibilities for personalized therapy have arisen in the rapidly developing area of genomics, which is reshaping healthcare. A promising method for guiding therapeutic decision-making, comprehensive genome profiling (CGP) can decipher the genetic composition of an individual. When compared to the present standard of care in oncology, several studies published from 2000 to 2023 show that incorporating CGP into routine care processes has proven beneficial (Ghosh, Lopes, and Chopra 2022).

Genomic profiling is increasingly recognized as a keystone of precision oncology, where therapies are personalized based on the genetic makeup of each type of cancer patient. This aims to

DOI: 10.1201/9781003542162-7

enhance treatment efficacy while minimizing adverse effects by matching patients with therapies most likely to be effective for their specific genetic alterations (Hatano and Nonomura 2021). As technology advances and the costs associated with genomic testing decrease, the amalgamation of genomic profiling into standard clinical practices is becoming more prevalent, allowing for earlier diagnoses and more targeted therapeutic interventions (Malone et al. 2020). Genomic profiling is a tool in modern medicine that utilizes advanced sequencing technologies to obtain genetic information of patients. Next-generation sequencing (NGS) is a product of technological novelties in the field of DNA sequencing that has allowed doctors to simultaneously mass sequence genes from various cancer kinds (Gasperskaja and Kučinskas 2017). Its applications span diagnosis, treatment planning, and risk assessment, making it an invaluable resource in the fight against cancer and other genetic disorders.

7.1.1 From Traditional Cancer Treatments to Precision Oncology

The evolution of cancer treatment has seen a significant shift from traditional methods to precision oncology, marking a paradigm change in how oncologists approach cancer therapy. Historically, cancer treatments were largely nonspecific and focused on the type of cancer rather than the individual characteristics of a patient's tumor (Tsimberidou et al. 2020). Standard treatments included chemotherapy, which utilized broad-spectrum cytotoxic agents that target rapidly dividing cells, often resulting in significant side effects and variable efficacy. Radiation therapy aimed at destroying cancer cells through high-energy radiation but similarly lacked specificity, affecting healthy tissues as well (Chakravarthi, Nepal, and Varambally 2016). Surgery was often employed to physically remove tumors without accounting for the underlying genetic makeup of the cancer. This "one-size-fits-all" model frequently led to ineffective treatments and unnecessary side effects. The concept of precision oncology began to take shape in the late 1990s and early 2000s, driven by key developments such as molecular targeting, genomic sequencing, and biomarker discovery. The sanction of imatinib (Gleevec) in 2001 for CML marked a crucial moment, demonstrating that targeting specific genetic mutations could lead to dramatic clinical outcomes (Coyle, Boudreau, and Marcato 2017). The completion of the HGP and advancements in NGS technologies allowed for comprehensive profiling of tumors at a genetic level, enabling the identification of specific mutations that drive cancer progression. The discovery of biomarkers like HER2 in breast cancer illustrated how certain genetic alterations can predict responses to targeted therapies, leading to more informed treatment decisions (Abbasi and Masoumi 2020). Today, precision oncology is recognized as a foundational component of cancer care, emphasizing the importance of understanding the unique genetic profile of a patient to guide treatment effectively. Key advancements include liquid biopsies, which analyze circulating tumor DNA (ctDNA) from blood samples for insights into tumor dynamics and potential resistance mutations without invasive tissue biopsies (Krzyszczyk et al. 2018). Treatments are increasingly targeted based on specific genomic alterations, improving outcomes while minimizing adverse effects associated with traditional therapies. Additionally, advancements in immunotherapy are enabling the development of therapies that harness the control of the immune system on order to target malignant cells more effectively (Krzyszczyk et al. 2018). Despite these advancements, challenges remain in ensuring broad access to precision medicine and integrating it into standard care practices. Issues such as healthcare disparities, insurance coverage for genomic testing, and the need for ongoing education among healthcare providers are critical areas that require attention as precision oncology continues to evolve (Berger and Mardis 2018). The journey from traditional cancer treatments to precision oncology reflects a significant transformation in medical science, driven by technological advancements and knowledge about cancer biology.

7.1.2 Importance and Relevance of Genomic Profiling in Modern Oncology

Modern oncology uses genetic profiling to increase cancer treatment precision and efficacy. This method analyzes the tumor DNA of the patient to find mutations and changes that can guide targeted therapy. Genomic profiling allows physicians to customize cancer therapy depending on genetic makeup of patient (Del Giacco and Cattaneo 2012)

Next-Generation Sequencing (NGS) allows simultaneous gene analysis, a major achievement in this field whose approach has transformed actionable mutation identification, delivering insights that older methods could not. For instance, comprehensive genomic profiling (CGP) can detect single nucleotide variants, copy number changes, insertions and deletions and gene fusions. This thorough analysis improves clinical decision-making and patient outcomes by selecting targeted medicines with minimal side effects that are more likely to work (Del Giacco and Cattaneo 2012; Pankiw, Brezden-Masley, and Charames 2024).

Moreover, genomic profiling is instrumental in identifying hereditary cancer risks. Tumor genomic profiling (TGP) can reveal inborn mutations in cancerous genes like BRCA1/2, which has significant implications for both treatment planning and family screening (Garofalo et al. 2016). As costs for genomic testing decline and its accuracy improves, access to these critical diagnostic tools has expanded, further solidifying their role in routine clinical practice. The integration of genomic profiling into oncology also supports the development of innovative clinical trial designs that match patients with therapies based on their genetic profiles rather than traditional histological classifications. This shift towards molecular characterization allows for a more empathetic tumor biology and enhances the efficacy of treatment options available to patients (Peleg Hasson et al. 2023).

Genomic profiling transforms current oncology and is a diagnostic tool. Early diagnosis, individualized treatment strategies, and better patient outcomes are possible while tackling genetic complexity of the cancer. Genomic profiling in oncology will likely become increasingly important as research advances, enabling more targeted cancer treatments.

7.2 THE SCIENCE BEHIND GENOMIC PROFILING

Genomic profiling identifies genetic variants that impact attributes, illness risk, and treatment response by interpreting the genetic fingerprint. Researchers can now scan and analyze vast quantities of genetic data with astounding accuracy with the help of modern technology. Understanding genetic predispositions to complicated diseases including cancer, heart disease, and neurological disorders will be aided by technology (Tarride, Gould, and Thomas 2022). The initiation of genomic profiling has opened the door to customized medicine, which improves results while decreasing adverse effects by allowing physicians to customize preventative measures and treatments to each patient's specific genetic composition (Butow et al. 2022).

7.2.1 Basics of Genomics and Cancer Biology

Genomic alterations are critical changes in genetic material that significantly aids to the initiation and proliferation of tumor, and they can be broadly categorized into three main types: mutations, copy number variations (CNVs), and translocations (Del Giacco and Cattaneo 2012).

DNA mutations are closely related to the development of cancer and fall into two main categories: somatic mutations, which happen during the lifespan of a person and germline mutations, which are inherited from parents. These mutations are essential in turning healthy cells into malignant ones because they interfere with regular cellular processes shown in Figure 7.1. There are permanent changes in the DNA sequence of a gene, which can arise during normal DNA replication or be induced by environmental factors such as chemicals or radiation (Previs et al. 2016).

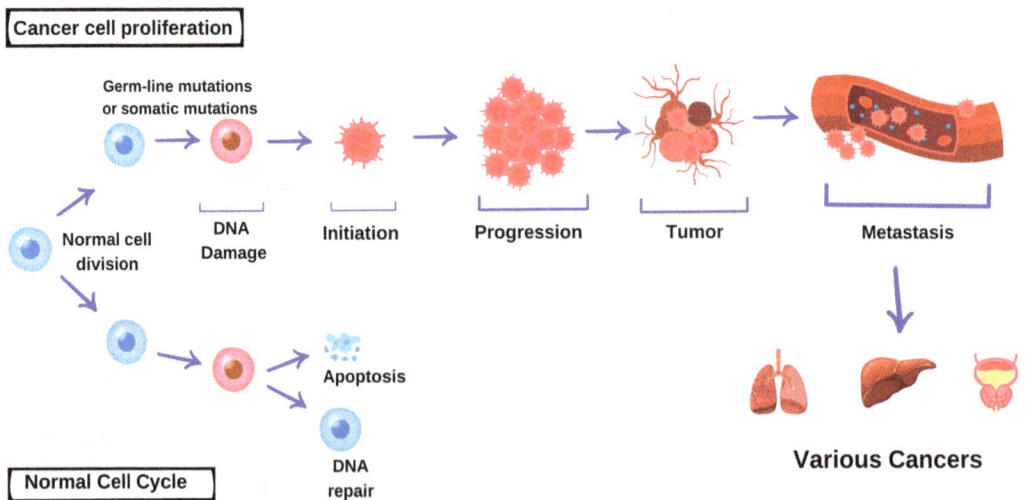

Figure 7.1 DNA mutation and damage lead to various cancers.

They include missense mutations, which result in the replacement of one amino acid for another; nonsense mutations, which create a premature stop codon leading to shortened proteins; and insertions and deletions that can disrupt the reading frame, resulting in frameshift mutations that alter protein function (Ostroverkhova, Przytycka, and Panchenko 2023).

The variations in the number of copies of specific genes or genomic regions, encompassing duplications that lead to gene overexpression and deletions that can cause loss of function, are referred to as copy number variations (Espinoza Pereira et al. 2023). These changes can drive tumorigenesis by either promoting uncontrolled cell proliferation through amplification of oncogenes or removing critical regulatory functions by deleting tumor suppressor genes. Translocations occur when chromosomal segments break off from one chromosome and attach to another, often resulting in the fusion of previously separate genes (Coyle, Boudreau, and Marcato 2017).

Oncogenes are genes that are normally involved in cell proliferation and division, but whenever they undergo mutation, their activity is increased multifold, which leads uncontrolled cell proliferation (Kontomanolis et al. 2020). This transformation can occur through various mechanisms, such as point mutations, gene amplification (where multiple copies of an oncogene are produced), or chromosomal translocations (where segments of DNA are rearranged). A single mutation in one copy of an oncogene is often sufficient to drive cancer development due to its dominant effect (Martincorena and Campbell 2015).

In contrast, tumor suppressor genes function to inhibit cell growth and promote apoptosis (programmed cell death). Mutations in these genes typically require both copies to be affected for cancer to develop, reflecting a recessive effect. The TP53 gene, which encodes the P53 protein that regulates the cell cycle and maintains genomic stability, has mutations found in over 50% of all human cancers (Morris and Chan 2015).

DNA repair genes such as BRCA1 and BRCA2 are accountable for amending errors that occur during DNA replication. When mutations occur in these genes, the ability to repair DNA damage diminishes, leading to an accumulation of mutations in both oncogenes and tumor suppressor genes. This accumulation significantly increases the risk of cancer development (Turgeon, Perry, and Poulogiannis 2018).

The progression from normal cells to cancerous cells is typically gradual and involves multiple mutations accumulating over time. Gene mutations associated with cancer include BRCA1 and BRCA2, linked to malignancies in the breast and ovaries, while TP53, a critical tumor suppressor gene, is found mutated in many cancers (Previs et al. 2016). Inherited mutations can accelerate this process; individuals with germline mutations start with one defective gene copy, making it easier for additional mutations to lead to cancer at an earlier age compared to those who acquire all mutations somatically (Hall et al. 2021). The protagonist of these genetic changes in cancer development is essential for identifying targeted therapies that can effectively combat various forms of cancer. As research advances, these mechanisms will lead to improved prevention strategies and treatment for patients.

7.2.2 Techniques in Genomic Profiling

Genomic profiling is a transformative approach that comprises the analysis of DNA to identify genetic differences associated with diseases, particularly cancer. This process begins with DNA extraction, where genetic material is isolated from biological samples such as tumor biopsies or blood, followed by library preparation for sequencing (Alkhateeb, Alshomali, and Dalain 2023). The core of genomic profiling lies in advanced sequencing technologies like NGS, Sanger, microarray, RNA sequencing, etc., as shown in Figure 7.2. The sequencing is followed up by bioinformatics analysis, which manage the vast amount of data generated; this involves aligning sequences to a reference genome, identifying variants, and interpreting their biological significance using advanced algorithms that classify variants, helping to pinpoint actionable mutations that inform targeted therapies. Additionally, genomic profiling often includes epigenetic analyses to understand how modifications like DNA methylation affect gene expression without making any alterations to the nucleotide sequence of DNA (Eifert et al. 2017). Developing technologies like long-read sequencing enhance the ability to capture complex structural variations, while optical genome mapping identifies large structural variants through high-resolution imaging techniques. The implications of genomic profiling for cancer treatment are profound, as it enables the identification of actionable mutations that aid in selecting the right treatment plans for individual patients.

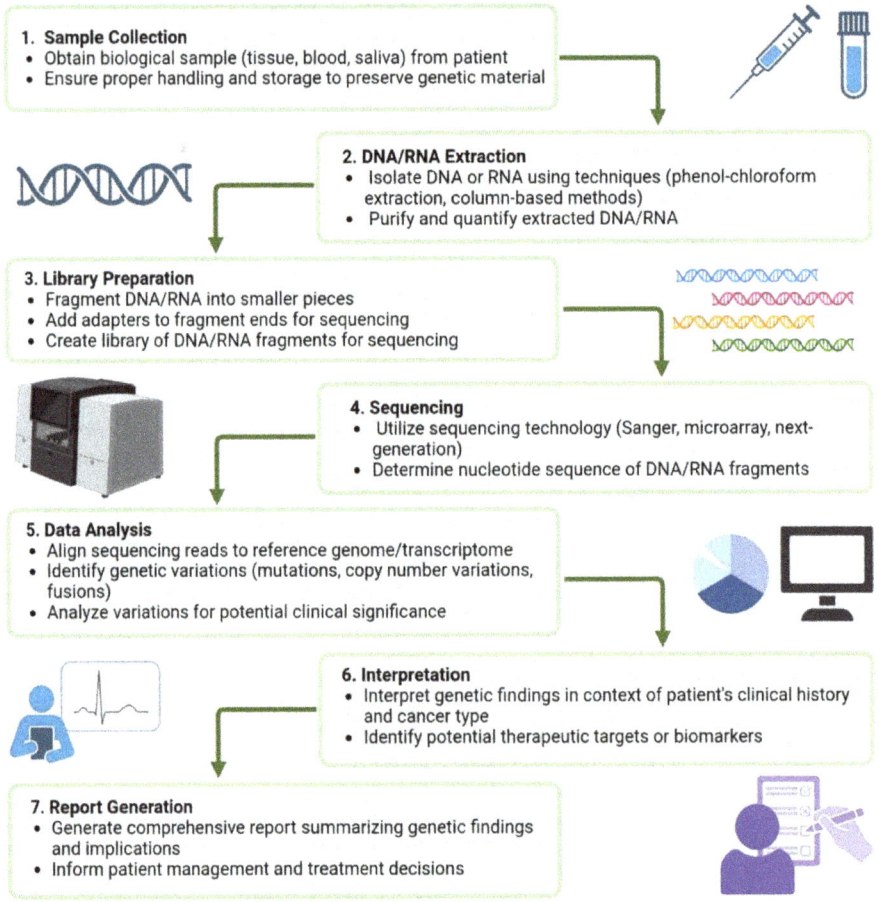

1. Sample Collection
- Obtain biological sample (tissue, blood, saliva) from patient
- Ensure proper handling and storage to preserve genetic material

2. DNA/RNA Extraction
- Isolate DNA or RNA using techniques (phenol-chloroform extraction, column-based methods)
- Purify and quantify extracted DNA/RNA

3. Library Preparation
- Fragment DNA/RNA into smaller pieces
- Add adapters to fragment ends for sequencing
- Create library of DNA/RNA fragments for sequencing

4. Sequencing
- Utilize sequencing technology (Sanger, microarray, next-generation)
- Determine nucleotide sequence of DNA/RNA fragments

5. Data Analysis
- Align sequencing reads to reference genome/transcriptome
- Identify genetic variations (mutations, copy number variations, fusions)
- Analyze variations for potential clinical significance

6. Interpretation
- Interpret genetic findings in context of patient's clinical history and cancer type
- Identify potential therapeutic targets or biomarkers

7. Report Generation
- Generate comprehensive report summarizing genetic findings and implications
- Inform patient management and treatment decisions

Figure 7.2 General mechanism of genomic profiling for clinical implications.

7.2.2.1 Next-Generation Sequencing (NGS)

NGS allows for high-throughput sequencing of multiple genes simultaneously followed by the detection of multiple genetic modifications, encompassing single nucleotide variants (SNVs), insertions and deletions, copy number variants (CNVs), gene fusions, and larger structural variants. Comprehensive Genomic Profiling (CGP) utilizes targeted NGS to detect cancer biomarkers across a wide range of genes, providing information about genomic alterations and characterizing tumors more accurately than single-gene assays (Slatko, Gardner, and Ausubel 2018).

When compared to traditional diagnostic methods, next-generation sequencing (NGS) provides a number of benefits due to its high throughput. Even though PCR, RT-PCR, and FISH are reliable and relatively inexpensive methods for identifying genomic changes, they have a limitation: they can only detect a small number of targets at a time due to the need for specialized primers or probes. By comparison, next-generation sequencing efficiently analyzes several targets using sophisticated sequencing methods (Slatko, Gardner, and Ausubel 2018). Clinicians can choose medications based on thorough diagnoses and tumor features with the help of NGS, which provides a more detailed tumor profile for every patient.

It is believed that NGS-based identification of unique molecular signatures would assist in effective therapeutic matching to patients, hence decreasing and/or preventing needless treatment delays (Rolfo et al. 2020). New genetic sequencing (NGS) technology has made it feasible to use circulating tumor DNA for cancer genomic status testing with minimal invasiveness; this method is also sensitive enough to be used with liquid biopsies (Gu, Miller, and Chiu 2019).

Molecularly personalized treatment selection, early cancer diagnosis of asymptomatic patients, and recurrence prediction by detection of residual cancer are only a few of the numerous clinical applications of liquid biopsy (Rolfo et al. 2020). There are various choices for next-generation sequencing (NGS), such as whole-genome sequencing, targeted or whole-transcriptome sequencing, small to large gene panels, and whole-exome sequencing (WES). Due to their sensitivity in detecting low-level molecular alterations, focus on clinically actionable changes, cost-effectiveness, quick turnaround times, and extensive coverage of genomic regions of interest, targeted gene panels have become the most widely used method in adult oncology (Satam et al. 2023). There have been few cost-effectiveness assessments of NGS, and the results have been inconsistent. However, this is expected to change when more biomarkers are discovered, which will make it more cost-effective to use a single test that perceives several targets rather than several tests that identify fewer targets (Buermans and den Dunnen 2014).

7.2.2.2 Whole-Genome Sequencing (WGS)

WGS is a wide-ranging method used for the analysis of the entire genome of an organism, providing insights into genetic variations across all regions, including coding and non-coding sequences. Unlike targeted approaches such as exome sequencing, which only focus on protein-coding regions, WGS captures the complete genetic makeup, allowing for the detection of SNVs, insertions/deletions, copy number changes, and LSVs (Nakagawa and Fujita 2018). The advent of next-generation sequencing (NGS) technologies has revolutionized WGS by significantly reducing costs and increasing throughput.

It aids in diagnosing inherited disorders by identifying causative mutations that may not be detectable through traditional methods. It is also instrumental in cancer genomics, where it helps characterize mutations driving tumor progression and can inform personalized treatment strategies (Kwong et al. 2015). Moreover, WGS is increasingly utilized in infectious disease research to track outbreaks and understand pathogen evolution by providing detailed genomic data on microbial species. These technologies enhance the ability to resolve complex genomic regions that are challenging for short-read methods, thereby improving the accuracy of genome assembly and variant detection (Ekblom and Wolf 2014). Additionally, improvements in bioinformatics tools have streamlined data analysis, enabling researchers to interpret vast amounts of genomic data more effectively. As WGS continues to evolve, it holds great promise for advancing personalized medicine and enhancing our understanding of genetic diseases and their underlying mechanisms (Rossing et al. 2019). The ongoing reduction in sequencing costs and improvements in technology suggest that WGS will become an integral part of routine clinical practice in the near future.

7.2.2.3 Whole-Exome Sequencing (WES)

The protein-coding sections of genes, called exons, make up around 1% of the human genome but include around 85% of the known disease-related variations. WES is presently accessible for clinical application and differs from WGS in that it exclusively examines the exons, or portions of the genome responsible for coding proteins (Bartha and Győrffy 2019). The approximately 22,000 genes that make up exons constitute 1.5% of the genome's DNA. The majority of the genes that have been linked to Mendelian diseases relate to the exons (Diderich et al. 2021). As an affordable alternative to whole-genome sequencing (WGS), this method focuses on the area's most likely to have genetic variations associated with certain diseases. Furthermore, the present significant limitation in the ability to understand intronic portions of the genome, WES is chosen (Iglesias et al. 2014).

It has ability to detect new genetic variants across all protein-coding genes at once makes it ideal for the diagnosis of rare genetic illnesses. More efficient and accurate sequencing has been made possible by recent developments in WES technology, which include target-enrichment strategies such in-solution capture approaches. Additionally, advances in high-throughput sequencing have slashed turnaround times for clinical diagnostics by facilitating quicker library preparation and data processing(Rabbani, Tekin, and Mahdieh 2014). Researchers and clinicians are able to better understand results and find important genetic variations associated with particular phenotypes because to the inclusion of sophisticated bioinformatics tools that make it easier to analyze the vast data sets produced by WES.

In addition, WES is finding more and more applications in customized medicine, namely in the area of adapting treatment plans to each individual patient's mutation profile. The method is finding more and more uses in both the lab and the clinic, and it is even being used in large-scale studies to find genetic links to diseases like diabetes and malignancies (Shi et al. 2018). In sum,

WES is a crucial technique in genomics that is always improving and shedding light on hereditary illnesses and their treatments.

It is outside the purview of WES to use microarray technology to detect differences in copy number. It does not have the capability to identify low-level mosaicism, translocations, trinucleotide repeats (repeat expansions, tandem repeat size), polyploidy (e.g., trisomy 21), or aneuploidy. Not enough of the genome has been sequenced using WES due to its inadequate depth/coverage, especially in GC rich areas (Yang et al. 2013). To ensure the accuracy of the results, Sanger sequencing is advised.

7.2.2.4 RNA Sequencing

RNA sequencing (RNA-seq) uses next-generation sequencing (NGS) technology to examine the transcriptome, giving gene expression patterns, RNA species, and the functions they play in different biological activities (Hong et al. 2020). By observing which genes are actively expressed in a cell at specific periods, RNA-seq enables researchers to identify dynamic changes linked to cellular activities and disease states, in contrast to traditional DNA sequencing that concentrates on genetic differences. Long non-coding RNAs, circular RNAs, microRNAs, and messenger RNAs are all detectable using this method, which allows for a thorough comprehension of gene regulation and expression (Baran-Gale, Chandra, and Kirschner 2018).

It is vital in cancer research for discovering biomarkers, describing tumor heterogeneity, and treatment resistance mechanisms. RNA-seq has become an important method for studying tumor microenvironments and cellular interactions by analyzing gene expression profiles at the single cell level (Kim et al. 2023). The ability of RNA-seq to detect gene fusions and differential transcript expression, which may signal the presence or progression of disease, is also making it a popular tool in the clinical diagnosis of infectious diseases and transplant medicine. The massive volumes of data produced by RNA-seq experiments can now be more accurately interpreted because of advancements in bioinformatics that have improved data processing capabilities (Ergin, Kherad, and Alagoz 2022). In sum, RNA-seq is an indispensable resource for genomics and molecular biology, opening up new vistas for the study of intricate biological systems and the development of targeted therapeutic approaches (Wang et al. 2023).

7.2.2.5 Comparative Genomic Hybridization (CGH)

A potent molecular cytogenetic tool for analyzing chromosomal copy number variations (CNVs) without cell culture is CGH. This approach is highly beneficial in cancer research and genetic diagnostics since it allows researchers to detect chromosomal increases and losses across the whole genome (Kahl 2015). Competitive fluorescence in situ hybridization (FISH) is the basic principle on which CGH functions. The method involves taking DNA samples from two different places: the tumor DNA and a normal DNA. Before being mixed in a 1:1 ratio, these samples are labeled with distinct fluorochromes. The test sample is usually green, while the reference sample is red. The final product is a hybrid that competes for binding sites on normal human metaphase chromosomal preparations using the tagged DNA (Smail 2022).

CGH has great utility in preimplantation genetic screening for the detection of chromosomal anomalies in embryos and onco cytogenetics for the detection of cancers with imbalanced chromosomes. Array CGH is a newer version of the technology that uses microarrays to do more in-depth genomic analyses at better resolutions. But there are several drawbacks to CGH, like the fact that it needs at least 50% abnormal cells to be reliable and that it cannot detect balanced rearrangements (Gajjar et al. 2023). Notwithstanding these obstacles, CGH is still a vital resource for molecular genetics, shedding light on chromosomal aberrations linked to cancer and other hereditary diseases.

New developments in CGH technology have greatly improved the accuracy and usefulness of this method for genetic diagnoses. Recent advances include High Resolution CGH, an improvement over traditional CGH that makes use of dynamic standard reference intervals established from normal karyotype's naturally occurring fluctuations in fluorescence intensities (Cokyaman and Silan 2022). Compared to conventional CGH techniques, this one is more sensitive, allowing for a resolution of about 4–5 megabases and the detection of abnormalities at 20–30% clonal representation. Another development that has made CGH a high-throughput method is array CGH (Sheidley et al. 2022). By using microarrays that include hundreds of unique DNA sequences, array CGH may identify differences in copy number down to the kilobase level. This development makes it possible to detect genetic abnormalities in diseases like cancer by analyzing amplifications and deletions across numerous genes all at once (Nowak et al. 2007) (Table 7.1).

Table 7.1: Comparative Analysis of Different Techniques with Their Advantages and Disadvantages

Technique/Method	Description	Application in Oncology	Tools/Resources Used	Advantages	Limitations	Cancer Types	Clinical Significance	References
Whole Genome Sequencing (WGS)	Sequencing the entire genome to identify mutations	Identifying genomic alterations across all cancers	Illumina, Oxford Nanopore	Comprehensive view of the genome	Expensive, time-consuming	Breast, lung, leukemia	Identifies driver mutations and targets	(Bagger et al. 2024)
Whole-Exome Sequencing (WES)	Sequencing of protein-coding regions (exome)	Detects somatic mutations in cancer-driving genes	Illumina, Agilent SureSelect	Cost-effective, focuses on clinically relevant mutations	Misses non-coding regions	Colorectal, breast cancer	Identifies actionable mutations	(Rabbani, Tekin, and Mahdieh 2014)
Liquid Biopsy (cfDNA, ctDNA)	Analyzing ctDNA or cfDNA from blood samples	Monitors tumor progression, treatment response	NGS, PCR-based assays	Non-invasive, real-time monitoring	Sensitivity issues, may miss some mutations	Breast, lung, prostate	Real-time therapy adjustments	(Nikanjam, Kato, and Kurzrock 2022; Gorgannezhad et al. 2018)
RNA Sequencing (RNA-Seq)	Sequencing of RNA to analyze gene expression	Detects aberrant gene expression and gene fusions	Illumina, PacBio, STAR	Functional insight into genomic alterations	Complex data analysis, RNA instability	Hematologic, sarcomas	Novel biomarker discovery	(Ozsolak and Milos 2011; Wilhelm and Landry 2009)
Targeted Gene Panels	Focused sequencing of cancer-related genes	Identifies actionable mutations in known cancer genes	Foundation One, OncoPanel	Cost-effective, faster than WGS or WES	Misses mutations outside the panel	Breast, ovarian, lung	Directs targeted therapy selection	(Fancello et al. 2019; De Koning et al. 2015)
Copy Number Variation Analysis	Detects changes in gene or chromosomal copy number	Identifies gene amplifications or deletions	aCGH, NGS	Insight into tumor growth and therapy resistance	Misses balanced structural rearrangements	Breast, glioblastoma	Identifies therapeutic targets	(Li and Olivier 2013; Coughlin, Scharer, and Shaikh 2012)
Epigenomic Profiling	Assesses DNA methylation patterns	Identifies epigenetic modifications in cancer	Bisulfite sequencing, ChIP-Seq	Detects regulatory changes in gene expression	Dynamic and reversible changes	Leukemia, colon cancer	Early detection, prognosis	(Mehrmohamadi et al. 2021; Gargiulo and Minucci 2009)

7.3 BENEFITS AND IMPACT ON TREATMENT OUTCOMES

Integrating genomic profiling into cancer treatment has significantly pushed forward personalized medicine, transforming how treatments are chosen and improving outcomes. This approach uses personalized treatment plans, predictive biomarkers, and real clinical case studies to match therapies with the specific genetic characteristics of each person's cancer, making treatments more effective. Personalized plans involve targeted therapies that focus on specific genetic mutations found through comprehensive genomic profiling (CGP). For instance, patients with RAS mutations can avoid anti-EGFR therapies that wouldn't be effective for them, while those with HER2-positive breast cancer may benefit from drugs like trastuzumab (Verdaguer, Saurí, and Macarulla 2017). Genomic insights are also enhancing immunotherapy by evaluating factors like tumor mutational burden (TMB), which helps predict how likely patients are to respond to immune checkpoint inhibitors—especially promising for cancers like melanoma and lung cancer (Hayashi et al. 2024). Genomic data is even helping to create combination therapies; for example, BRCA mutations in gastrointestinal cancers are guiding the use of platinum-based therapies and PARP inhibitors (Tarighati, Keivan, and Mahani 2023). Predictive biomarkers are essential to understanding which treatments are likely to work. They also help distinguish between prognosis and prediction. For example, prognostic biomarkers can identify patients who may need aggressive treatment due to a high risk of their disease progressing, as in some cases of metastatic colorectal cancer where elevated levels of circulating tumor DNA (ctDNA) are linked to lower survival rates (Čerina et al. 2023). Predictive biomarkers, on the other hand, show the likelihood of response to certain treatments, cutting down on the trial-and-error approach. Testing for specific biomarkers in metastatic non-small cell lung cancer (mNSCLC), for instance, helps ensure that targeted therapies are used effectively, improving survival rates (Nimeiri et al. 2022).Clinical case studies highlight the impact of genomic profiling. For example, HER2-positive breast cancer patients treated with trastuzumab have shown better survival and quality of life compared to those receiving only standard chemotherapy (Tarighati, Keivan, and Mahani 2023). Still, not every patient responds predictably, as factors like tumor variety and unidentified mutations can affect treatment success. This underscores the need for ongoing research to improve genomic testing and refine predictions (Tjota, Segal, and Wang 2024).

7.4 CHALLENGES AND LIMITATIONS

As we have seen till now, genomic profiling shows a lot of promise for tailoring cancer treatments, but it comes with a fair share of technical, clinical, and biological challenges. On the technical side, one of the main issues is getting consistent, reliable results across different labs. Variability can lead to different recommendations for patients, which can throw off the whole precision approach (Čerina et al. 2023). Another tricky area is interpreting what are called "variants of unknown significance" (VUS). These are genetic markers that researchers haven't fully figured out yet in terms of how they affect cancer or how a patient might respond to treatment. As a result, doctors may feel uncertain about basing treatment plans on them (Christofyllakis et al. 2022). Processing and analyzing all the genomic data also require considerable computational power; when there are delays, patients may face a longer wait to start the best-suited therapies (Tjota, Segal, and Wang 2024). On the clinical side, integrating genomic profiling into everyday medical practices isn't straightforward. Doctors might need to adapt their routines to fit in these complex tests, which may require some extra training and adjustments to their usual processes (Mayekar and Bivona 2017). Financial cost is another big factor; with limited insurance coverage, many people may struggle to afford these tests, particularly those in underserved communities. This often exacerbates existing healthcare inequalities (Chan, Chin, and Low 2022). Ethical and legal considerations add further complexity—doctors and patients alike must consider issues like consent, privacy, and the impact genetic findings could have on patient's family members. Handling these areas carefully is essential to help patients make informed choices and feel comfortable with genomic testing (Lonardi et al. 2022). Biologically, tumors themselves can vary a lot within a single patient—this is called tumor heterogeneity. Different sections of a tumor might have different mutations, which can lead to unpredictable treatment responses (Lee and Ross 2017). On top of that, cancer cells often evolve over time, building resistance to treatments, which means doctors need to be prepared to adjust therapies as needed (Gorgannezhad et al. 2018). Some tumors even have overlapping or conflicting mutations, which can create challenges when it comes to choosing a treatment since different mutations might suggest different therapeutic approaches (Tjota, Segal, and Wang 2024). To get the most out of genomic profiling in cancer treatment and make precision medicine a viable option for more people, these challenges need ongoing attention and improvement.

7.5 FUTURE PERSPECTIVES

Precision oncology and genomic profiling are on the cusp of a paradigm shift in cancer care and it pinpoints the specific genetic changes and mutations that cause cancer by doing a thorough analysis of DNA of the individual (Nero et al. 2022). To accurately detect genetic alterations in tumor DNA, techniques like next-generation sequencing (NGS), whole-genome sequencing (WGS) and whole-exome sequencing (WES) are currently in use. This allows for the development of individualized treatment programs that concentrate on particular discrepancies, boosting therapy efficacy while decreasing adverse effects (Lassen et al. 2021).

Precision oncology describes this targeted strategy for cancer therapy which focuses on combining patients with treatments developed to target their particular genetic makeup. It is still not easy to interpret variations of unknown significance or deal with tumor heterogeneity, in which different tumor cells contain different mutations (Malone et al. 2020). These genetic findings can only be clarified and put to clinical use with the help of standardized procedures and strong data analysis tools.

A significant amount of scientific research shows that genomic profiling has the ability to enhances patient outcomes through the use of genetic information to guide drug selection. Implications for healthcare systems as entirety include the need for more international consensus on best practices and better communication and coordination among scientists, doctors, and geneticists (Thapa et al. 2023). Genomic profiling will need to be further established as an essential constituent of clinical oncology by ongoing research, new technologies, and collaborative efforts. This study will provide patients globally with renewed optimism by improving cancer treatments and creating a healthcare system more efficient and personalized to the need of each individual (Kokkali et al. 2023).

7.6 CONCLUSION

Genomic profiling is leading an effort for transforming precision oncology by bringing light to the genetic origins of several cancers. The development of advanced sequencing technologies such as whole-genome sequencing (WGS), next-generation sequencing (NGS), and whole-exome sequencing (WES) has allowed doctors to track down specific mutations and genetic changes that promote tumor development and progression. By precisely mapping cancer genes, we can develop aimed treatments that improve treatment efficacy while minimizing side effects by tackling the specific genetic makeup of each patient's tumor. But there are obstacles to this method, and tumor heterogeneity is among them. This is because various cells in the same tumor can have different mutations, which makes treatment techniques challenging. Furthermore, in order to make correct clinical decisions based on variations of unknown significance, strong analytical tools and established methods are necessary. Multiple studies have shown that genetic profiling can be effectively used to create aimed cancer treatments, which could significantly impact patient care. It promotes a larger movement towards globally healthcare standardization and improved interdisciplinary cooperation, in addition to individual benefits. With the rapid progression of science and technology, genomic profiling has the capacity to transform the cancer therapy by providing patients with more targeted and individualized treatments. This might lead to a new era of adaptive and personalized medicine and completely change the way cancer is treated in the future.

REFERENCES

Abbasi S, Masoumi S. 2020. Next-Generation Sequencing (NGS). *Int J Advanced Sci Technol* 29(3):6364–6377.

Alkhateeb A et al. 2023. Prostate Cancer Bioinformatics Analysis: Emerging Genomic Profiling Techniques. *Translat Cancer Res* 12(1):4–7.

Bagger FO et al. 2024. Whole Genome Sequencing in Clinical Practice. *BMC Medical Genom* 17(1):39.

Baran-Gale J et al. 2018. Experimental Design for Single-Cell RNA Sequencing. *Brief Funct Genom* 17(4).

Bartha Á, Győrffy B. 2019. Comprehensive Outline of Whole Exome Sequencing Data Analysis Tools Available in Clinical Oncology. *Cancers* 11(11):1725.

Berger MF, Mardis ER. 2018. The Emerging Clinical Relevance of Genomics in Cancer Medicine. *Nature Rev Clin Oncol* 15(6):353–365.

Buermans HPJ, den Dunnen JT. 2014. Next Generation Sequencing Technology: Advances and Applications. *Biochim Biophys Acta* 1842(10):1932–1941.

Butow PN et al. 2022. Psychological Impact of Comprehensive Tumor Genomic Profiling Results for Advanced Cancer Patients. *Patient Educat Counsel* 105(7).

Čerina D et al. 2023. The Challenges and Opportunities of the Implementation of Comprehensive Genomic Profiling in Everyday Clinical Practice with Non-Small Cell Lung Cancer: National Results from Croatia. *Cancers* 15:13.

Chakravarthi BSVK et al. 2016. Genomic and Epigenomic Alterations in Cancer. *Am J Pathol* 186(7):1724–1735.

Chan HT et al. 2022. Circulating Tumor DNA-Based Genomic Profiling Assays in Adult Solid Tumors for Precision Oncology: Recent Advancements and Future Challenges. *Cancers* 14(13):3275.

Christofyllakis K et al 2022. Cost-Effectiveness of Precision Cancer Medicine-Current Challenges in the Use of next Generation Sequencing for Comprehensive Tumour Genomic Profiling and the Role of Clinical Utility Frameworks (Review). *Molec Clin Oncol* 16(1):21.

Cokyaman T, Silan F. 2022. Diagnostic Utility of Array Comparative Genomic Hybridization in Children with Neurological Diseases. *Fetal Pediat Pathol* 41(1).

Coughlin CR et al. 2012. Clinical Impact of Copy Number Variation Analysis Using High-Resolution Microarray Technologies: Advantages, Limitations and Concerns. *Genome Med* 4(10):80.

Coyle K et al. 2017. Genetic Mutations and Epigenetic Modifications: Driving Cancer and Informing Precision Medicine. *BioMed Res Int* 2017:9620870.

De Koning TJ et al. 2015. Targeted Next-Generation Sequencing Panels for Monogenetic Disorders in Clinical Diagnostics: The Opportunities and Challenges. *Expert Rev Molec Diagnost* 15(1):61–70.

Del Giacco L, Cattaneo C. 2012. Introduction to Genomics. *Meth Molec Biol* 823:79–88.

Diderich KEM et al. 2021. The Potential Diagnostic Yield of Whole Exome Sequencing in Pregnancies Complicated by Fetal Ultrasound Anomalies. *Acta Obstetr Gynecolog Scandinav* 100(6).

Eifert C et al. 2017. Clinical Application of a Cancer Genomic Profiling Assay to Guide Precision Medicine Decisions. *Personal Med* 14(4):309–325.

Ekblom R, Wolf JBW 2014. A Field Guide to Whole-Genome Sequencing, Assembly and Annotation. *Evol Appl* 7(9):1026–1042.

Ergin S et al. 2022. RNA Sequencing and Its Applications in Cancer and Rare Diseases. *Mol Biol Rep* 49(3):2325–2333.

Espinoza Pereira KN et al. 2023. Histone Mutations in Cancer. *Biochem Soc Trans* 51(5):1749–1763.

Fancello L et al. 2019. Tumor Mutational Burden Quantification from Targeted Gene Panels: Major Advancements and Challenges. *J ImmunoTher Cancer* 7(1):183.

Gajjar K et al. 2023. Array Comparative Genomic Hybridization Analysis of Products of Conception in Recurrent Pregnancy Loss for Specific Anomalies Detected by USG. *Reprod Fertil* 4(2).

Gargiulo G, Minucci S. 2009. Epigenomic Profiling of Cancer Cells. *Int J Biochem Cell Biol* 41(1):127–135.

Garofalo A et al. 2016. The Impact of Tumor Profiling Approaches and Genomic Data Strategies for Cancer Precision Medicine. *Genome Med* 8(1).

Gasperskaja E, Kučinskas V. 2017. The Most Common Technologies and Tools for Functional Genome Analysis. *Acta Med Litu* 24(1):1–11.

Ghosh J et al. 2022. Are We Right on Target? Is Comprehensive Genomic Profiling Ready for Prime Time in Resource-Constrained Settings? *JCO Global Oncol* 8.

Gorgannezhad L et al. 2018. Circulating Tumor DNA and Liquid Biopsy: Opportunities, Challenges, and Recent Advances in Detection Technologies. *Lab on a Chip* 18(8):1174–1196.

Gu W et al. 2019. Clinical Metagenomic Next-Generation Sequencing for Pathogen Detection. *Ann Rev Pathol Mech Dis* 14:319–338.

Hall MJ. et al. 2021. Oncologists' Perceptions of Tumor Genomic Profiling and the Communication of Test Results and Risks. *Public Health Genomics* 24(5–6).

Hatano K, Nonomura N. 2021. Genomic Profiling of Prostate Cancer: An Updated Review. *World J Men's Health*. 40(3):368–379.

Hayashi R et al. 2024. Molecularly Matched Therapies Identified by Comprehensive Genomic Profiling before the First-Line Setting to Provide Alternative Treatment Outcomes in Patients with Solid Tumors: 1-Year Follow-up of the Prospective FIRST-Dx Study. *J Clin Oncol* 42(16_suppl):3137–3137.

Hong M et al. 2020. RNA Sequencing: New Technologies and Applications in Cancer Research. *J Hematol Oncol* 13(1):166.

Iglesias A et al. 2014. The Usefulness of Whole-Exome Sequencing in Routine Clinical Practice. *Genet Med* 16(12).

Kahl, G. 2015. Array Comparative Genomic Hybridization (aCGH, Matrix Comparative Genomic Hybridization, Matrix CGH, Matrix-based Comparative Genomic Hybridization, Array CGH, Array-based Comparative Genomic Hybridization, CGH Chip). In The Dictionary of Genomics, Transcriptomics, and Proteomics (5th ed., 4-volume set; pp. 2742). Wiley-Blackwell. ISBN-13: 978-3-527-67867-9.

Kim N et al. 2023. Perspectives on Single-Nucleus RNA Sequencing in Different Cell Types and Tissues. *J Pathol Translat Med* 57(1).

Kokkali S et al. 2023. Genomic Profiling and Clinical Outcomes of Targeted Therapies in Adult Patients with Soft Tissue Sarcomas. *Cells* 12(22):2632.

Kontomanolis E et al. 2020. Role of Oncogenes and Tumor-Suppressor Genes in Carcinogenesis: A Review. *Anticancer Res* 40(11):6009–6015.

Krzyszczyk P et al. 2018. The Growing Role of Precision and Personalized Medicine for Cancer Treatment. *Technol* 06(03n04):79–100.

Kwong JC et al. 2015. Whole Genome Sequencing in Clinical and Public Health Microbiology. *Pathol* 47(3).

Lassen UN et al 2021. Precision Oncology: A Clinical and Patient Perspective. *Future Oncol* 17(30):3995–4009.

Lee H, Ross JS. 2017. The Potential Role of Comprehensive Genomic Profiling to Guide Targeted Therapy for Patients with Biliary Cancer. *Therapeut Adv Gastroenterol* 10(6):507–520.

Li W, Olivier M. 2013. Current Analysis Platforms and Methods for Detecting Copy Number Variation. *Physiol Genom* 45(1).

Lonardi S et al. 2022. Comprehensive Genomic Profiling (CGP)-Informed Personalized Molecular Residual Disease (MRD) Detection: An Exploratory Analysis from the PREDATOR Study of Metastatic Colorectal Cancer (MCRC) Patients Undergoing Surgical Resection. *Int J Molec Sci* 23(19).

Malone ER et al. 2020. Molecular Profiling for Precision Cancer Therapies. *Genome Med* 12(1):8.

Martincorena I, Campbell PJ. 2015. Somatic Mutation in Cancer and Normal Cells. *Science* 349(6255):1483–1489.

Mathew A et al. 2022. Clinical Benefit of Comprehensive Genomic Profiling for Advanced Cancers in India. *JCO Glob Oncol* 8:e2100421.

Mayekar MK, Bivona TG. 2017. Current Landscape of Targeted Therapy in Lung Cancer. *Clin Pharmacol Therapeut* 102(5).

Mehrmohamadi M et al 2021. A Comparative Overview of Epigenomic Profiling Methods. *Front Cell Development Biol* 9:714687.

Morris LGT, Chan TA. 2015. Therapeutic Targeting of Tumor Suppressor Genes. *Cancer* 121(9):1357–1368.

Nakagawa H, Fujita M. 2018. Whole Genome Sequencing Analysis for Cancer Genomics and Precision Medicine. *Cancer Sci* 109(3):513–522.

Nero C et al. 2022. Integrating a Comprehensive Cancer Genome Profiling into Clinical Practice: A Blueprint in an Italian Referral Center. *J Personal Med* 12(10):1746.

Nikanjam, M et al. 2022. Liquid Biopsy: Current Technology and Clinical Applications. *J Hematol Oncol* 15(1):131.

Nimeiri H et al. 2022. Comprehensive Genomic Profiling (CGP)-Informed Personalized Molecular Residual Disease (MRD) Detection: An Exploratory Analysis from the PREDATOR Study of Metastatic Colorectal Cancer (MCRC) Patients Undergoing Surgical Resection. *J Clin Oncol* 40(4_suppl).

Nowak NJ et al. 2007. Challenges in Array Comparative Genomic Hybridization for the Analysis of Cancer Samples. *Genet Med* 9(9).

Ostroverkhova D et al. 2023. Cancer Driver Mutations: Predictions and Reality. *Trends Molec Med* 29(7):554–566.

Ozsolak F, Milos PM. 2011. RNA Sequencing: Advances, Challenges and Opportunities. *Nature Rev Genet* 12(2):87–98.

Pankiw M et al. 2024. Comprehensive Genomic Profiling for Oncological Advancements by Precision Medicine. *Med Oncol* 41(1):1.

Peleg Hasson S et al. 2023. Implementation of Comprehensive Genomic Profiling in Ovarian Cancer Patients: A Retrospective Analysis. *Cancers* 15(1).

Previs RA et al. 2016. The Rise of Genomic Profiling in Ovarian Cancer. *Expert Rev Molec Diagnost* 16(12):1337–1351.

Rabbani B et al. 2014. The Promise of Whole-Exome Sequencing in Medical Genetics. *J Hum Genet* 59(1):5–15.

Rolfo C et al. 2020. Challenges and Opportunities of CfDNA Analysis Implementation in Clinical Practice: Perspective of the International Society of Liquid Biopsy (ISLB). *Crit Rev Oncol Hematol* 151:102978.

Rossing M et al. 2019. Whole Genome Sequencing of Breast Cancer. *APMIS* 127(5):303–315.

Satam H et al. 2023. Next-Generation Sequencing Technology: Current Trends and Advancements. *Biology* 12(7).

Sheidley BR et al. 2022. Genetic Testing for the Epilepsies: A Systematic Review. *Epilepsia* 63(2).

Shi W et al. 2018. Reliability of Whole-Exome Sequencing for Assessing Intratumor Genetic Heterogeneity. *Cell Rep* 25(6).

Slatko BE et al. 2018. Overview of Next-Generation Sequencing Technologies. *Curr Prot Molec Biol* 122(1).

Smail HO. 2022. The Roles of the Fluorescent In Situ Hybridization (FISH) and Comparative Genomic Hybridization (CGH) Techniques in the Detection of the Breast Cancer. *Biol Med Natural Product Chem* 11(1).

Tarighati E et al. 2023. A Review of Prognostic and Predictive Biomarkers in Breast Cancer. *Clin Experiment Med* 23(1):1–16.

Tarride JE et al. 2022. Challenges of Conducting Value Assessment for Comprehensive Genomic Profiling. *Int J Technol Assess Health Care* 38(1):e57.

Thapa B et al. 2023. Comprehensive Genomic Profiling: Does Timing Matter? *Front Oncol* 13.

Tjota MY et al. 2024. Clinical Utility and Benefits of Comprehensive Genomic Profiling in Cancer. *Appl Lab Med* 9(1):76–91.

Tsimberidou AM et al. 2020. Review of Precision Cancer Medicine: Evolution of the Treatment Paradigm. *Cancer Treat Rev* 86:102019.

Turgeon MO et al. 2018. DNA Damage, Repair, and Cancer Metabolism. *Front Oncol* 8:15.

Verdaguer H et al. 2017. Predictive and Prognostic Biomarkers in Personalized Gastrointestinal Cancer Treatment. *J Gastrointest Oncol* 8(3):405–417.

Wang S et al. 2023. The Evolution of Single-Cell RNA Sequencing Technology and Application: Progress and Perspectives. *Int J Molec Sci* 24(3):2943.

Wilhelm BT, Landry JR. 2009. RNA-Seq-Quantitative Measurement of Expression through Massively Parallel RNA-Sequencing. *Methods* 48(3):249–57.

Yang Y et al. 2013. Clinical Whole-Exome Sequencing for the Diagnosis of Mendelian Disorders. *New Engl J Med* 369(16).

8

Pharmacogenomics and Personalized Cancer Treatment

Rituparna Choudhury, Chandan Kumar Bahadi, and Kumar Nikhil

8.1 INTRODUCTION TO PHARMACOGENOMICS

8.1.1 Historical Context of Pharmacogenomics

8.1.1.1 Early Foundations: Archibald Garrod (1909)

A British physician "Archibald Garrod" made an early contribution to the understanding of genetic influences on disease in the year 1909. He proposed the concept of inborn errors of metabolism—an idea that genetic defects can lead to metabolic disorders. Garrod's work laid the foundation for future research on how genetic variations might affect drug metabolism and response. He was the first to suggest that some individuals could have unique genetic profiles that might cause them to have unusual reactions to some chemicals, including drugs. A famous quote of his stated, "Every active drug is a poison when taken in large enough doses, and in some subjects, a dose which is innocuous to the majority of people has toxic effects, whereas others show exceptional tolerance to the drug." This concept predicted the eventual emergence of pharmacogenetics and pharmacogenomics (Figure 8.1) [1].

8.1.1.2 Arthur L. Fox (1932)

After Garrod, an American geneticist, Arthur L. Fox, made an important discovery that linked genetics to the perception of taste in the year 1932. In this discovery, he found that some individuals could not taste phenylthiocarbamide (PTC), a compound with a bitter taste that is present in certain foods like broccoli. This lack of sensitivity was shown to be linked to polymorphisms in the TAS2R38 gene, which codes for a bitter taste receptor. His discovery was one of the earliest demonstrations that genetic variations can influence how people interact with and respond to certain dietary components. This eventually contributed to the broader field of pharmacogenetics, where both food and drugs are foreign substances (xenobiotics) that our bodies must metabolize (Figure 8.1) [1].

8.1.1.3 Genetic Factors in Drug Metabolism: 1950s–1960s

Friedrich Vogel in 1959 coined the term pharmacogenetics, which marked the formation of the field (Figure 8.1). His work was influenced by several key observations of how genetic factors influence the metabolism of certain drugs:

N-acetyltransferase: N-acetyltransferase (an enzyme involved in the metabolism of drugs like isoniazid used to treat tuberculosis) was discovered with genetic defects. Some individuals were found to be slow acetylators. These individuals have a slow pace of drug metabolism. Slow acetylators possess a greater risk of drug toxicity.

Glucose-6-phosphate dehydrogenase (G6PD) deficiency: Hemolysis, i.e., the destruction of red blood cells, can be found in patients with defects in G6PD, a genetic condition when these individuals are exposed to certain drugs like primaquine, a drug used to treat malaria. This phenomenon showed how genetic deficiencies could result in adverse drug reactions.

Plasma cholinesterase deficiency: The inability to break down succinylcholine—a muscle relaxant used in anesthesia—causing prolonged apnea (difficulty in breathing) in some individuals. This discovery illustrated how genetic variations could affect the efficacy and safety of anesthesia agents.

CYP2D6 deficiency: In the 1960s, certain individuals were found to have a deficiency in the enzyme CYP2D6, which metabolizes various drugs. This finding showed that genetic differences in drug-metabolizing enzymes could lead to either toxic effects or reduced therapeutic efficacy in different individuals [1].

8.1.1.4 Expansion into Pharmacogenomics (1970s–present)

The above-mentioned discoveries led to the expansion of the field of pharmacogenetics. Researchers initiated exploring the genetic basis for the variation in drug metabolism and response on a broader scale, leading to the emergence of pharmacogenomics, including the study

DOI: 10.1201/9781003542162-8

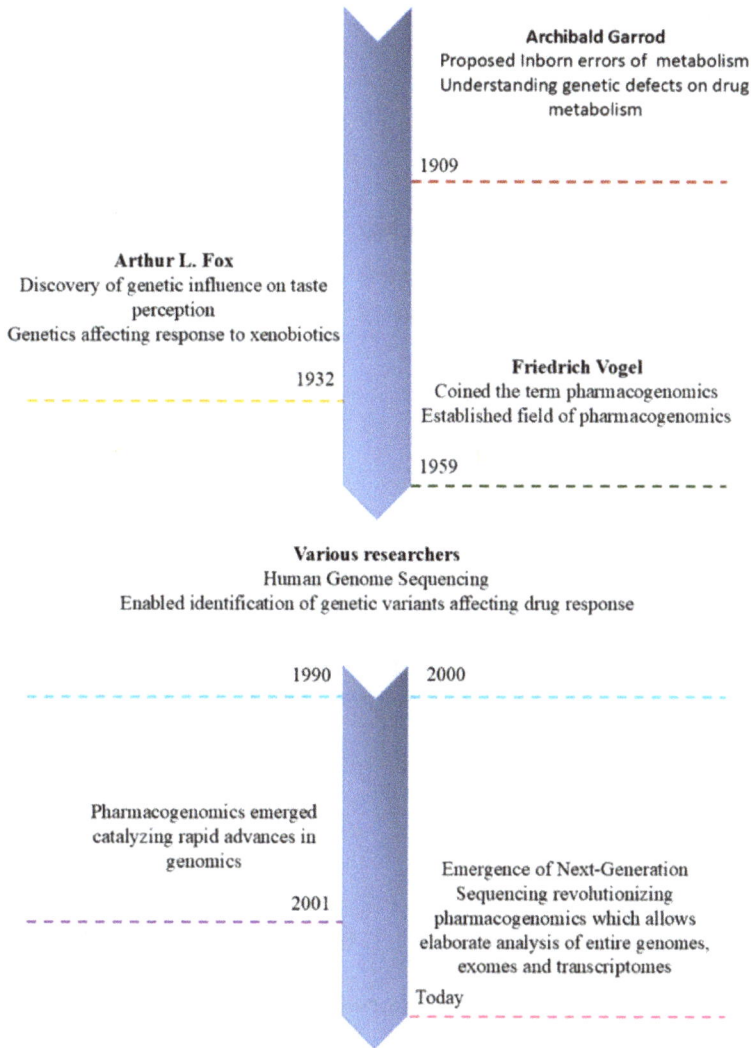

Figure 8.1 Key milestones in pharmacogenomics.

of the entire genome to understand drug interactions. This field gained more recognition as the genetic foundation of drug response became clearer, and as advances in molecular biology paved the way for the identification of specific genes involved in drug metabolism by the 1990s. During the early 2000s, human genome sequencing provided further momentum for pharmacogenomics, which made it possible to identify genetic variants that affect drug responses in populations. Pharmacogenomics had started moving from a niche area of research into clinical practice, with the ability to personalize medicine and optimize drug therapy based on an individual's genetic profile (Figure 8.1) [1].

8.1.2 Overview of Pharmacogenomics: Definition and Importance in Modern Medicine

Pharmacogenomics is a branch of pharmacology concerned with using DNA and amino acid sequence data to inform drug development and testing. This field plays a crucial role in modern medicine by integrating genomic data into drug development, testing, and treatment strategies to tailor therapies to individual patients. Following the human genome sequencing in 2001, this field emerged, catalyzing rapid advances in genomics and highlighting the importance of understanding the complex correlation between genes, health, and disease [1]. Pharmacogenomics provides the niche to design more effective and safer drugs tailored to an individual's genetic makeup by understanding the genetic variations that influence drug responses (Figure 8.2). This

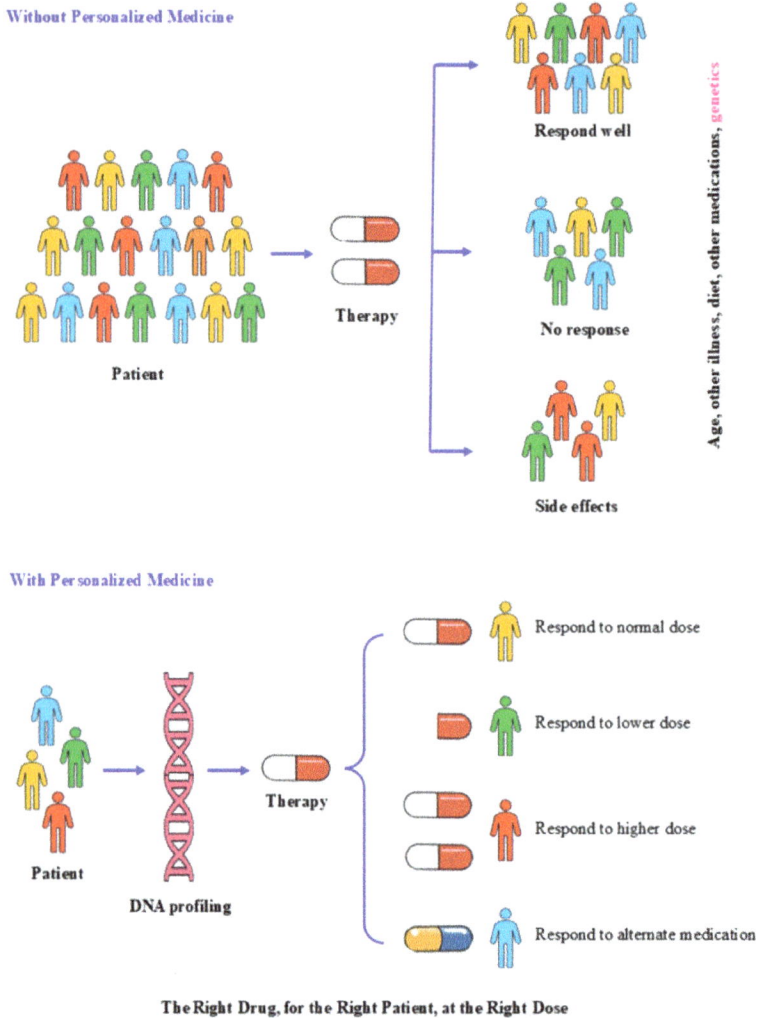

Figure 8.2 Pharmacogenomics and drug response in individuals with different genotypes.

can eventually help optimize drug dosages, avoid adverse drug reactions, and improve treatment outcomes. This unique approach has been applied to complex diseases such as cardiovascular disorders, diabetes, psychiatric conditions, and cancer. Pharmacogenomics aids in the development of targeted therapies in cancer, where somatic mutations in oncogenes and germline mutations in drug-metabolizing genes can dictate the success of treatments. Advances in technologies such as Next-Generation Technologies have now revolutionized pharmacogenomics by allowing the elaborate analysis of entire genomes, exomes, and even transcriptomes. These data can help identify genetic factors that influence disease risk and treatment responses, providing the foundation for more personalized therapies. However, the integration of such large-scale data into clinical practice remains challenging due to the complexity of genome-phenome relationships [2]. Pharmacogenomics is also about newer treatment strategies, such as RNA-based therapies, gene editing, and gene therapy. These therapies can be designed based on an individual's genetic profile. For example, mRNA vaccines, antisense RNAs, and micro RNAs hold promise for treating inherited disorders, cancer, cardiovascular disease, and infectious diseases [1].

8.2 BIOMARKERS IN PHARMACOGENOMICS

8.2.1 Drug-Metabolizing Enzyme and Transporters

Pharmacogenomics examines how genetic variations affect drug absorption, distribution, metabolism, and excretion. Genetic variants in enzymes, transporters, and receptors can significantly influence drug metabolism (Table 8.1). For instance, cytochrome P450 (CYP) enzymes, involved in phase 1 drug metabolism, metabolize a wide range of drugs. Genetic variations in these enzymes can alter drug efficacy and toxicity. ABCB1 (MDR1), a transporter, plays crucial role in drug absorption and elimination. Understanding these genetic factors is essential for personalized medicine. Assessing whether genetic variants enhance or reduce enzyme activity impacts drug responses. Age, sex, and conditions like smoking can also affect enzyme activity, further complicating pharmacogenomic assessments [1].

8.2.2 Adverse Drug Reactions (ADRs)

Certain genetic variations in drug-metabolizing enzymes or transporters lead to Adverse Drug Reactions (ADRs). For example, the drug irinotecan, activated by an esterase and inactivated by UGT1A1 (a glucuronidation enzyme), can cause toxicity in individuals with certain UGT1A1 gene variants. These genetic biomarkers can be used to predict adverse reactions and guide dosing. However, factors like drug-drug interactions, age, or liver function can influence the severity of ADRs. Thus, pharmacogenetic testing must take into consideration both genetic and environmental factors to optimize drug therapy and minimize side effects [1].

8.3 PHARMACOGENOMICS IN CANCER TREATMENT

Pharmacogenomics plays a key role in the development of targeted therapies for cancer. Molecular biomarker identification has approved several treatments that target specific genetic mutations or overexpressed proteins in tumors [1]. For example, trastuzumab (Herceptin) targets the HER2 protein, which is overexpressed in certain breast cancers. Breast cancers being the fifth leading cause of cancer among women throughout the world marks a global concern due to the lack of effective therapeutic approaches [3]. Next-Generation Sequencing (NGS) has enabled precise identification of mutations and other biomarkers such as Tumor Mutational Burden (TMB) or microsatellite instability, leading to revolution in cancer treatment. This can predict responses to therapies like immune checkpoint inhibitors [4]. Along with tumor-specific mutations, targeted therapies have evolved to include broader genetic signatures like BRCAness, which can predict response to drugs like PARP inhibitors. However, the effectiveness of targeted therapies can be limited by cancer resistance mechanisms like secondary mutations or tumor heterogeneity. This has led to the development of combination therapies and the use of liquid biopsies to monitor tumor evolution and therapeutic resistance in real time [5].

8.4 GENETIC VARIABILITY IN DRUG RESPONSE

Pharmacogenomics is known to have transformed cancer treatment by introducing advances in genomic science. The paradigm shift from a one-size-fits-all approach to precision medicine has brought significant change in cancer care. Genetic factors play a major role in how different patients metabolize cancer drugs, influencing both their effectiveness and potential for toxicity. By understanding these genetic variations, clinicians can design treatments for individual patients, optimizing drug dosages, selecting the most effective therapies, and minimizing side effects. Drugs like irinotecan impart significant variability in patient response in colorectal cancer. Hence, understanding the genetic variations in this context is particularly important in cancers like colorectal cancer (CRC). Genetic screening and personalized treatment strategies are becoming essential in oncology, improving outcomes by reducing side effects, enhancing drug efficacy, and ensuring more cost-effective care [6].

Table 8.1: Drug-Metabolizing Enzymes and Transporters Involved in Pharmacogenomics

	Enzyme / Transporter	Function	Genetic Variations Impact	Example Drug Affected
1	Cytochrome P450 (CYP) enzymes	Phase 1 drug metabolism (oxidation, reduction, hydrolysis)	Variations can alter drug efficacy and toxicity	Warfarin, Clopidogrel, Diazepam
2	ABCB1 (MDR1)	Drug absorption and elimination	Variants effect drug absorption and elimination rates	Digoxin, Tacrolimus, Vincristine
3	UGT1A1	Inactivation of certain drugs via glucuronidation	Variants can reduce drug inactivation, increasing toxicity	Irinotecan, Bilirubin

8.4.1 Genetic Factors Affecting Drug Metabolism

Genomic science, proteomics, and pharmacogenomics have undergone various recent advancements that have transformed cancer care. With the integration of NGS and companion diagnostics, more targeted treatments have been developed, drifting away from the traditional chemotherapy approach. This medical approach, along with improving treatment efficacy, also helps in managing drug toxicities, tailoring dosages to individual patient metabolism. Pharmacogenomic research enables clinicians to predict potential side effects or treatment failures based on individual genetic variations. This knowledge supports personalized treatment plans aiming to reduce toxicity and enhance the effectiveness of drugs like chemotherapy and immunotherapies. Colorectal cancer, one of the most common and deadly cancers worldwide, has ongoing improvements in early detection and treatment leading to better survival rates. Targeted therapies and biologic agents, e.g., bevacizumab, cetuximab, are now core to treating metastatic colorectal cancer, offering improved response rates and survival benefits. Pharmacogenomics, specifically genetic testing of variations such as UGT1A1*28 and KRAS status, plays a critical role in optimizing the use of drugs like irinotecan, reducing toxicities and adjusting dosages based on the patient's genetic makeup [6]. Irinotecan, a chemotherapy drug used in colorectal cancer treatment, can cause severe toxicities, especially neutropenia and diarrhea. These toxicities vary due to genetic differences between patients, including ethnic variations. Genetic screening for variations in genes like UGT1A1 helps guide treatment decisions. This allows for tailored dosing to reduce toxicity while maintaining therapeutic effectiveness [6]. The integration of genetic screening before administering chemotherapy, including irinotecan, is key to personalizing treatment regimens. By considering genetic factors, alongside patient specific characteristics (e.g., liver function, medications), healthcare providers can optimize therapy to reduce side effects and improve treatment outcomes [6]. Personalized medicine approaches could lower chemotherapy related toxicity and associated healthcare costs while enhancing the effectiveness of treatment.

Cancer treatment decisions are more complex than ever, requiring the integration of molecular data, genetic testing and patient specific factors such as co-morbidities, medications and lifestyle. With the rise of genomic technologies and AI, clinicians are better equipped to make informed decisions, although the complexity of this data can overwhelm individual oncologists. AI tools can help manage and interpret vast amounts of molecular and clinical data, ensuring the consistent application of evidence-based practices in oncology care. The cost of genetic and genomic tests has significantly decreased in recent years, making them more accessible for routine use in clinical practice. These tests are not only essential for improving patient outcomes but also for reducing the cost of ineffective treatments or severe drug toxicities which could lead to costly emergency visits or hospitalizations. The broader use of genetic testing is expected to enhance decision-making in cancer care, providing more precise and effective treatments for patients.

8.4.2 Pharmacodynamics and Pharmacokinetics

Pharmacodynamics and pharmacokinetics are the two fundamental components of drug development, particularly in oncology. These two disciplines help determine how a drug interacts with the body (pharmacodynamics) and how the body affects the drug (pharmacokinetics). Both the areas are crucial for understanding the efficacy, safety and therapeutic potential of new drugs, including those used in cancer treatment [1].

8.4.3 Pharmacodynamics: Mechanisms of Action and Drug-Target Interactions

Pharmacodynamics refers to the study of the effects of drugs on the body, especially at the molecular and cellular levels. It focuses on how drugs interact with biological targets, such as proteins, enzymes, receptors and ion channels to produce their therapeutic effects [1]. Pharmacodynamics is the central focus to be understood how cancer therapies exert their anticancer effects in oncology, which can involve inhibition of cancer cell proliferation, induction of apoptosis, interference with DNA repair or modulation of signaling pathways [1, 7].

8.4.3.1 Key Aspects of Pharmacodynamics in Oncology
8.4.3.1.1 Mechanism of Action

Many cancer drugs particularly targeted therapies and biologics are designed to interact with specific molecular targets in cancer cells. These targets include oncogenic proteins, signaling pathways, and mutated genes that drive tumor growth.

ALK inhibitors: Anaplastic lymphoma kinase is a protein involved in several cancers, particularly non-small-cell-lung cancer (NSCLC). Drugs like crizotinib, ceritinib, alectinib, brigatinib and lorlatinib target ALK, which is often mutated or fused with ALK (e.g., EML4-ALK) in cancer cells. These inhibitors block the activity of the mutated ALK protein leading to reduced tumor cell proliferation and increased apoptosis [8].

Targeted inhibition and downstream effect: Some ALK inhibitors like ceritinib and brigatinib affect downstream signaling pathways such as STAT3 and AKT. These are involved in cell survival and growth. Inhibition of these pathways can lead to reduced tumor cell proliferation, tumor shrinkage and complete regression [8].

8.4.3.1.2 Cytotoxicity and Apoptosis

Maximum cancer drugs have the capability to induce cell death through various form of cytotoxicity. Some of them might induce DNA damage leading to the activation of apoptotic pathways. Others interfere with the cellular division therein inducing mitotic catastrophe and apoptosis [1].

8.4.3.1.3 Resistance Mechanisms

A critical issue involved in cancer treatment is drug resistance. The evolution of cancer cells to evade drug action is often included in pharmacodynamic studies. Some mutations in the ALK gene can reduce drug binding and efficacy, promoting the development of 2nd and 3rd generation ALK inhibitors (Table 8.2) [8].

8.4.4 Pharmacokinetics

The reaction of the body towards the action of a drug is what called as pharmacokinetics. Determining the appropriate dosing, frequency and duration of treatment is very crucial along with the understanding of the drug's potential for toxicity or therapeutic failure. Pharmacokinetics is a major tool in cancer treatment as it can help optimize the efficacy of drugs and minimize side effects [7].

8.4.4.1 Key Aspects of Pharmacokinetics in Oncology

Absorption: The process by which a drug enters the bloodstream. Every drug varies based on factors such as solubility, formulation, and gastrointestinal conditions.

Blood-brain barrier penetration: Few cancer drugs behold the need to penetrate the blood-brain barrier to treat brain metastases. Drugs such as ceritinib and lorlatinib have some ability to cross the blood-brain barrier. Among the two, lorlatinib has shown efficacy in patients with ALK-positive NSCLC and brain metastases [7].

Table 8.2: Mechanisms of Action of ALK Inhibitors in Cancer Therapy

	Mechanism	Details	Drugs Example	Therapeutic Effects	Resistance Mechanisms
1	Targeted inhibition of ALK	ALK inhibitors target the mutated or fused ALK protein, such as EML-4, ALK in cancer cells	Crizotinib, Ceritinib, Alectinib, Brigatinib, Lorlatinib	Reduces tumor cell proliferation, promotes apoptosis	ALK gene mutations reducing drug binding and efficacy
2	Downstream signaling pathways	Inhibition of downstream pathways such as STAT3 and AKT which are involved in cell survival and growth	Ceritinib, Brigatinib	Reduced tumor cell proliferation, tumor shrinkage, or regression	Mutation in the ALK gene or other compensatory signaling pathways
3	Cytotoxicity and apoptosis	Induction of DNA damage and mitotic catastrophe leading to apoptosis	All ALK inhibitors	Cell death, tumor regression	Resistance can occur through mutations preventing DNA damage or apoptosis induction
4	Pharmacokinetics (Blood-brain barrier penetration)	Some ALK inhibitors cross the blood–brain barrier to treat brain metastases.	Lorlatinib, Ceritinib	Effective against brain metastases in ALK-positive NSCLC	Resistance mechanism in the brain microenvironment.

Metabolism: These drugs primarily undergo metabolism in the liver where enzymes such as cytochrome P450 is involved. This metabolic process is responsible for activating or deactivating the drug, affecting its efficacy and potential toxicity. Drug metabolism is also influenced by enzyme polymorphism, leading to variations in drug response among individuals.

Excretion: This marks the final phase of pharmacokinetics which is done primarily via the kidneys or the liver.

Drug interactions and personalized medicine: The field of pharmacokinetics is also extended to the exploration of how drugs interact with other medications. For example, the interaction of ALK inhibitors with other therapies such as chemotherapy and immunotherapy when used in combination with it. This enables the understanding of potential drug-drug interaction which could highly impact the efficacy and toxicity of treatments [1]. Personalized medicine deals with the genetic variations in enzymes and transporters to design treatments for individual patients. Thus, pharmacodynamics and pharmacokinetics play a vital role for the development and optimization of cancer therapies [1]. Therapeutic efficiencies can be increased along with minimizing side effects only by understanding how drugs interact with biological targets and how the body processes these drugs. Personalized approaches are becoming increasingly important, offering hope for more effective cancer treatments. They account for genetic variations in drug targets metabolism and transport [1, 5].

8.5 ADVANCES IN CANCER CARE AND THE ROLE OF PHARMACOGENOMICS

In the past few years, cancer care has evolved drastically due to the advances in genomic sciences. There has been the emergence and development of targeted therapies and immunotherapies along with the application of pharmacogenomics to personalize treatment regimens. This chapter focuses on the evolving complexity of cancer care paying attention to the treatments that are selected and optimized for individual patients. Traditional chemotherapy treatments are being replaced by more precise therapies that consider genetic makeup, drug metabolism and response to specific treatments.

8.5.1 Advances in Cancer Treatments

Targeted therapies and immunotherapies: These treatments particularly target cancer cells or improve the body's immune response to fight cancer. This offers a more effective alternative to conventional chemotherapy. However, they hold some unique toxicity profiles that require specialized management.

Next-Generation Sequencing: This technology provides detailed genetic analysis of tumors which enables the identification of specific mutations and help chose a therapy.

Companion diagnostics: These tests are performed to help determine that whether a patient is likely to benefit from a particular treatment being prescribed for them based on their genetic and molecular profile.

8.5.2 The Role of Pharmacogenomics

Personalized medicine: Designing of treatments by understanding how a patient's genetic variations affect drug metabolism, response and side effects. Pharmacogenomics allows clinicians to design personalized cancer treatments. This plays a crucial role in optimizing drug dosing and selection, reduces the risk of adverse reactions or treatment failures.

Toxicity management: Pharmacogenomics help predict who may experience toxic effects based on their genetic makeup. Here, cancer treatments are more targeted, managing their specific toxicities shows up to be an important part of cancer care [1, 5].

Pharmacokinetics and dosing: The relationship between drug dose, blood concentration, and treatment response is very essential as some drugs might not follow the expected dose response curve and a higher dose may not always lead to better outcomes. These could increase toxicity. Hence, pharmacokinetics guided dosing, which is using the drug concentration monitoring to guide dosing is exemplified by the use of busulfan in hematopoietic cell transplantation. To adjust the dosage to optimize therapeutic outcomes and reduce risks the drug's pharmacokinetic properties are to be monitored [1, 4].

8.5.3 Challenges and Opportunities in Supportive Care

Pharmacogenomics is important in selecting and dosing supportive care drugs, such as antinausea agents or pain management medications. These can have varying effects based on the individual genetic profiles. Despite these advances, translation of pharmacogenomics research into routine clinical practice remains a challenge. Integrating and implementing pharmacogenomics into everyday cancer care requires infrastructure, training, and clearer guidelines for oncologist's help. Clearly, more research and refinement are needed to make pharmacogenomic testing and pharmacokinetic guided dosing standard practice across different cancer treatments. Enhancement of precision medicine can also be achieved by integrating pharmacogenomics data into clinical workflows (Table 8.3) [1, 2].

8.6 PERSONALIZED MEDICINE IN ONCOLOGY: Revolutionizing Cancer Treatment

Traditionally, cancer therapies were applied to cancer populations keeping in mind the cancer type and stage. There was limited individual patient characteristics consideration but, with advances in genomics and molecular biology, the focus has drifted from the traditional cancer therapies to individualized treatment approaches. Personalized medicine's main aim is to design cancer treatment based on the unique genetic makeup of an individual patient, focusing on more targeted and effective therapies reducing adverse effects and improve outcomes.

Table 8.3: **Advances in Cancer Care and the Role of Pharmacogenomics**

	Category	Description	Examples
1	Advances in cancer treatment	Evolving therapies offering more precision, reducing side effects, compared to traditional methods.	Targeted therapies, immunotherapies, Next-Generation Sequencing, Companion diagnostics
2	Targeted therapies	Therapies designed to target cancer cells, based on genetic makeup, often reducing collateral damage to healthy cells.	Trastuzumab (HER2 positive breast cancer), Erlotinib (EGFR mutations in lung cancer)
3	Immunotherapies	Enhances the immune system's ability to fight cancer	Pembrolizumab, Nivolumab (immune checkpoint inhibitors for melanoma and NSCLC)
4	Next-Generation Sequencing	Technology allowing for detailed genetic analysis of tumors to identify specific mutations, enabling more precise treatment selection.	Used to identify mutations like EGFR, BCR-ABL fusion protein.
5	Companion diagnostics	Tests that determine whether a patient will benefit from a specific treatment based on their genetic or molecular profile	KRAS testing for EGFR targeted therapy in lung cancer.
6	Pharmacogenomics	The study of how genetic variations affect drug metabolism, response and toxicity allowing for personalized cancer treatment regimens.	Reduces adverse reactions and optimizes drug dosing based on genetic variations.
7	Personalized medicine	Treatment strategies designs based on the individual's genetic profile, aiming for more effective therapies with fewer side effects.	EGFR targeted therapies in lung cancer, HER-2 targeted therapies in breast cancer.
8	Toxicity management	Use of pharmacogenomics to predict and manage drug toxicity based on patient's genetic makeup.	Busulfan dosing in hematopoietic cell transplantation.
9	Pharmacokinetics and Dosing	Monitoring drug concentrations to adjust dosing for optimal therapeutic outcomes and to reduce risks of toxicity.	Busulfan concentration monitoring during transplantation.
10	Challenges in Supportive Care	Despite advances, integrating pharmacogenomics into routine clinical practice is still a challenge due to infrastructure and training needs.	Pharmacogenomics in supportive care for pain management and anti-nausea medications.
11	Traditional Cancer Treatments	Traditional approaches like chemotherapy, radiation, and surgery, though effective, have limitations in efficacy and side effects.	Chemotherapy, radiation therapy, surgery.
12	Limitations of Traditional Treatments	Chemotherapy can cause collateral damage and treatment resistance, surgery is not viable for all tumors, and radiation can damage healthy tissues.	Severe side effects like immunosuppression, nausea, hair loss, fibrosis, organ damage.

8.6.1 The Limitations of Traditional Cancer Treatment Approaches

Cancer treatment has relied on the three preliminary pillars for decades: surgery, radiation therapy, and chemotherapy. These treatment approaches have made significant contributions to improving cancer, but they come with their own limitations, especially in terms of efficacy, toxicity and the development of treatment resistance.

Surgery: For localized tumors, surgery is the most promising treatment but with metastases it becomes less viable [9]. Tumors located near vital organs cannot be removed completely. Successful surgeries also inherit the risk of infections, bleeding and complications that can arise due to incomplete excision [10].

Radiation therapy: One of the most essential and promising treatment for various cancers. It beholds a limitation by often causing collateral damage to surrounding healthy tissues [11]. It is highly effective in shrinking tumors but is associated with long-term side effects. It can cause fibrosis, organ damage and in some cases may also cause secondary malignancies [12].

Chemotherapy: For decades, chemotherapy has been the systemic cancer treatment even after being a non-specific approach as it targets all rapidly dividing cells and not only cancer cells. Chemotherapy's lack of specificity has always led to severe side effects including immunosuppression, nausea, and hair loss [9]. Many cancers have been found to develop resistance to chemotherapy over time. This could diminish its long-term efficacy. These limitations of the traditional treatment's available underscore the need for more precise treatment options where comes the personalized medicine with more promising solutions [12].

8.7 EMERGENCE OF PERSONALIZED MEDICINE IN ONCOLOGY

Unlike the one-size-fits-all approach of the traditional therapies, the emergence of personalized treatment has given a paradigm shift in cancer treatment. Personalized medicine has its own unique strategy of using genetic and molecular profiling to identify specific mutations driving a patient's cancer [9]. This understanding of personalized medicine has allowed oncologists to select the most appropriate and effective treatment strategies designed to the unique characteristics of the tumor. Personalized medicine has offered a more precise, effective and less toxic cancer care.

With the completion of the Human Genome Project in 2003, a milestone had been marked in the field of personalized medicine by providing the foundation for understanding the genetic makeup of cancer. Since then, researchers had found out a range of mutations and genetic alterations for example, EGFR (Epidermal Growth Factor Receptor) in lung, breast and ovarian cancer. These have become now target for specific therapies. These therapies have led to a new era of cancer treatment. Therapy is now no longer based on tumor type alone, but also on the molecular profile of the tumor itself [13].

8.7.1 Key Components of Personalized Medicine in Oncology

Genetic Profiling and targeted therapy: Targeted therapies can be developed by identifying specific genetic mutations or alterations that drive tumor growth and progression. These targeted therapies block the activity of the proteins or in some cases the pathways responsible for cancer occurrence and progression. For instance, trastuzumab for HER2-positive breast cancer and erlotinib for EGFR mutated lung cancer have caused significant improvement in patients. They precisely focused on the underlying molecular causes of cancer rather than the tumor's location [14].

Immunotherapy: This form of therapy for cancer particularly harnesses the body's immune system and recognizes the cancer cells to destroy them. This treatment has shown remarkable success in some known aggressive cancers such as melanoma and non-small cell lung cancer (NSCLC). Immunotherapeutic agents such as checkpoint inhibitors, e.g., pembrolizumab, has an important role in revolutionizing cancer treatment. It reactivates the immune cells that were previously suppressed by the tumor [15].

8.7.2 Distinguishing Personalized Medicine from Traditional Oncology

The most distinct and significant difference between traditional oncology and personalized medicine is specificity. The age-old traditional cancer therapies such as chemotherapy and radiation do not differentiate among the cancerous cells and the healthy cells. This inability of differentiation often leads to substantial side effects [10]. For instance, chemotherapy can be administered to all patients with lung cancer but personalized medicine would differ in treatment based on whether a patient's tumor carries an EGFR mutation or not. This aims to give more effective treatment with fewer side effects [13]. Personalized oncology often employs for advanced diagnostic tools such as liquid biopsies. These technologies promise to monitor treatment response in real time. Liquid biopsies primarily allow for non-invasive detection of genetic mutations or alterations from a blood sample. This detection provides dynamic insights into tumor evolution and enables oncologists to tailor treatment plans accordingly [16].

8.8 PERSONALIZED TREATMENT APPROACHES IN ONCOLOGY

8.8.1 Targeted Therapy

Targeted therapies are the center of attraction to the personalized oncology paradigm. Targeted therapies focus on disrupting specific molecules or pathways that are crucial for the growth and survival of cancer cells.

8.8.1.1 Mechanisms of Targeted Therapies

The basis of targeted therapy includes the identification of cancer-related genetic mutations or alterations that could contribute to tumorigenesis. The two main classes of targeted therapies are

1. Tyrosine Kinase Inhibitors.

2. Monoclonal Antibodies.

Tyrosine Kinase Inhibitors (TKIs): These are small molecules blocking the action of specific enzymes, called tyrosine kinases, which play a crucial role in cell signaling that drive tumor growth. Imatinib (Gleevec) is a TKI that targets the BCR-ABL fusion protein in chronic myeloid leukemia (CML). On the other hand, Erlotinib (Tarceva) targets EGFR mutations in non-small cell lung cancer (NSCLC).

Monoclonal Antibodies: They are some laboratory-engineered molecules tailored to bind to specific antigens found on the surface of cancer cells. They either directly inhibit tumor growth or mark the cells for destruction by the immune system. Trastuzumab (Herceptin) is a monoclonal antibody that targets HER2-positive breast cancer. It is a revolutionizing treatment for this subset of breast cancer patients.

8.8.2 Success Stories of Targeted Therapies

After the era of traditional treatments available, targeted therapies have shown transformative change in the field of cancer care. Several drugs have contributed to it by demonstrating substantial benefits for patients. The success of Imatinib in CML turned a once-terminal disease into a manageable chronic condition for many patients. Trastuzumab in HER2-positive breast cancer similarly revolutionized outcomes in patients by reducing recurrence rates and improving survival by targeting the specific overexpression of the HER2 receptor [17]. Targeted therapies like them underline the power of precision medicine. They technically offer patients with specific mutations the potential for significantly better treatment outcomes, fewer side effects, and improved quality of life.

Immunotherapy: Immunotherapy, one of the most leveraging advances in cancer treatment has been offering new hope to patients with cancers. Immunotherapy works by enhancing the body's own immune system to recognize and destroy cancer cells. This section will be covering the key immunotherapeutic strategies, particularly immune checkpoint inhibitors and CAR-T cell therapy, that has paved the way for personalized cancer treatment [15].

Immune Checkpoint Inhibitors: The immune checkpoint inhibitors block the "brakes" that the tumors put on the immune system. This mechanism allows T-cells to attack cancer cells more effectively. The most prominent of these are inhibitors of the PD-1/PD-L1 pathway, including drugs like Pembrolizumab (Keytruda) and Nivolumab (Opdivo). These drugs have shown remarkable efficacy in treating aggressive cancers such as melanoma, NSCLC, and bladder cancer [18]. This has dramatically improved survival rates in patients having cancers that were previously resistant to conventional therapies.

CAR-T Cell Therapy: An immunotherapy that attacks cancer cells by modifying a patient's own T-cells. In hematologic cancers like leukemia and lymphoma, CAR-T cell therapy has transformed treatment options for patients who have relapsed to other therapies [19]. Kymriah (tisagenlecleucel) have shown success in achieving remission in patients with acute lymphoblastic leukemia (ALL). However, CAR-T therapy bears its own challenges, like the risk of cytokine release syndrome (CRS) and some neurotoxicity. Precise monitoring and patient selection are needed for these side effects to ensure that the patients are suitable candidates for this therapy [15].

Hormonal Therapy: A new approach of therapies called the hormonal therapy is widely used in cancers that are driven by hormonal signals, such as breast cancer and prostate cancer. These block the effects of hormones (such as estrogen or testosterone) or reduce their levels which in turn slows down or completely stops the growth of hormone dependent tumors.

Breast Cancer and Estrogen Receptor (ER) Blockade: Some breast cancers bear estrogen receptor positive tumors. For these cancers, Tamoxifen (an estrogen receptor antagonist) and aromatase inhibitors like Anastrozole are commonly used [20]. These therapies have the ability to significantly reduce the recurrence rates and improve survival in both premenopausal and postmenopausal women. Hormonal therapy is an excellent example of personalized treatment, as it depends on the tumor's expression of hormone receptors. This therapy ensures that only those patients who have the probability of benefiting from this treatment receives it [20].

Prostate Cancer and Androgen Deprivation Therapy (ADT): Androgen deprivation therapy (ADT) is the cornerstone of treatment in prostate cancer for tumors that are dependent on androgens (male hormones) for growth. Certain agents like Leuprolide (LHRH agonists) and Enzalutamide (androgen receptor antagonists) blocks androgen signaling. This can ultimately lead to significant survival benefits for patients even with advanced or metastatic disease [20].

8.9 THE IMPACT OF PERSONALIZED MEDICINE ON PATIENT CARE AND OUTCOMES

8.9.1 Improved Patient Outcomes

The shift away from the one-size-fits-all model, particularly in the context of oncology, has significantly improved patient outcomes, offering more precise treatments that increase survival rates, enhance the quality of life, and reduce adverse effects.

Enhanced Survival Rates and Quality of Life: Personalized medicine showed the most important impact in oncology. Here, treatments are designed to target specific genetic mutations or molecular features of tumors, not only improving the survival rates but also contributing to a better quality of life. Personalized medicine has been taken into account because the traditional cancer treatments even though involve killing of fast-growing cells, but they also harm some healthy cells. In contrast, personalized medicine, focuses on the genetic drivers of cancer and also minimizing damage.

8.9.2 Targeted Therapy in Breast Cancer

The most evident example for patients with HER2-positive breast cancer patients of how personalized medicine plays an important role in improving outcomes is Trastuzumab (Herceptin). This drug specifically targets the HER2 protein, an over expressive protein in some breast cancers. Adding trastuzumab to chemotherapy in HER2-positive patients significantly improved disease-free survival rates, reducing the risk of recurrence by 46% demonstrated by Piccart-Gebhart et al. (2005) [21]. By designing treatment to the genetic profile of the tumor, the approach ensures that therapies are more effective. This can avoid unnecessary exposure to drugs that might not be beneficial to patients.

8.9.3 EGFR Mutations in Lung Cancer

Lung cancer has also seen transformations due to personalized treatments. Mutations are very common in the epidermal growth factor receptor (EGFR) gene especially in non-small cell lung cancer (NSCLC) patients. Targeted therapies like gefitinib and erlotinib have been shown to improve survival rates and quality of life for these patients. Mok et al. [22] in his study found that patients with EGFR mutations when treated with gefitinib gave higher responses and survived longer compared to those receiving traditional chemotherapy. This particularly highlighted the effectiveness of targeting specific molecular alterations.

8.9.4 Immunotherapy in Melanoma and Other Cancers

Certain cancers, even after having limited efficacy, showed enhanced patient outcomes upon treatment with the emergence and rise of immunotherapy. Immunotherapies, such as nivolumab and pembrolizumab, work by stimulating the patient's own immune system to recognize and attack cancer cells. Snyder et al. (2014) [23] in their study showed that certain patients with some kinds of tumor mutations showed better response to immune checkpoint inhibitors. Thus, immunotherapy has shown that it not only extends survival but also improves the quality of life as it ensures fewer side effects than other treatments [24]. These innovations bring us to the conclusion that personalized medicine allows for a more effective approach to cancer care as it offers treatments that are more in line with the individual's specific disease characteristics and also less harmful to healthy cells. This ultimately ensures in both better survival and a better quality of life.

8.9.4.1 Reduction in Adverse Effects Compared to Traditional Treatments

Among many, one of the most important benefits of personalized medicine is the reduction of side effects which is often associated with conventional treatments. The traditional therapies like chemotherapy and radiation are designed to target rapidly dividing cells, which include cancer cells but also affect healthy cells, leading to side effects such as nausea, fatigue, and hair loss [25]. Personalized treatments, however, use genetic and molecular information to select therapies that specifically target cancer cells, sparing healthy tissues and thereby reducing the frequency and severity of side effects [26].

8.9.5 Pharmacogenomics in Drug Dosing

Another area where personalized medicine minimizes adverse effects is in the field of pharmacogenomics, which examines how genetic variations influence drug metabolism. For example, the metabolism of tamoxifen, a widely used drug in the treatment of breast cancer, can vary depending on genetic variants in the CYP2D6 gene. Some individuals have genetic variants that make them poor metabolizers of tamoxifen, leading to less effective treatment. By screening for these genetic variations, clinicians can adjust dosing or choose alternative treatments to ensure both efficacy and safety (Jukic et al., 2017). By matching patients with the right treatments based on their genetic profiles, personalized medicine helps to reduce the incidence of adverse effects while also optimizing therapeutic efficacy [27].

8.9.6 Role of Personalized Medicine in Treatment Decisions

Personalized medicine is revolutionizing the way treatment decisions are made in clinical practice. By incorporating genetic profiling and molecular diagnostics, healthcare providers can make more informed decisions, choosing therapies that are most likely to be effective based on the patient's unique genetic makeup. This enables a more precise and individualized approach to care, leading to better outcomes [28].

8.9.7 Genetic Profiling to Guide Treatment Decisions

Genetic profiling involves analyzing a patient's DNA to identify genetic mutations or variations that influence both disease risk and response to treatments. This approach allows clinicians to select therapies that target specific genetic alterations, rather than using a generic treatment plan. For example, in the case of non-small cell lung cancer (NSCLC), genetic testing for EGFR mutations allows oncologists to choose EGFR inhibitors like gefitinib or erlotinib for patients whose tumors harbor these mutations, leading to improved outcomes compared to traditional chemotherapy [29]. Similarly, for breast cancer patients, genetic testing for mutations in BRCA1 and BRCA2 can guide decisions about the use of PARP inhibitors, which have shown effectiveness in cancers with these mutations. This type of precision oncology allows for more informed and personalized treatment regimens that are tailored to the individual patient, maximizing the chances of success while minimizing unnecessary or ineffective treatments.

8.9.8 Genetic Counseling and Risk Assessment

In addition to guiding treatment selection, genetic profiling can also be instrumental in assessing the risk of developing certain conditions. Genetic counseling helps patients understand their genetic predispositions, enabling them to make informed decisions about preventive measures, surveillance, and treatment options [30]. For instance, patients with a family history of hereditary cancers (such as BRCA mutations in breast and ovarian cancer) can undergo genetic testing to determine their own risk. If mutations are found, these individuals might opt for more aggressive screening, chemoprevention, or even prophylactic surgeries to reduce their cancer risk. By integrating genetic information into decision-making, personalized medicine not only helps in selecting the most effective treatments but also empowers patients to take a more active role in managing their health, based on a comprehensive understanding of their genetic risks [31].

8.10 CHALLENGES AND LIMITATIONS OF PERSONALIZED MEDICINE IN ONCOLOGY

While personalized medicine has transformed the landscape of oncology, offering more targeted and effective treatments, it is not without its challenges. Despite the remarkable advances in genetic testing, molecular diagnostics, and tailored therapies, there remain several hurdles that must be overcome before personalized medicine can be fully integrated into routine clinical practice. These challenges span technical, biological, and logistical domains, each of which can impact the effectiveness, accessibility, and reliability of personalized treatments. This chapter explores these issues in detail, discussing the current limitations and the potential solutions needed to maximize the benefits of personalized medicine for cancer patients.

8.10.1 Technical and Logistical Challenges

The core of personalized medicine lies in its ability to leverage genetic information to guide treatment decisions. In oncology, the ability to profile tumor genomes through advanced genetic testing methods like next-generation sequencing (NGS) has revolutionized how cancers are diagnosed and treated. NGS enables the identification of mutations, gene amplifications, fusions, and other genomic alterations that drive cancer progression, and has led to the development of targeted therapies that directly address these changes. However, while NGS offers the promise of comprehensive tumor profiling, there are several technical limitations that currently hinder its widespread use in clinical oncology:

8.10.1.1 Accuracy of Genetic Testing

Accuracy is paramount when using genetic testing to inform treatment decisions. Inaccurate results—whether false positives or false negatives—can have serious consequences. A false positive may lead to unnecessary treatment with targeted therapies that could cause adverse effects without benefiting the patient, while a false negative could result in the missed opportunity to provide a more effective, personalized treatment. For example, if a tumor's genetic profile is incorrectly interpreted, a patient may be denied access to targeted therapies that could have significantly improved their prognosis. A study by Mardis [14] highlighted that discrepancies in the accuracy of NGS results often arise from variations in sample preparation, sequencing techniques, and the bioinformatics pipelines used to analyze genetic data. Tumors are inherently heterogeneous, meaning that genetic mutations can vary not only between patients but also within different regions of the same tumor. This biological complexity further complicates the interpretation of genetic data, contributing to the potential for misdiagnosis. The development of more standardized and reliable sequencing technologies, as well as improved bioinformatics tools, is essential to mitigate these issues and ensure that genetic testing results are accurate and actionable.

8.10.1.2 Coverage of Genetic Tests

Another significant limitation is the coverage of genetic testing panels. While NGS allows for the analysis of multiple genes simultaneously, the panels used in clinical practice may not cover all relevant mutations, particularly in complex or rare cancers. Some genetic tests may only examine a subset of the most common mutations associated with specific cancers, leaving out less well-characterized but potentially actionable alterations [32]. This can limit the identification of all the genetic factors contributing to the tumor and reduce the potential for identifying optimal targeted treatments. Comprehensive tumor profiling is especially important in cancers such as non-small cell lung cancer (NSCLC), where mutations in genes like EGFR, ALK, ROS1, and BRAF can significantly influence treatment outcomes. However, the genetic landscape of tumors is constantly evolving, and new mutations may be discovered over time. As a result, current testing panels may not be up to date with the latest scientific discoveries [33]. This underscores the need for ongoing research to expand genetic testing panels and for standardized testing protocols that cover a wider array of clinically relevant mutations.

8.10.1.3 Cost of Genetic Testing

The cost of genetic testing, particularly comprehensive genomic profiling, remains a significant barrier to its widespread adoption. While the price of NGS has decreased over the years, the cost of testing remains prohibitive for some healthcare systems and patients. This is particularly challenging in countries where healthcare access is limited, or in settings where insurance coverage may not fully reimburse the costs associated with genetic testing [32]. Furthermore, the financial burden of repeated or follow-up testing—particularly in cases where a patient's tumor evolves over time—can compound the problem. Cost-effective solutions, such as the development of less expensive testing platforms or insurance models that provide broader coverage for genetic tests, will be essential to ensure that personalized medicine can be made available to all patients, not just those who can afford the upfront costs [33].

8.11 PERSONALIZED CANCER VACCINES

8.11.1 Development and Potential of Cancer Vaccines Tailored to Individual Patients

One of the most exciting prospects in personalized oncology is the development of personalized cancer vaccines, which leverage the body's immune system to target and destroy tumor cells. Unlike traditional vaccines that stimulate a broad immune response, personalized cancer vaccines are designed to elicit a targeted immune response against neoantigens, which are unique to each patient's tumor. Neoantigens arise from mutations in tumor cells and are not present in normal tissues, making them ideal targets for immunotherapy. Recent advancements in genomic sequencing and proteomics have enabled researchers to identify these tumor-specific mutations and develop vaccines tailored to individual patients. Personalized cancer vaccines have shown promising results in clinical trials. For instance, Sahin et al. (2017) [34] developed a personalized mRNA vaccine for patients with metastatic melanoma, targeting neoantigens identified in each patient's tumor. The study demonstrated robust immune responses and improved progression-free survival among patients who received the vaccine, suggesting that personalized cancer vaccines have significant potential in enhancing the efficacy of immunotherapy [34, 35].

8.11.2 Challenges and Future Directions in Personalized Cancer Vaccines

Despite their promise, several challenges remain in the development and implementation of personalized cancer vaccines. One of the major hurdles is the identification of suitable neoantigens, as tumors vary greatly in their mutation profiles, and not all mutations generate immunogenic antigens. Additionally, producing personalized vaccines on a large scale is logistically complex, time-consuming, and expensive. Manufacturing delays and the cost of developing individualized vaccines could limit their accessibility and widespread use. To overcome these challenges, future research should focus on improving the identification of neoantigens, optimizing vaccine formulation, and enhancing delivery methods to ensure robust immune responses. Furthermore, combining personalized vaccines with other treatments, such as checkpoint inhibitors, could create a synergistic effect that enhances the overall immune response and improves therapeutic outcomes. This combination approach could prove to be a key strategy in addressing treatment resistance and reducing relapse rates.

8.12 ROLE OF ARTIFICIAL INTELLIGENCE IN GENETIC DATA INTERPRETATION

As molecular diagnostics generate increasingly complex datasets, artificial intelligence (AI) has the potential to transform the interpretation of genetic data. AI algorithms, particularly machine learning and deep learning, can analyze vast amounts of genetic information quickly and accurately, identifying patterns and connections that might elude human experts. AI can also facilitate the integration of multi-modal data from various diagnostic tools, such as genomic, proteomic, and imaging data. By synthesizing these diverse datasets, AI can create a comprehensive profile of a patient's tumor, which can guide treatment decisions. As AI technologies continue to evolve, their integration into personalized oncology will become more widespread, potentially leading to more effective patient stratification, optimized treatment regimens, and better overall outcomes.

8.13 INTEGRATION OF MULTI-OMICS APPROACHES

8.13.1 Role of Integrating Genomics, Proteomics, and Metabolomics in Personalized Cancer Care

As the understanding of cancer biology becomes more nuanced, multi-omics approaches are gaining prominence in personalized oncology. By integrating data from multiple biological layers—genomics, proteomics, and metabolomics—researchers and clinicians can obtain a more comprehensive picture of tumor behavior, progression, and response to treatment (Figure 8.3).

Genomics focuses on identifying genetic alterations, including mutations, copy number variations, and structural rearrangements. These alterations provide key insights into tumorigenesis and guide the selection of targeted therapies.

Proteomics examines the expression and modifications of proteins in tumor cells. Since proteins are the functional molecules that drive cellular processes, understanding the proteomic landscape can reveal signaling pathways and cellular interactions that drive cancer growth and metastasis.

Metabolomics analyzes the metabolites produced by tumors, which are often altered in cancer cells due to changes in metabolic processes. These alterations can provide insights into tumor aggressiveness, treatment response, and potential therapeutic targets.

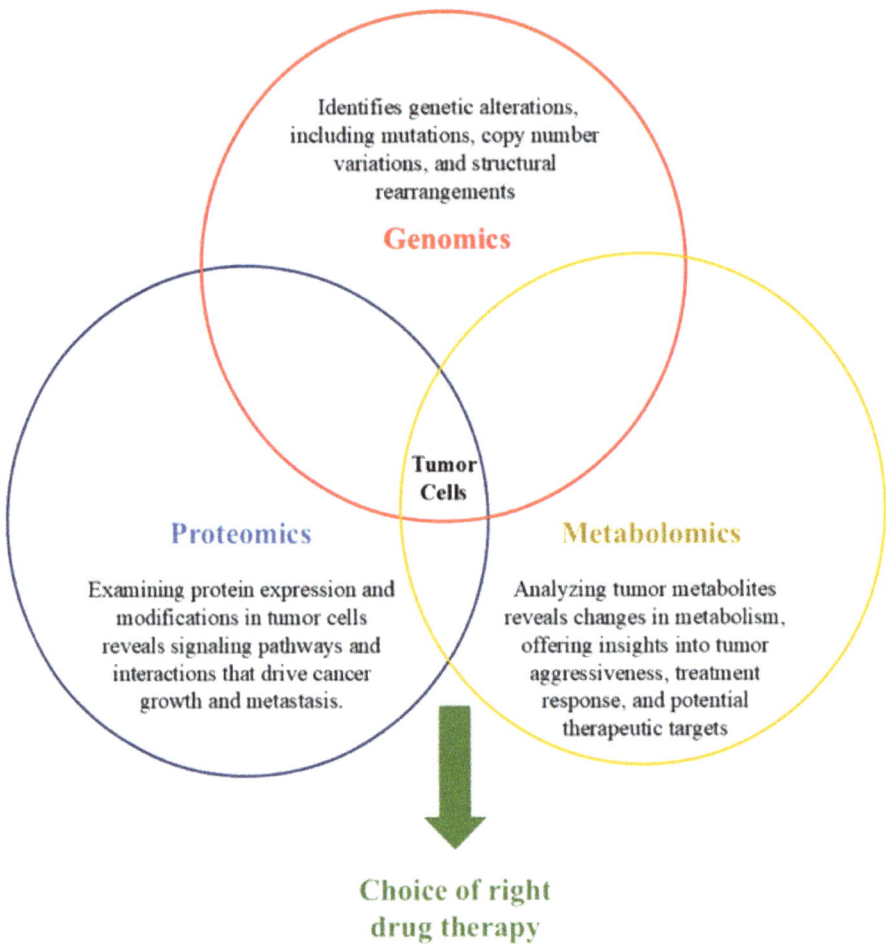

Figure 8.3 Multi-omics approaches.

By integrating these layers of biological data, multi-omics approaches allow for a more comprehensive understanding of cancer and provide a more robust framework for personalized treatment planning (Figure 8.3). For example, Duran et al. (2021) [36] identified metabolic signatures in glioblastoma patients that correlated with treatment outcomes, highlighting the potential for metabolomics to inform treatment decisions [36, 37].

8.13.2 Future Directions for Multi-Omics Integration in Oncology

The future of multi-omics integration lies in computational biology and machine learning techniques that enable the analysis of complex datasets. By combining genomic, proteomic, and metabolomic data, researchers can identify patterns and biomarkers associated with treatment response, resistance, and disease progression. These insights could lead to the development of predictive models that forecast a patient's response to specific therapies and provide a basis for more accurate patient stratification.

Furthermore, multi-omics data could inform the development of combination therapies that target multiple pathways simultaneously, addressing issues like treatment resistance and tumor heterogeneity. For instance, combining targeted therapies with immune checkpoint inhibitors or metabolic modulators could overcome resistance mechanisms and enhance treatment efficacy.

8.14 THE ROLE OF PERSONALIZED MEDICINE IN PREVENTATIVE ONCOLOGY

8.14.1 Genetic Screening for Cancer Risk and Early Interventions

Personalized medicine is not only transforming cancer treatment but also playing a crucial role in preventive oncology. By identifying individuals at high risk for certain cancers through genetic

Table 8.4: **Integration of AI and Multi-omics in Preventive Oncology and Personalized Cancer Therapy**

	Category	Description
1	AI in Genetic Data Interpretation	AI, particularly machine learning and deep learning, analyzes complex genetic data, aiding in faster, more accurate interpretation and treatment decisions.
2	Personalized Cancer Vaccines	Tailored vaccines target unique tumor neoantigens, showing promising results in clinical trials, but challenges remain in production and scalability.
3	Multi-Omics Integration	Integrating genomics, proteomics, and metabolomics provides a comprehensive view of tumor behavior and response, enabling more personalized treatment planning.
4	Preventative Oncology	Genetic screening identifies high-risk individuals for early interventions, reducing cancer risk and improving early detection.
5	Future of Personalized Oncology	Continued advancements in AI, multi-omics, and genetic testing will enhance treatment precision, prevention strategies, and overall cancer care.

screening, healthcare providers can implement early interventions that reduce the risk of developing cancer or catch it at an early, more treatable stage. Genetic tests, such as those for mutations in BRCA1 and BRCA2, can identify individuals at high risk for breast and ovarian cancers. In such cases, personalized prevention strategies, including enhanced surveillance, prophylactic surgeries, or targeted lifestyle modifications, can be recommended to significantly reduce cancer risk (Table 8.4) [38].

8.15 CONCLUSION

As personalized oncology continues to evolve, it holds the potential to revolutionize cancer care by offering more precise, effective, and individualized treatment options. The integration of emerging technologies, such as liquid biopsies, single-cell sequencing, and artificial intelligence, combined with advancements in personalized cancer vaccines, multi-omics approaches, and preventive oncology, will be key to realizing the full promise of personalized medicine in oncology. While challenges remain, particularly in terms of cost, accessibility, and the identification of biomarkers, the future of personalized oncology is bright. With continued research, collaboration, and innovation, personalized oncology will not only improve treatment outcomes but also pave the way for more effective prevention strategies, ultimately leading to a future where cancer is more manageable and, in some cases, preventable. Preventive oncology holds the potential to significantly reduce the burden of cancer by identifying individuals at high risk and providing them with the tools to prevent cancer or detect it early when it is most treatable. However, substantial challenges remain, particularly in terms of public awareness, access to genetic screening, and addressing disparities in healthcare. As we look to the future, advancements in genetic testing, AI-driven predictive models, personalized prevention strategies, and the development of new interventions will continue to shape the landscape of cancer prevention. For personalized preventive oncology to reach its full potential, efforts must be made to educate the public, ensure equitable access to genetic services, and integrate these strategies into routine healthcare. By addressing these challenges, we can work towards a future in which cancer prevention is as personalized and accessible as the treatment of the disease itself, ultimately improving outcomes and reducing cancer-related morbidity and mortality worldwide.

REFERENCES

1. Sadee W et al. Pharmacogenomics: driving personalized medicine. *Pharmacol Rev* 2023;75(4):789–814.

2. Patel JN et al. Pharmacogenomics in cancer supportive care: key issues and future directions. *Support Care Cancer* 2021;29:6187–91.

3. Jeibouei S et al. Personalized medicine in breast cancer: pharmacogenomics approaches. *Pharmacogen Personal Med* 2019;12:59–73.

4. Zhou Y et al. Review of personalized medicine and pharmacogenomics of anti-cancer compounds and natural products. *Genes* 2024;15(4):468.

5. Kumar RM, Joghee S. Enhancing breast cancer treatment through pharmacogenomics: a narrative review. *Clin Chim Acta* 2024;562:119893.

6. Paulík A et al. Irinotecan toxicity during treatment of metastatic colorectal cancer: focus on pharmacogenomics and personalized medicine. *Tumori J* 2020;106(2):87–94.

7. Belle DJ, Singh H. Genetic factors in drug metabolism. *Am Fam Physic* 2008;77(11):1553–60.

8. Iragavarapu C et al. Novel ALK inhibitors in clinical use and development. *J Hematol Oncol* 2015;8:1–9.

9. Herbst RS et al. The biology and management of non-small cell lung cancer. *Nature* 2018;553(7689):446–54.

10. Ellis LM, Fidler IJ. Finding the tumor copycat: therapy fails, patients don't. *Nature Med* 2010;16(9):974–5.

11. DeVita Jr VT, Rosenberg SA. Two hundred years of cancer research. *New Engl J Med* 2012;366(23):2207–14.

12. Chabner BA, Roberts Jr TG. Chemotherapy and the war on cancer. *Nature Rev Cancer* 2005;5(1):65–72.

13. Schwaederle M et al. Impact of precision medicine in diverse cancers: a meta-analysis of phase II clinical trials. *J Clin Oncol* 2015;33(32):3817–25.

14. Mardis ER. Next-generation DNA sequencing methods. *Ann Rev Genomics Hum Genet* 2008;9(1):387–402.

15. Robert C et al. Nivolumab in previously untreated melanoma without BRAF mutation. *New Engl J Med* 2015;372(4):320–30.

16. Walko C et al. Precision medicine in oncology: New practice models and roles for oncology pharmacists. *Am J Health Syst Pharm* 2016;73(23):1935–42.

17. Jabbour E et al. Characteristics and outcomes of patients with chronic myeloid leukemia and T315I mutation following failure of imatinib mesylate therapy. *Blood* 2008;112(1):53–5.

18. Slamon DJ et al. Use of chemotherapy plus a monoclonal antibody against HER2 for metastatic breast cancer that overexpresses HER2. *New Engl J Med* 2001;344(11):783–92.

19. Baccarani M et al. European LeukemiaNet recommendations for the management of chronic myeloid leukemia. *Blood* 2013;122(6):872–84.

20. Chodak GW et al. Results of conservative management of clinically localized prostate cancer. *New Engl J Med* 1994;330(4):242–8.

21. Piccart-Gebhart MJ et al. Trastuzumab after adjuvant chemotherapy in HER2-positive breast cancer. *New Engl J Med* 2005;353(16):1659–72.

22. Mok TS et al. Gefitinib or carboplatin–paclitaxel in pulmonary adenocarcinoma. *New Engl J Med* 2009;361(10):947–57.

23. Snyder A et al. Genetic basis for clinical response to CTLA-4 blockade in melanoma. *New Engl J Med* 2014;371(23):2189–99.

24. Brauch H et al. Pharmacogenomics of tamoxifen therapy. *Clin Chem* 2009;55(10):1770–82.

25. Van Cutsem E et al. Cetuximab and chemotherapy as initial treatment for metastatic colorectal cancer. *New Engl J Med* 2009;360(14):1408–17.

26. Tanaka K et al. Osimertinib versus osimertinib plus chemotherapy for non–small cell lung cancer with EGFR (T790M)-associated resistance to initial EGFR inhibitor treatment: an open-label, randomised phase 2 clinical trial. *Eur J Cancer* 2021;149:14–22.

27. Patel JN, Villadolid J. Cancer drug delivery: pharmacogenetics, biomarkers, and targeted therapies. In: Pharmaceutical Sciences: Breakthroughs in Research and Practice. Publisher; 2017:185–228.

28. Kris MG et al. Using multiplexed assays of oncogenic drivers in lung cancers to select targeted drugs. *JAMA* 2014;311(19):1998–2006.

29. Paik S et al. A multigene assay to predict recurrence of tamoxifen-treated, node-negative breast cancer. *New Engl J Med* 2004;351(27):2817–26.

30. Chassevent AK. *Is It Feasible? Self–Affirmation for Hereditary Breast and Ovarian Cancer Genetic Counseling.* Doctoral dissertation, Johns Hopkins University, 2018.

31. Berliner JL, Fay AM. Risk assessment and genetic counseling for hereditary breast and ovarian cancer: recommendations of the National Society of Genetic Counselors. *J Genet Counsel* 2007;16:241–60.

32. Lin JS et al. Evaluating genomic tests from bench to bedside: a practical framework. *BMC Med Inform Decis Mak* 2012;12:1–9.

33. Chakravarty D, Solit DB. Clinical cancer genomic profiling. *Nature Rev Genet* 2021;22(8):483–501.

34. Sahin U, Türeci Ö. Personalized vaccines for cancer immunotherapy. *Science* 2018;359(6382):1355–60.

35. Uppu S, et al. Towards deep learning in genome-wide association interaction studies. In: Proceedings of the 20th Pacific Asia Conference on Information Systems (PACIS 2016). Pacific Asia Conference on Information Systems; 2016:20. ISBN 978-9860491029.

36. Wishart DS. Emerging applications of metabolomics in drug discovery and precision medicine. *Nature Rev Drug Disc* 2016;15(7):473–84.

37. Ghose A et al. Applications of proteomics in ovarian cancer: dawn of a new era. *Proteomes* 2022;10(2):16.

38. Ludwig KK et al. Risk reduction and survival benefit of prophylactic surgery in BRCA mutation carriers, a systematic review. *Am J Surg* 2016;212(4):660–9.

9

Genetic Counseling in Oncology

Depanshi Pandit, Ambica Koul, Sneha S. Kagale, and Ravindranath B.S

9.1 INTRODUCTION

Genetic counseling is a process that involves communication related to the diagnosis and the importance of factors related to genetics, helping determine the risk of recurrence of the disorder, and ultimately ensuring psychological support for patients undergoing or at risk of genetic disorders. According to the World Health Organization (WHO), genetic counseling is the act of providing patients or people with heritable disorders or those who are at a higher risk of developing a disorder or disease, or of passing it on to their unborn children, with information on the genetic components of that disease. A specific genetic service for families with a suspected or confirmed high genetic risk of cancer, as well as the need to create family-specific surveillance programs, has become necessary as a result of growing knowledge of hereditary risk factors in common cancers and advancements in molecular biology. This service is provided by genetic counselors, who help patients understand the importance of testing, associated risk factors, and guide patients through their hardships.

Although genetic counseling as a service has been available for much longer, the profession of genetic counseling was founded in the United States in 1969 (Heimler, 1997). In the last 30 years, the field of genetic counseling has expanded globally, having started over 50 years ago in the United States (Abacan et al., 2019). Genetic counseling as a therapeutic profession has its roots in the now-discredited field of eugenics, which attempted to improve human populations via selective breeding. The provision of genetic counseling is not limited to genetic counselors; it is also carried out by a range of medical and allied health professionals, including clinical and human geneticists, physicians pursuing ongoing genetic education, and medical social workers. This highlights the necessity for a standardized approach to genetic counseling. The establishment of the Board of Genetic Counseling, India (BGC) in the Global State of the Genetic Counseling Profession in 2014 was an attempt to uphold professional standards and give respectability to the field (Abacan et al., 2019). According to a survey, the number of genetic counselors in India is approximately 76, and two degrees can be awarded for genetic counseling (Shah et al., 2023; Global Hallyu Status, 2023).

Oncology certainly has a genetic basis, as the risk of mutations in genes will have a profound and increased risk of cancer. Identification of the risks and communication of the same with patients is important, as there is a possibility of preventing cancer by analyzing the known mutations. It is estimated that 5–10% of tumors are associated with hereditary cancer syndromes, which are mostly defined by autosomal dominant and, less frequently, autosomal recessive heredity. Around 15% of cancer cases are familial and are caused by a multifactorial inheritance process, which results from genetic, environmental, and possibly carcinogenic variables interacting to raise an individual's susceptibility to their effects. The remaining 75% of cancer cases are sporadic (Garber & Offit, 2005).

In India, oncologists usually offer counseling. However, they might not have the time or knowledge to provide patients the level of genetic counseling necessary to enable and empower them to choose the kind of testing that suits their family. When genetic counselors are available, referring patients with a personal or family history of cancer who fit the criteria for hereditary cancer syndromes is a crucial part of cancer care (Mikkelson & Odunsi, 2019). Before and following the administration of a molecular test, genetic counseling is a crucial and required procedure in oncology clinics, particularly those that treat hereditary cancer. There are reports which reveal that, in India, genetic testing in Hereditary Breast and Ovarian Cancer (HBOC) is still underutilized despite recent advancements. Genetic counseling entails an effort by one or more suitably qualified individuals to assist the individual or family in diagnosing the disorder's likely trajectory, and the available treatment options, to recognize the role that hereditary plays in the condition and the likelihood of recurrence in relatives who have first-degree mutations, to make a decision based on their risk tolerance and family objectives, and also to help you adapt to the disorder as best you can (Sąsiadek et al., 2020). A patient or a healthy person may be referred by a medical, surgical, or

DOI: 10.1201/9781003542162-9

community oncologist if they come across clinical situations that might indicate hereditary malignancies. However, a genetic counseling center or clinic can be recommended to any practitioner who sees a patient who may be at risk for a rare or family cancer (Ulhaq et al., 2023).

9.1.1 Overview of Genetic Counseling Protocol

To assist people and families in understanding and managing the risks of hereditary illnesses like cancer, genetic counseling is an organized approach. The methodology typically takes a clear, sequential approach, as do the types of genetic counseling (Ulhaq et al., 2023). The first step is pre-test counseling, during which the counselor collects a thorough medical and family history, determines the person's risk, and goes over the possible advantages, restrictions, and ramifications of genetic testing. Before starting the genetic test, informed permission is acquired. Following the results, post-test counseling is conducted, during which the counselor analyses the data, discusses the implications, and goes over potential next steps, such as treatment, prevention, or surveillance. Along with assisting the patient and their family, the counselor also tackles the psychological and emotional components of the diagnosis. The overview of the genetic counseling procedure is given in Figure 9.1.

The protocol emphasizes confidentiality, ethical considerations, and a non-directive approach, respecting the patient's autonomy. Following is the stepwise protocol followed by the counselor (Ulhaq et al., 2023).

a) *Identifying symptoms*: To determine the likelihood of a disease developing or recurring, a family tree is created by interpreting the medical history, family history, and physical examination.

b) *Examining the possibilities*: Variant inheritance education, a discussion of the various genetic tests and testing labs, and, if necessary, setting them up are followed by information on cancer prevention, management, and surveillance techniques.

c) *Risk assessment*: advice to assist in making wise decisions and adjusting to the risk or condition.

d) *Conversation*: Assisting individuals in comprehending the disease they are concerned about during pre-test counseling meetings and in understanding and interpreting the genetic testing results once the test is completed.

e) *Follow-up and support*: To enable the person and their family to access services and support groups if they are diagnosed with an inherited disease, such as cancer.

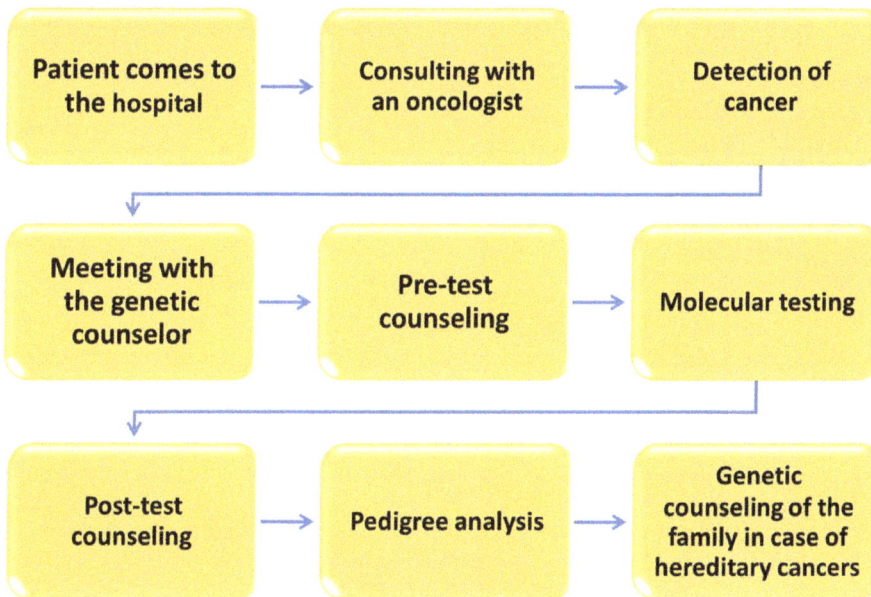

Figure 9.1   Framework of the genetic counseling procedure.

9.2 ROLE AND IMPORTANCE OF GENETIC COUNSELING AND COUNSELORS IN ONCOLOGY

Genetic counseling aids consultants in assessing the likelihood of acquiring and/or passing on genetic diseases, as well as the options available to them after genetic testing is completed and the results are known (e.g., essential treatments, need-to-know essentials, etc.). A competent professional figure has no say in the choice, which is always left to the doctors and consultants. Genetic counseling is bound by some ethical principles, providing unbiased and accurate information with respect for families and individuals, preserving the integrity of the family, complete health-related information to be provided to the individual and family, confidentiality needs to be maintained during the process of counseling, informing individuals to reveal their genetic status, using non-directive techniques, etc. (Pina Neto J., 2008).

Genetic counselors are the pillars of the process involved in genetic counseling. They could collaborate with the medical geneticist or operate alone in patient care settings. The ability to communicate effectively is frequently the strongest suit of genetic counselors. This includes gathering information from the patient and explaining the risk, presenting genetic test results to the patient, placing them within the larger context of the patient's family, and offering support and direction based on the diagnosis. A genetic counselor needs to have strong cooperation among the different medical care areas like medical geneticist, laboratory geneticist, and the genetic counselor themselves. The expertise and skill sets that genetic counselors need to have are: the genetic counselor should be able to identify the medical and family history of the patient, should be capable of facilitating the decision-making ability, should also communicate the results of the tests appropriately by quantifying the chance of recurrence, and finally, long-term support and guidance should be given to the patients (Schaaf et al., 2021).

Genetic counselors have important responsibilities and roles, some of which are as follows:

1. To collect the patient information also including the psychological factors, medical history, family history, and genetic information with its interpretation.

2. A genetic counselor to make accurate and appropriate genetic risk assessment.

3. A genetic counselor should build a network and trust with the patient, healthcare professionals, and support groups for different inherited conditions.

4. Guiding and supporting the patient is an integral part of the service rendered by the genetic counselor.

5. Genetic counselors also enable the patient to make an informed decision by keeping the information confidential.

6. A genetic counselor needs to convey all the necessary information about the disease and the potential treatment strategy, if available (Ulhaq et al., 2023).

9.3 METHODS INVOLVED IN GENETIC COUNSELING FOR ONCOLOGY

Genetic counseling for cancer can be structured into pre-test, test, and post-test phases, outlining the tools, methodology, and documentation pertinent to each stage. By methodically directing patients through this process, healthcare providers can optimize risk management, elevate patient outcomes, and advance the rapidly developing domain of personalized cancer care.

9.3.1 Pre-test Counseling

Cancer patients need pre-test genetic counseling to make educated decisions. Patients and their families must understand the scope, purpose, and potential effects of any genetic test before it is done. This phase helps patients make complex health decisions in oncology, where genetic abnormalities might affect cancer risk, early identification, and therapy. The counselor engages closely with the client to examine personal and family medical history, assess hereditary cancer syndrome risk, facilitate informed consent, and explain testing alternatives during the pre-test. In addition to genetic risk assessment, emotional and psychosocial readiness for testing is examined. Genetic counselors inform patients about the technical elements of genetic testing, such as the possibility of identifying harmful mutations, single nucleotide polymorphisms (SNPs), variants of unknown significance (VUS), or negative results, and how these may affect future medical decisions. The counselors also give patients the chance to pose queries, promoting open communication. They employ the "non-directive counseling" technique that empowers the patient's autonomy in making choices without providing any direct guidance, and sometimes, this technique may involve guiding the patient on various "what if" situations in pre-test counseling (Garber et al., 2008). Therefore, hypothetical discussions allow the patients to think about the possible answers to varied test findings to make better-informed decisions (Garber et al., 2008; American Society of Clinical Oncology, 2003).

The following are the components essential to the pre-test counseling phase:

a) *Cancer history review and risk assessment*

Individuals qualify for cancer screening based on personal and family backgrounds (Table 9.1), including early-onset cancer, multiple primary cancers, bilateral cancer, familial clustering of cancer, rare tumors, and specific high-risk ethnic groups, which may indicate a potential hereditary cancer predisposition (PDQ Cancer Genetics Editorial Board, 2024). Collecting family history, ancestry, and consanguinity data is essential (Trepanier et al., 2004). This process includes documenting health, carcinogen exposure, alcohol or tobacco consumption information for both the proband and family, as well as recording the cause of death and age of deceased relatives (Trepanier et al., 2004) (Table 9.2).

A family tree or pedigree provides the best representation of a family's health background. This standardized graphic depiction of familial links aids in the identification of disease transmission patterns, the recognition of clinical features related to various hereditary cancer syndromes, and the development of optimal risk assessment methodologies and tools (PDQ Cancer Genetics Editorial Board, 2024; Bennett et al., 2008; Bennett et al., 1995). A three-generation pedigree is used to chronicle a thorough family cancer history, including first- and second-degree relations from both maternal and paternal sides, highlighting hereditary cancer inheritance patterns. It also records the race, provenance, and ethnicity of all grandparents, which can influence genetic testing decisions because certain harmful mutations are more common in certain populations (Malhotra et al., 2020; Lu et al., 2014). It also includes information on seemingly unrelated health issues, adoption, non-paternity, consanguinity, pregnancies, assisted reproductive technology, and half-siblings (PDQ Cancer Genetics Editorial Board, 2024; Lu et al., 2014; Malhotra et al., 2020), alongside gender and sex distinctions when they differ (Bennett et al., 2022).

A pedigree's detailed information not only exposes inherited tendencies but also serves as the foundation for risk assessment in genetic counseling. Risk assessment models in oncology are crucial for anticipating an individual's risk of getting various tumors. These models use personal and family history, genetic data, and additional risk variables to deliver individualized screening and preventive recommendations. For example, the Gail Model evaluates a woman's 5-year and lifetime risk of breast cancer, taking into account characteristics such as age and family history, and informs mammography decisions (Gail et al., 1989). Similarly, models such as BOADICEA and Tyrer-Cuzick concentrate on BRCA-related risks for breast and ovarian cancer (Antoniou et al., 2008; Tyrer et al., 2004), whereas PREMM5 determines the likelihood of Lynch syndrome mutations, and guides in assessing colorectal and endometrial cancer prevention methods (Kastrinos et al., 2017). These techniques enable tailored risk management in clinical practice. Table 9.3 illustrates a few risk assessment tools.

Predictive genetic assessments are evaluations conducted on seemingly healthy persons, hence on healthy persons aimed at assessing their potential risk of developing diseases in the future These tests are of two types:

Table 9.1: **Individuals Qualifying for Cancer Screening**

1. People who want to inquire about the hereditary of a cancer.

2. People who have had first-degree relatives with cancer and want to check for the germline status of the cancer.

3. People who meet the clinical criteria of various cancers including the hereditary ones.

4. People with childhood cancers.

5. Families with pedigree data that suggests a high probability of a germline mutation.

6. Women with numerous cancer types detected in the family, especially triple-negative breast cancer or those with a clinical history and investigations suggestive of HNPCC or Lynch Syndrome.

7. Rare cases of cancer presentation such as retroperitoneal schwannoma, ocular melanoma.

8. Discrepancy between the results obtained from two or more laboratories.

Table 9.2: Comprehensive Clinical Information: Gathering Essential Medical History and Family Background Information Regarding Cancer and Non-Cancer Conditions

Clinical Information

Personal		Family	
Cancer	**Non-Cancer**	**Cancer**	**Non-Cancer**
Current age	Age	Race/ethnicity	Race/ethnicity
Race/ancestry/ ethnicity	Race/ancestry/ethnicity	Primary cancer site	Current age or age at death
Pre-cancerous history	Personal history of benign or malignant tumors	Medical documentation (e.g., pathology reports)	Cause of death
Screening practices or last screening date	Major illnesses Hospitalizations	Age at diagnosis	Surgeries/treatment history
Tumor organ	Surgeries	Tumor count	Cancer screening practices
Age at diagnosis	Biopsy history	Diagnosis/treatment location	Non-malignant features
Tumor count	Reproductive history	Risk-reducing surgery or treatment history	Carcinogenic exposures or risk factors
Malignant and benign pathology	Cancer surveillance Carcinogenic exposures or risk factors	Treatment regimen	Germ line genetic testing
Treatment regimen and toxicity		Current age (if living)	Tumor testing or genomic profiling
Reproductive history		Age at death and cause of death	Significant health problems
Carcinogenic exposures or risk factors		Carcinogenic exposures Germ line genetic testing	
Multifocal or bilaterality of disease		Significant health problems	
Current surveillance plan			
Cancer detection (e.g., self-exam/screening)			
Germ line genetic testing			
Tumor testing/Genomic profiling			

Source: From Trepanier et al. (2004). With permission.

9.3.2 Presymptomatic Testing

It refers to the search for genetic alterations that exhibit high penetrance, generally associated with autosomal dominant inheritance. Concerning such disorders, tests ought to be extremely sensitive and specific, minimizing the possibility of false negatives or false positives. For example, genetic analysis for Huntington's Disease and early-onset Alzheimer's disease. These tests may be able to recognize individuals who are healthy but are almost certainly (practically 100%) bound to suffer future from severe and crippling diseases which are so far unknown to have any practical remedy or cure (Schienda & Stopfer, 2020).

Testing protocols involved in the presymptomatic testing include:

1. Neurological examination of the patient.

2. Pre-genetic test counseling.

3. Procurement of informed consent after thoroughly explaining the outcomes and the probability.

4. Results especially negative are given in person.

5. Follow-up including therapy.

Table 9.3: Examples of a Few Disease Risk Assessment Tools

Model	Disease	Gene Mutations	Features	Limitations	Website
Gail/ BCRAT (The Breast Cancer Risk Assessment Tool)	Invasive Breast Cancer	None	Five-year/ lifetime risk Personal medical history First-degree family history Five-minute completion time	Genetic exclusion (BRCA mutation carriers) Excludes prior cancer Predictive uncertainty Risk estimate variability Limited subgroup applicability	https://bcrisktool.cancer .gov/
CanRisk Tool (Uses BOADICEA v6 model)	Breast Cancer & Ovarian Cancer	BRCA1 BRCA2 PALB2 CHEK2 ATM RAD51D RAD51C BARD1 BRIP1	Personal risk factors Family cancer history Genetic testing (high/ moderate-risk genes) Polygenic scores Mammographic density User-friendly Textual and graphical risk presentation User-friendly	Tailored communication needed No patient-facing interface Feasibility still untested Limited clinical adaptation	https://canrisk.org
PREMM₅ Model (Prediction of MMR Gene Mutations v.5)	Lynch syndrome	*MLH1 MSH2 MSH6 PMS2 EPCAM*	Germline mutation probability Lynch syndrome-associated cancer Personal cancer history Family history data Second-degree relatives User-friendly	Exclusion of lifestyle or environmental exposure	https://premm.dfci.harvard .edu/
Tyrer-Cuzick Risk Assessment Calculator	Invasive Breast Cancer	BRCA1 BRCA2	Lifetime risk probability Menarche and menopause details Personal /Family medical history Hormone replacement therapy Mammographic density Biopsy details User-friendly	Limited subgroup applicability Exclusion of lifestyle or environmental exposure	https://magview.com/ibis -risk-calculator/

Ethical Issues in Presymptomatic Testing:

1. Does a positive genetic test affect the quality of life?

2. Valuing personal autonomy is essential.

3. Informed consent.

4. Right to "not to know."

5. Reluctance to test patients, especially children.

6. Costs for the tests especially psychological ones.

7. Late onset disorders often require testing in pre-natal cases.

9.3.3 Susceptibility Testing

Susceptibility testing deals with studies on genetic defects that predispose to disease. Disorders are broadly considered multifactorial conditions. Tests can vary in sensitivity and specificity. Examples include testing for Apo-E4-Alzheimer's disease, BRCA1 and BRCA2-breast cancer. Such test results do not predict disease occurrence nor the absence of it; rather, they substitute an individual's risk previously calculated based on population or familial data with risks determined by genotype (Evans et al., 2019).

Following are the ethical issues in susceptibility testing:

1. Educating and counseling for patients at risk.

2. The interpretation of tests can be complex.

3. Potential for increased monitoring and possible treatment.

4. What constituents are the useful information requisite for the testing?

Risk is described as the probability of occurrence of a specific event within a fixed time limit. In other words, the probability or chance of an event is called risk (Park, 2007). This concept is one of the most important epidemiological tools, as it provides a numerical estimate of the amount of evidence required for prudent public health action choices.

Risks can be quantified using a 2 × 2 table or a contingency table where the x-axis describes the disease, or the outcome and the y-axis describes the exposure or intervention.

	+	-
+	a	b
-	c	d

Relative risk: It is defined as the risk of developing disease in the exposed group divided by the risk in the unexposed group. It is usually used in cohort studies.

If relative risk (RR) = 1 → it indicates no association between the exposure and the disease or inversely that both groups have the equal likelihood of developing cancer.

If RR >1 → exposure associated with disease or inversely the risk of acquiring cancer in the group is higher when compared to general populace.

If RR<1 → it indicates that the exposure is associated with decreased disease occurrence or inversely that the risk of developing cancer in the group is less when compared to general populace.

For example, if 10/20 individuals subjected to radiation are diagnosed with cancer, and 2/20 individuals who were not subjected to radiation develop cancer, the relative risk can be expressed as the following:

	Cancer (+)	Cancer (−)
Radiation (+)	a = 10	b = 10
Radiation (−)	c = 2	d = 18

Relative risk = $\frac{a/(a+b)}{c/(c+d)}$ = 5

Hence, a relative risk of 5 indicates that the individuals exposed to radiation have a 5 times higher likelihood of developing cancer compared to those not exposed to radiation.

Absolute risk: It refers to the likelihood of getting a particular disease such as breast cancer or colon cancer, within a given time frame.

Odds ratio: It is the odds of exposure among cases compared to the odds of exposure among control. This measure is used mainly for case-control studies

OR = 1→The odds of exposure are equal in both cases and controls.

OR>1 →The odds of exposure are higher in cases.

OR<1 → odds of exposure are higher in controls

Example: In a case-control study, 30/40 lung cancer patients and 15/75 healthy individuals report smoking, the odds ratio can be calculated as:

	Smoker (+)	Smoker (–)
Cases	a = 30	b = 10
Controls	c = 15	d = 60

$$OR = \frac{a/c}{b/d} = 12$$

Therefore, it indicates that lung cancer patients are 12 times more likely to have smoking history.

Empiric risk: it is defined as the probabilistic risk about the chance of an event occurring based on experiential data rather than the cause of the mechanism.

b) *Patient education and informed consent*

Patient education and informed consent in genetic counseling is to equip counselees with the necessary knowledge to make sound decisions regarding genetic testing. Education covers the testing method, implications for health, and ethical issues. Informed consent ensures that patients readily agree to tests after fully understanding the risks, benefits, and alternatives. Both go hand in hand and are crucial for patients and healthcare professionals to build trust and collaborative decision-making skills. In genetic counseling education, it is imperative to ensure that the patients comprehend their risk assessment by correctly describing key genetic concepts such as penetrance, inheritance patterns, variable expressivity, moderate and high-risk genes, and genetic heterogeneity. Patients should also be informed about their treatment options, whether they choose to do genetic testing or not, and what the results (positive, negative, or variations of unknown significance) may imply for them (Schneider et al., 2023). This conversation often includes evidence on the effectiveness of cancer prevention, early detection strategies, and limits.

Informed consent for cancer susceptibility testing is an organized method that ensures patients make informed decisions while maintaining their autonomy. Initial informed consent can be oral or written. However, it usually ends with the signing of an informed consent agreement, which is required by law in many countries (Schneider et al., 2023). Genetic counselors help patients make decisions by giving essential information before testing and ensuring that patients understand their options after completing the test. For instance, patients can choose to defer or decline results when available, while counselors provide time for patients to evaluate their thoughts and concerns, adding to the overall informed nature of the process (PDQ Cancer Genetics Editorial Board, 2024). Following are the elements of informed consent in genetic counseling for oncology (Lu et al., 2014; PDQ Cancer Genetics Editorial Board, 2024; Trepanier et al., 2004).

i) **Purpose of the Testing**: Explain why the genetic test is being conducted.

ii) **Specific genetic mutation(s)**: Identify the specific gene variant(s) being tested and how they may affect medical care.

iii) **Implications of test results**: Discuss potential outcomes like true positives, negatives, VUS, and false positives/negatives.

iv) **Possibility of non-informative results**: Inform that the test may not provide conclusive information.

v) **Risk to family members**: Explain the potential for relatives to inherit the genetic condition.

vi) **Technical accuracy**: Clarify the accuracy of the test, and mention laboratory licensure when required.

vii) **Fees and counseling:** Provide information about the cost of testing and counseling, including direct-to-consumer (DTC) services.

viii) **Psychological implications:** Discuss the possible emotional benefits and risks of getting test findings.

ix) **Genetic discrimination risks:** Discuss safeguards against genetic bias by employers or insurers.

x) **Confidentiality:** Maintain privacy by employing data security processes, especially during DTC testing.

xi) **Future research use:** Determine whether the DNA samples can be used in future research.

xii) **Medical surveillance strategies:** Explain the various medical monitoring and preventative strategies available after testing.

xiii) **Sharing results with family**: Highlight the significance of sharing genetic test results to at-risk family members.

xiv) **Disclosing results and follow-up**: Outline how results will be communicated and what follow-up support will be provided.

xv) **Patient expectations**: Discuss the individual's goals, beliefs, and motivations regarding testing.

xvi) **Inheritance explanation**: Clarify how genetic inheritance may influence cancer susceptibility.

xvii) **Alternatives to testing**: Present options like risk assessment without genetic testing or tissue banking.

Traditionally, genetic counselors imparted this teaching component in one-on-one meetings. Nevertheless, there is a rising preference for other models to improve scalability and accessibility (Schneider et al., 2023). Group counseling and technology-based alternatives such as chatbots and instructional films have been explored to communicate this critical knowledge (Schienda et al., 2020). While these alternatives offer intriguing possibilities to improve access, they must not jeopardize the patient's experience or ability to give informed consent (Schneider et al., 2023).

9.3.2 Test Phase

The testing phase is a crucial stage in genetic counseling, particularly in the context to oncology, as it bridges pre-test discussions with the provision of actionable data. This phase reveals genetic mutations that may raise an individual's cancer risk. It converts the theoretical risks outlined during pre-test counseling into tangible, scientifically proven data, allowing genetic counselors to provide individualized advice and support. The results of genetic testing impact the patient's medical management and their family members, who may have comparable hereditary risks. As a result, the test phase is essential in genetic counseling because it ensures patients obtain precise, evidence-based information to help them make healthcare decisions.

It incorporates the possible recommendations from counselors related to sample collection, laboratory, and test selection.

a) *Sample collection and laboratory selection*

Biological samples used for testing should be clarified on the limitations of these samples; for instance, while blood and saliva are popularly used for germline genetic testing, these can sometimes detect somatic alterations, especially among patients with blood malignancies (Schienda et al., 2020). It leads to misinterpretation whereby a patient is somatically misdiagnosed as suffering from germline mutations or even misses actual cases of germline mutations. Further, individuals with blood cancers who have been diagnosed non-verifiably may also display somatic changes, for example, clonal hematopoiesis, which may obscure the scenario more (Steensma DP. 2018; Weitzel et al., 2018). Counselors can also offer alternative sources of DNA, such as cultured skin fibroblasts, and advise against cheek swabbing or saliva collection for DNA preparation as white blood cells may contaminate (Weitzel et al., 2018). This counseling assists the patient in understanding what the test entails and helps to set expectations for what could be discovered. After a client has decided to advance on molecular testing, it is vital to arrange the collection and transport of samples while providing an estimated turnaround for results (Trepanier et al., 2004). In addition, counselors should prepare a plan for disclosure of findings, encourage clients to bring a support person to disclose results and advise the clients about the options to withdraw from the testing process or receive their results later (Trepanier et al., 2004).

Choosing the correct laboratory is an important part of cancer evaluation since the lab's experience and capabilities can have a substantial impact on the accuracy of genomic tests. Whether undertaking a single-gene study or a multigene panel, factors such as deep intronic variant coverage, gene rearrangements, and pseudogene regions differ between labs and can have a major impact on variant detection rates (Schienda et al., 2020). A careful assessment of the gene or disease most relevant to the patient is critical for getting the maximum sensitivity and detection rates (Richards et al., 2015). Furthermore, the lab's experience evaluating germline variations is critical, as interpretation is subjective and can vary depending on the lab's competence (Schienda et al., 2020; Kim et al., 2019; Amendola et al., 2016). In the USA, the labs must adhere to standards established by the Clinical Laboratory Improvement Act (CLIA). Clinical genetic tests should only be ordered from CLIA-approved laboratories to ensure compliance and reliability (Trepanier et al., 2004).

b) *Test selection*

Genetic testing for cancer screens for mutations in genes that are associated to cancer. To achieve accurate and valuable results, test selection considers various parameters such as cancer kind, familial patterns, and the availability of specialized genetic tests. Following are a few examples of genetic testing methods.

i) **Single-gene testing**: Single-gene panel testing focuses on sequencing a single gene, usually when there is a strong clinical suspicion that it is responsible for an individual's cancer risk. This technique is precise and commonly used for well-defined hereditary cancer syndromes, offering several advantages, including high sensitivity, precision, straightforward interpretation, and cost-effectiveness, as only one gene is sequenced. For instance, testing BRCA1/BRCA2 mutations is primarily conducted for ovarian and breast cancer risk or TP53 for Li-Fraumeni syndrome, which predisposes individuals to various cancers.

ii) **Multigene panel testing**: It detects mutations in multiple genes at once and can be beneficial if an individual is at risk of a familial cancer syndrome with several genes or has a personal or familial history of cancer, and single-gene testing has not revealed a mutation or the outcome is ambiguous. Furthermore, it is recommended if the patient is at risk for several cancers or if the practitioner wants to investigate a broader spectrum of hereditary reasons. For example, multigene panels thoroughly assess risk for diseases such as colorectal cancer, which may contain several genes (e.g., MLH1, MSH2, MSH6, PMS2). According to certain studies that use multigene panels, up to 17% of high-risk patients who test negative for BRCA pathogenic variations are likely to have a pathogenic variant found in another gene (Walsh et al., 2006; Walsh et al., 2010; Pilarsk. 2021). Multigene panels frequently produce Variants of Uncertain Significance (VUS), making interpretation more challenging and requiring specialized genetic counseling, while their higher cost and complexity demand advanced bioinformatics tools. Furthermore, testing multiple genes increases the risk of over-diagnosis, with some findings lacking clear clinical relevance that could lead to inappropriate medical interventions.

iii) **Next-generation sequencing**: NGS, commonly known as high-throughput sequencing, can concurrently sequence millions of DNA fragments either entire or particular genome of interest, yielding precise information on the copy number variations (CNVs), single nucleotide variants, insertions and deletions, gene fusions, structural variations, splice site mutations, mitochondrial DNA mutations, tumor mutational burden, microsatellite instability, epigenetic modifications, polygenic risk, transcriptome sequencing, somatic mutations, inherited genetic variant. The NGS platforms have broadened the breadth of genomic research, allowing for investigations on relatively rare genetic disorders, microbiome analysis, cancer genomics, infectious diseases, and genetic epidemiology (Satam *et al.*, 2023). Furthermore, NGS has allowed for the creation of tailored therapeutics, personalized healthcare approaches, and enhanced tests (Satam et al., 2023).

9.3.3 Post-test Counselling

Post-genetic counseling is the process that occurs after genetic testing is completed. It entails assisting patients in comprehending their test results and the medical, psychological, and familial consequences. This counseling provides recommendations on the subsequent steps, which may involve medical management, lifestyle changes, or further testing for the patient and their relatives. The general post-test counseling procedures are as follows:

a) *Disclosure and explanation of genetic test results*

Upon receiving the patient's approval, advise them of the outcome, usually done over the phone, via video calls, or in person. Results are rarely shared solely via fax, email, or letter, partly because of confidentiality considerations with these communication channels (Schneider et al., 2023). Nevertheless, electronic medical record portals are getting safer and thus could be an effective way of conveying data to counselees (Schneider et al., 2023). As the patient's reactions may differ, unanticipated, and change over time, the disclosure should be done prudently, taking time to evaluate psychological status, address queries, and provide supportive resources. Start by explaining the test outcomes accurately, objectively, and in a non-directive manner whether they are positive, negative, or VUS for the patient's disease risk or diagnosis.

1. **Positive result**: This means that there is an increased risk of cancer due to the gene mutation, but it does not mean that the person will get cancer. Epigenetic factors must also be taken into consideration.

2. **Negative result (no known mutation)**: This is uninformative again, especially if there is a strong family history; there may be an unrecognized mutation. Moreover, as with a positive result, repeat screening and strategies for risk reduction are required.

3. **Negative finding (familial mutation known)**: The client is not at a higher risk for familial cancer and has the same risk as the population, except for some ethnic groups with common mutations.

4. **Variant of unknown significance**: The impact of the gene mutation on the clinical condition is unknown and requires further research. However, family history and risk management should be used in the medical decisions up to the time of further research.

Furthermore, the counselor should address how the results impact their reproductive decisions. As an example, pathogenic variants in numerous breast cancer genes that involve BRCA are passed down in an autosomal dominant pattern, suggesting that offspring of BRCA carriers have a 50% likelihood of inheriting the cancer predisposition variant (Malhotra et al., 2020; Petrucelli et al., 2022). BRCA carriers receive reproductive counseling, which incorporates information on prenatal testing and assisted conception treatments (Paluch-Shimon et al., 2016).

b) *Psychosocial support and coping*

Clinicians must assess psychological difficulties to better understand the elements that influence risk estimation and the utilization of cancer genetic information (Trepanier et al., 2004; Biesecker BB. 1997; Croyle et al., 1997; Hopwood P. 1997). This method enables physicians to assess the possible effects of genetic information on a client's quality of life, reproductive choices, profession, and other life decisions (Trepanier et al., 2004). Bringing together genetic counseling, psychology, and psycho-oncology principles can help detect and resolve these problems (Trepanier et al., 2004; Baker et al., 1998).

An assessment of 30 international genetic counseling standards revealed the significance of psychological support and a sympathetic interaction between the counselor and the patient (Rantanen et al., 2008). Many guidelines emphasize that emotional support is just as crucial as providing facts, with some arguing that addressing emotional responses should come first (Rantanen et al., 2008). Support in genetic counseling is critical for patients to make educated decisions and effectively handle their test results. In a randomized controlled study of 100 female BRCA1/BRCA2 carriers, the 12-week Inquiry-Based Stress Reduction (IBSR) intervention improved psychological outcomes and sleep quality when results were evaluated 24 to 26 weeks after intervention (Landau et al., 2021).

Genetic testing is distinct from other medical tests because their outcomes might affect the patient and their family (Biggio & Ralston. 2017). Studies reveal that anomalous outcomes, such as mutations or VUS, can have a significant psychological impact on patients and families (Biggio et al., 2017). Even negative results, particularly in cancer susceptibility testing, can result in "survivor guilt" or alterations in family dynamics (Biggio et al., 2017; Offit & Thoml.,2007). Patients discovering a cancer-related mutation may feel distressed, especially if they lack support. Offering resources and guidance can help reduce worry by demonstrating how to handle the implications. Providers should also be prepared to aid patients in coping with "survivor guilt" (Biggio et al., 2017). Counselors can further recommend the patients to professionals or support groups depending on a case-to-case basis. Figure 9.2 gives some examples of topics to explore with patients.

c) *Risk assessment and management*

It includes thoroughly reviewing the patient's risk of developing specific disorders considering genetic test findings, family history, and lifestyle factors. As an example, a 40-year-old woman with breast cancer and a family history of Li-Fraumeni syndrome (LFS) would qualify for LFS guidelines, regardless of whether her testing was negative or revealed a VUS in TP53 (Schienda & Stopfer, 2020). Akin, a woman without a supportive family background, is unlikely to be given such recommendations (Schienda et al., 2020). The counselor should clearly describe the relevance of these findings, including individualized screening and monitoring techniques such as regular mammograms or magnetic resonance imaging (MRI) for people with hereditary breast cancer risk. Other screening methods for high individual risks:

9.3.3.1 Pre-natal Screening

It is a type of screening where the services focus on women before conception and during pregnancy, especially the high-risk women (Williams et al., 2008). The rough criteria for high-risk women include:

1. Maternal age (>35 years at the age of delivery).

2. Birth orders of more than 3.

3. Twins or triplets.

4. Gestational diabetes.

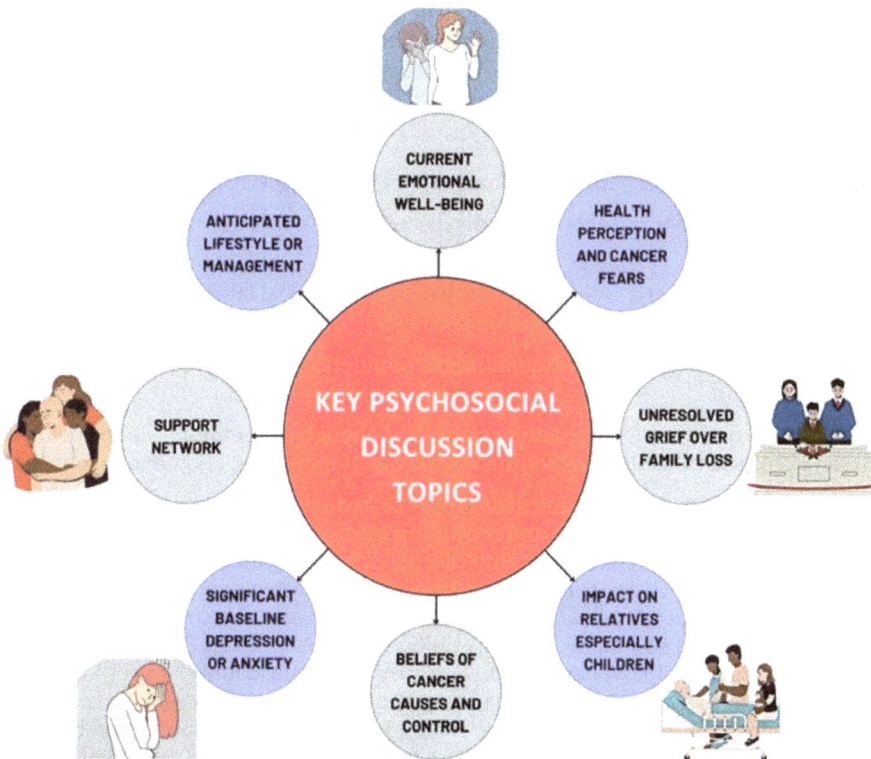

Figure 9.2 A few examples of the topics that can be discussed with patients to analyze the psychological or psychosocial impact.

5. Pre-eclampsia.

6. Maternal use of alcohol or smoking.

7. Previous child with a hereditary cancer syndrome or a congenital abnormality.

8. *In vitro* fertilization.

9. Consanguineous marriage.

10. History of abortion, miscarriage, stillborn.

Prenatal genetic counseling can assist patients in the process of deciding by guiding them through examples of how others have navigated similar situations, along with the reasoning behind their choices. Patients' decisions are influenced by various factors, including the timing of the counseling, the accuracy of the information provided by tests, and the associated risks and benefits of those tests (Angus, 2022). The American College of Obstetrics and Gynecology recommended that all gestating females must undergo various tests to rule out conditions like anencephaly, neural tube defects like spina bifida, etc. The most commonly practiced method of prenatal screening is amniocentesis, followed by chorionic villus sampling, followed by ultrasonography. For example, ultrasonography can be useful to determine conditions like spina bifida where the fetal skull shows:

1. Small biparietal diameter.

2. Ventriculomegaly.

3. Frontal bone scalloping.

4. Displacement of the cerebellum in the downward direction.

5. Elongation of the rhombencephalon.

9.3.3.2 Newborn Screening

Screening of newborns is often done soon after birth for the detection of genetic defects. Their purpose is the detection of treatable conditions so treatment may be initiated as early in life as possible to avoid severe mental or physical handicaps or disabilities (PDQ Cancer Genetics Editorial Board, 2024). Criteria for effective newborn screening programs:

1. Treatment is ubiquitous and for all.

2. Reduction or elimination of permanent damage by early treatment.

3. Screening is done in those patients where the disorder will not be revealed in newborns without a test.

4. One of the important criteria is the availability of an economical laboratory test that is rapid, available, highly sensitive, and reasonably specific.

5. The genetic condition is present in a quantifiable population and severe enough to rationalize the cost of screening.

6. The societal infrastructure is robust and established enough to communicate the results to parents and physicians, confirm and initiate subsequent treatment, and offer to counsel.

Lifestyle adjustments, such as restricting alcohol intake, reducing smoking, dietary changes, exercise, sustaining a balanced weight, and refraining from hormone replacement therapy should be encouraged to help reduce risks, along with discussions of pharmaceutical therapies or surgical options as needed. Risk-reduction contralateral prophylactic mastectomy is frequently provided for patients with or without previous experiences of breast cancers that contain a germline genetic variant that imparts a high risk for breast cancer BRCA1, BRCA2, STK11, PTEN, TP53, CDH1 mutations (Carbine et al., 2018; Wong et al., 2017). Furthermore, the counselor should emphasize the significance of alerting at-risk family members about the potential consequences of the results and encourage them to pursue genetic testing. A long-term monitoring plan should be developed to assess the patient's health and adjust care tactics when new studies and treatments become available.

d) *Legal and social considerations*

It includes several elements that can affect patients after genetic testing. Genetic diseases can cause social stigma and prejudice, leading to feelings of isolation or fear about one's identity. It is critical to address these emotional aspects during therapy, assisting patients in navigating family relationships and discussing shared inherited risks. Patients should also be informed about legislative protections against discrimination, such as the Genetic Information Non-discrimination Act (GINA), which bans health insurance companies and employers from using genetic information against them (Asmonga D, 2008). Understanding these safeguards can help people feel empowered and less concerned about the consequences of their test results.

Additionally, the anonymity of genetic test results is essential. Patients should be informed of their rights regarding informed consent and how their genetic data may be used in research or clinical settings. Discussions about insurance implications, such as potential changes in coverage or premiums due to genetic results, are also necessary. Encouraging patients to notify at-risk relatives about their genetic status is critical, as this may lead them to consider testing or preventive actions. Furthermore, it is critical to highlight community services and support choices, such as local or online support groups and advocacy organizations, as it can offer emotional support and knowledge. These services can help patients feel less isolated and more connected to others facing similar issues, thus improving their overall well-being.

e) *Follow-ups and resources*

Any individual seeking cancer genetic risk evaluation and counseling assistance, irrespective of their risk category, should receive follow-up services that include discussing cancer screening specifications, assessing limitations, identifying risk-reduction methods, and referring to competent medical practitioners for long-term management (Trepanier et al., 2004). Periodic check-ins allow for the reviewing of family history, lifestyle, and health status updates and the adaptation of care plans and recommendations accordingly. Thorough documentation supports continuity, while educational resources help patients understand and manage genetic risks. Regular follow-ups with genetic counselors or healthcare providers also enable medical or lifestyle adjustments as informed by advancements in genetic science. Sharing information with relatives and providing resources like support groups and advocacy organizations support emotional well-being and financial resources, which help address insurance concerns and enable preventive care. Coordinate with the oncology team during transitions and summarize key takeaways from each session to ensure patients are well-prepared for informed health management.

9.3.4 Documentation Across Phases

Documenting informed permission for genetic analysis is done subsequent to describing the genetic examination and gauging participant comprehension, which is crucial (Schneider et al., 2023). The informed approval document is usually divided into the information sheet and the consent certificate signed by the patient being examined and the person requesting authorization (Schneider et al., 2023). The individual acquiring consent certifies that they have informed the patient about the testing, that the participant is aware of it, and that the patient is undergoing the testing willingly by signing the consent form with a copy provided to the patient, and the signed document should be kept in the individual's health record (Schneider et al., 2023). This document also becomes significant because most laboratories require proof of informed consent before conducting genetic testing (Schneider et al., 2023).

Documenting is critical for establishing accurate communication between the counselor and the counselee, making it necessary throughout the genetic counseling process. Traditional forms of clinical recordkeeping comprise the clinical appointment note (including follow-up visit entries), a letter to the recommended physician and patient, and a result report to the patient and the referring clinician (Hunt Brendish et al., 2021). The increased numbers of patients, emerging genetic counseling methods, switching to electronic medical records (EMR), new genetics-trained professional clinics, and innovations in genetic assessment technologies all pose complications to drafting various clinical papers (Hunt Brendish et al., 2021). Therefore, to address these problems, practice resource (PR) aims to contain the best guidelines for U.S.-based genetic advisers in writing compelling and exhaustive clinical paperwork utilizing a hybrid clinical document intended to promote interactions among individual providers, clients or families, and payers (Hunt Brendish et al., 2021).

9.4 CURRENT PRACTICE OF GENETIC COUNSELING IN ONCOLOGY IN INDIA

Cancer is an atrocious disease that has tormented humankind for ages. As shown in the 2020 publication from the World Health Organization, cancers accounted for almost one in six deaths. The Global Cancer Observatory, GLOBOCAN, estimated astonishing numbers of 19.3 million new cases with a total number of almost 10 million people losing their lives due to this disease within the same year (Sathishkumar, 2022). In this compilation, it's estimated that 5–10% of cases can be traced back to genetic factors; these factors are encrypted in the very blueprint of our genetic material called deoxyribonucleic acid, or DNA. Carriers of these genetic mutations responsible for hereditary cancer face serious issues, from being diagnosed early to intensive treatments with remarkably devastating long-term effects. It is, therefore, crucial to identify such individuals at the early stages of cancer, a critical step in preventing the devastating consequence of being diagnosed with terminal cancer.

According to the National Society of Genetic Counselors, genetic counseling is a complex procedure that not only assesses the risk of a genetic disorder occurring within a family lineage but offers individuals and their family's important information necessary during times of great uncertainty. It includes facets of testing and management, thus creating a setting through which families can come to terms with the threat of sickness. Therefore, genetic counseling involves much more than the dissemination of simple information; it becomes a demanding process of adjustment, which includes continuous psychological support that enhances resilience while individuals and families navigate the complexities of medical information. Genetic counseling has emerged as an important conversation within human life, where the characteristics inherited merge with the living experience. It becomes a way to understand how our genes interact with possible health issues that might affect us. According to the World Health Organization, this process serves as a quintessential tool to illuminate the genetic facets of afflictions that negatively affect individuals with hereditary disorders, or those standing on the border of potential genetic risks for themselves or their future progeny.

In the field of oncology, genetic components in DNA intertwine, and it is therein that genetic counseling plays a very pertinent role. Genetic counseling is conducted in both pre- and post-molecular testing phases. This teaching module is designed to educate the practicing clinician, basic and translational researcher, and layperson about the important role genetic counseling plays and its pivotal function in combating cancer. In the year 1947, Sheldon Clark Reed introduced the term "genetic counseling," later expanding upon the concept in his seminal work, Counseling in Medical Genetics, published in 1955. During its nascent stages, many of the early genetic clinics were operated by non-medical scientists or individuals lacking substantial clinical experience. However, as the understanding of genetic disorders evolved and the field of medical genetics emerged as a distinct discipline in the 1960s, genetic counseling gradually underwent a transformation, becoming an integral aspect of clinical genetics. It was only after some time that the significance of a solid psychological foundation was acknowledged, with the work of Seymour Kessler playing a pivotal role in this recognition. In 1969, Sarah Lawrence College in Bronxville, New York, established the first master's degree program in genetic counseling in the United States. Ten years later, in 1979, the National Society of Genetic Counselors (NSGC) was founded, with Audrey Heimler serving as its inaugural president.

9.4.1 Burden of Genetic Disorders in India

With India being the most populous country in the world, its staggering population with a crude birth rate of 16.27 live births per 1,000 people, and a country where there is a high prevalence of consanguineous marriage, it's no wonder that there is a high prevalence of genetic disorders. In a study done by I.C Verma, and S.Bijarnia, considering that India witnesses almost 24 million births every year, a significant proportion of such newborns will be affected by some form of genetic disorder. The Indian Genetic Disease Database (IGDD) release 1.0 (http://www.igdd.iicb.res.in), is a consolidated and curated library of numerous mutation data on prominent genetic illnesses that affect Indian populaces. The database has information on 5760 people who have the mutant alleles of the causative genes for 52 disorders. Based on published literature, information is provided regarding locus heterogeneity, mutation type, clinical and biochemical data, geographic location, and common mutations (Pradhan S., 2010).

9.4.2 The Current Scenario of Genetic Counselling in India

a) *Training and subsequent education*

The field of genetic counseling in India is relatively nascent compared to Western countries. However, several universities and institutions are beginning to offer specialized training programs. Organizations like the Indian Society of Human Genetics (ISHG) are working towards establishing guidelines and standards for genetic counseling practice. Increased awareness and educational initiatives are crucial to developing a skilled workforce in this field.

b) *Availability of services*

The availability of genetic counseling services differs markedly in urban and rural settings. For instance, cities like Mumbai, Delhi, and Bangalore have already put up genetic clinics and hospitals providing holistic genetic counseling services, whereas, in rural areas, such facilities are more often than not absent. However, mobile health initiatives and telemedicine could aid in addressing this challenge, thus enhancing accessibility to genetic counseling services.

c) *Healthcare system integration*

Incorporating genetic counseling into the larger healthcare system is critical for maximizing its benefits. This entails working with genetic counselors, doctors, and various other specialists. A multilateral system can improve patient outcomes and reinforce that genetic counseling is a medical treatment.

9.4.3 Future Prospects for Genetic Counselling in India

a) *Technological advancements*

The advancements observed in technologies and the onset of the genetic age will determine the future of genetic counseling in India. The advent of next-generation sequencing (NGS), and whole-exome sequencing (WES) among other technologies has created a platform that allows for in-depth genetic studies. Genetic counselors must keep up with these trends to counsel patients effectively.

b) *Research and development*

There is a need for more studies in genetics and genomics if we are to devise appropriate intervention methods for the Indian population. This is because academia, healthcare, and genetic research organizations can be used to propel policies and improve the services offered in genetic counseling.

9.4.3.1 Policy Development

As it stands, there is a great need to establish national parameters or policies concerning the practice of genetic testing and counseling in India. This can be achieved through lobbying for policymakers to develop appropriate ethical frameworks and availing resources for genetic research and counseling services (Verma & Bijarnia, 2002; Pradhan S., 2010).

9.5 CASE STUDIES IN INDIA

In 2022, the number of predicted cancer cases in India was 1,461,427, with an incidence rate of 100.4 per 100,000, suggesting that 1 in 9 Indians is likely to have cancer in their lifetime (Sathiskumar K et al., 2022). With lung and breast cancer quintessentially leading the cases in males, and females respectively, ALL (Acute Lymphoblastic Leukemia) was the leading cause of leukemia in children (0–14 years). Advances in our understanding of the genetic makeup and genotype-phenotype correlations would play an important role in refining current practices used in planning, monitoring, and evaluating cancer control activities.

9.5.1 Breast Cancer

This section focuses on the anatomy of the breast and its interlinking with metastasis and lymphatic spread.

The breasts are a pair of modified glands of sweat located over the pectoralis muscle. Vertically lying between the 2nd to 6th rib and horizontally between the sternum to the mid axillary line, in females, they contain mammary glands which are essential for lactation through the exudation of milk through nipples via a lactiferous duct. The lactiferous system consists of 15–20 lactiferous ducts, each draining a separate lobe of the mammary gland. The breast also contains a stroma of connective tissue which consists of a fibrous and a fatty part. The former condenses to form a suspensory ligament of Cooper which supports mostly the lower part of the breast. They also separate the secretory lobules of the breast. Moreover, if they're infiltrated during cancer, it pulls the ligaments inside resulting in dimpling of the skin, and subsequently subdermal lymphatics get blocked called *peau d'orange* (French: *orange skin*).

The functional unit in the breasts is called TDLU (Terminal Duct Lobular Unit) which acts as the site of origin for most breast cancers. Lymphatic and arterial supply to the breasts is essential for determining the extent of the spread of cancer and the route of administration.

Breast cancer can arise from epithelial cells anywhere in the ductal system, ranging from the area of the major lactiferous duct near the nipple to the terminal duct unit located in the breast lobule. The disease may be entirely in situ, a diagnosis that has increasingly become common with the discovery of screening for breast cancer, or it may be invasive cancer. The level of differentiation of the tumor is usually one of three grades: well differentiated, moderately differentiated, or poorly differentiated.

Usually, a scale of numerical grading is adopted that assesses three independent variables: nuclear pleomorphism, tubule formation, and mitotic rate. Tumors graded Grade III are usually classified in the poorly differentiated category. Traditionally, the cancer of the breast was broadly classified as 'scirrhous' (woody) or 'medullary' (brain-like). In modern practice, histologic descriptions are used to detail and classify types.

These correlations have been demonstrated to have clinical significance in the manner in which the tumor behavior and advancement. With the growing technologies and usage of molecular markers, there is anticipated to be a shift in the classification of breast cancers. According to the results from the immunohistochemistry testing of key proteins, it has been categorized into four distinct subgroups of breast cancer: Estrogen Receptor (ER), Progesterone Receptor (PR), Hormone Receptor (HR), HER2 proto-oncogene, and Proliferation Ki-67 antigen (Kumar et al., 2023). Breast cancer is categorized into four main groups based on the presence or absence of expressing factors, including hormone receptor (HR) and human epidermal growth factor receptor 2 (HER2): luminal A (HR+/HER2-), luminal B (HR+/HER2+), HER2 positive (HR-/HER2+), and triple-negative (HR-/HER2-) (Table 9.4). Due to the inherent resistance of this cancer to both endocrine and targeted treatments, the therapeutic alternatives for triple-negative breast cancer are limited. TNBC is characterized by an aggressive nature, higher rates of recurrence, and poor prognosis. Endocrine therapy constitutes one particular method in medical management for dampening the impact of estrogen on neoplastic cells within the breast.

9.5.1.1 Risk Factors and Assessment

One in every 21 Indian women developed breast cancer during her lifetime, being a hormone-driven cancer, here are some risk factors that contribute to the development and predisposition to breast cancer (Williams et al., 2008):

1. Increasing age.

2. Early menarche.

Table 9.4: Receptors and Their Receptor Modulation

	ER	PR	HER2/neu
Luminal A	+	+	-
Luminal B (majority)	+	+	+
Luminal B (minority)	+	+	_
Basal type (cytokeratin 5/6 +)	-	-	-
Claudin low (cytokeratin 5/6 -)	-	-	-
HER2/neu	-	-	+

Source: From Williams et al. (2008). With permission.

3. Late menopause.

4. Family history (both maternal and paternal).

5. Obesity.

6. Alcohol.

7. Smoking (pre-menopausal women).

8. Hormone Replacement Therapy.

9. Nulliparity.

10. Maternal age of >30 years at first live birth.

9.5.1.2 Triple Assessment

The triple assessment is a series of hierarchical/sequential steps that is used in the diagnosis and screening of breast cancer (Figure 9.3). It's considered one of the gold standard assessments and has a high sensitivity and specificity for a palpable breast mass.

9.5.1.2.1 Case Example

A 45-year-old homemaker from Bihar, Savita, comes to the hospital anxiously, complaining of a lump in her breast for the past six months. The onset was insidious, initially measuring 3×3cm but then rapidly progressed to the present size of 10×10cm. At first, the lump presented with no pain, but since the past month, she has complained of a dull aching continuous pain that is relieved by NSAIDs (non-steroidal anti-inflammatory drugs) prescribed by a local quack. On examination, an ulceration is found which is associated with foul-smelling discharge. Savita gives no history of discharge or retraction of the nipple. She has noticed no loss of weight, hemoptysis, or bone pain. Her serum bilirubin is within normal limits (Williams et al., 2008).

Savita says she must have been in 5th grade when she started menstruating and attained menopause 2 years ago, after having three kids: two daughters and one son. She is scared because her mother was the same age as her when she died of liver metastasis due to breast cancer. She says she is "terrified of dying and leaving her children alone."

During the initial genetic counseling session, the genetic counselor discovered that before her demise, Savita's mother underwent gene testing and was informed of a pathogenic variant in the BRCA1 gene. Savita's family history reveals that her maternal aunt had a double radical mastectomy when she was 60 years old and her maternal grandfather died from complications of chronic myeloid leukemia.

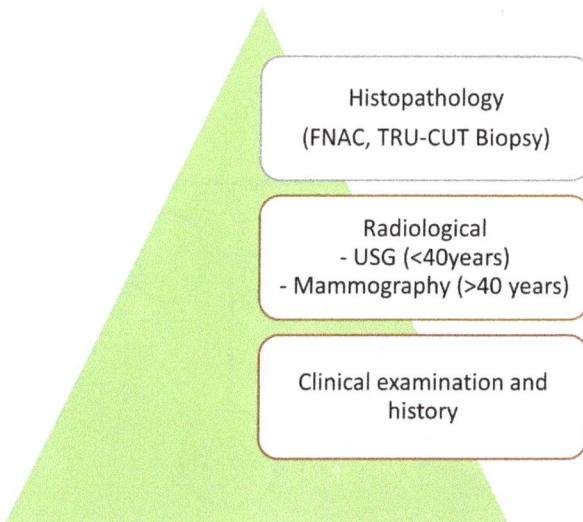

Figure 9.3 Three-tier diagnostic method for breast lesion evaluation.

After compiling all the data, the following pedigree chart was assigned for Savita's case illustrated in Figure 9.4 (see also Figure 9.5).

9.5.1.2.2 *Genetic Assessment*

When conducting a risk assessment, it is crucial to educate the patient about heredity patterns, penetrance, gene expression, and the risk of genetic variation, including the management of patients who choose to proceed with the testing versus those who do not. Many factors are taken into consideration when approaching the method of screening, treatment, and subsequent follow-ups (Table 9.5).

The genetic counselor gave detailed statistics and guidance informing the patient of the genetic testing. After digging in the record about her mother's positive *BRCA1* gene, and her maternal grandfather's death from CML, concluded that Savita should not only be tested for *BRCA1 and 2* but also for changes in the *TP53 gene*. Her genetic counselor introduced the idea of gene panel testing alluding to the prevalence of other members having cancers in the family. After mustering up enough courage, Savita proceeded with the testing.

Table 9.5: Questionnaire for Pre-genetic Counseling for Breast Cancer

Family history	1. At what ages were your relatives diagnosed?
	2. Do you know if any relatives have had genetic testing for cancer risk?
	3. Is there a family history of other cancers (ovarian, colon, sarcomas)?
Reproductive history	1. Did you attain menarche at a young age or menopause at an older age?
	2. At what age did you have your first child?
	3. Have you used hormone replacement therapy or oral contraceptive pills for extended periods?
	4. Were the kids breastfed or were other lactation sources used?
Lifestyle history	1. Do you smoke or drink alcohol recreationally?
	2. Have you had any radiation exposure or reside near any industrial region?
Miscellaneous history	1. How would you like to proceed with your screening?
	2. Do you have any questions regarding the treatment or the process?
	3. Are you concerned with the risk of your kids developing cancer?

Source: Adapted from Schneider et al. (2023).

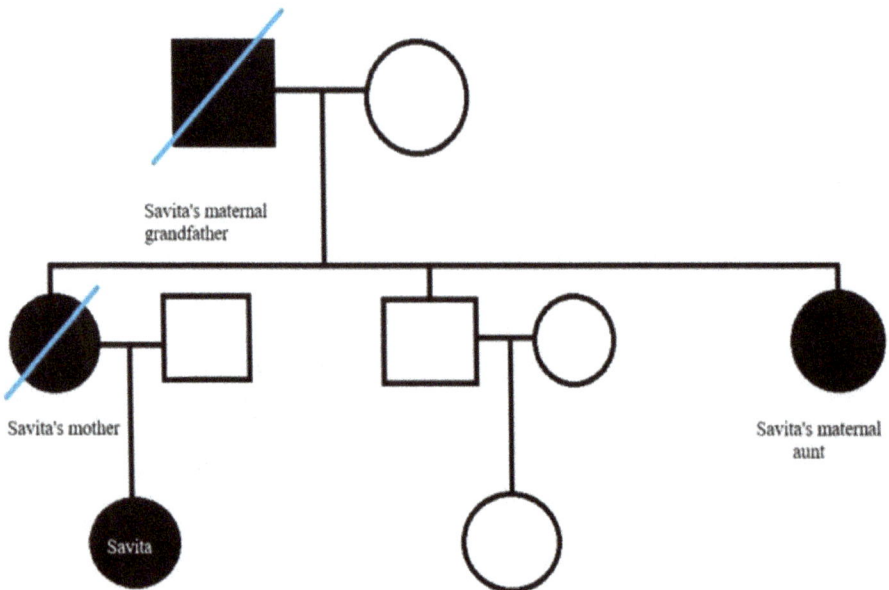

Figure 9.4 Savita's pedigree diagram.

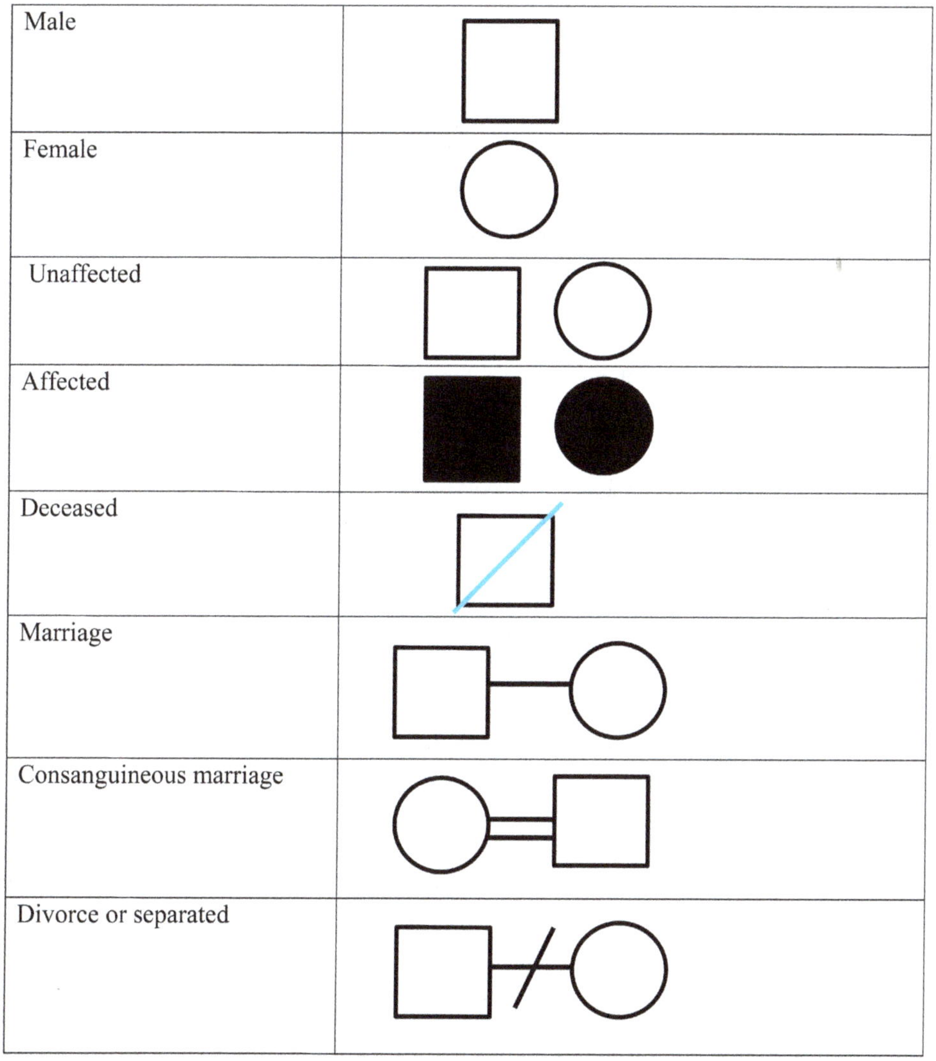

Male	
Female	
Unaffected	
Affected	
Deceased	
Marriage	
Consanguineous marriage	
Divorce or separated	

Figure 9.5 Pedigree analysis of breast cancer patients along with index for identification.

Four weeks later, genetic testing disclosed that Savita had a missense mutation in one of the most essential cell cycle genes, the *p53* gene located on chromosome 17p13, leading to a diagnosis of Li-Fraumeni syndrome. The aforementioned syndrome mainly consists of soft tissue/bone sarcomas, breast cancer coupled with leukemias, and adrenal cortical carcinomas. The counselor elaborated on the results and advised Savita to see an oncologist to discuss chemotherapies that reduce the risk of leukemias. After providing informed written consent and making an informed decision, Savita underwent a bilateral modified radical mastectomy and was placed on a prophylactic chemotherapy drug, Hydroxycarbamide.

9.5.1.2.3 Follow-up

In the follow-up visit, Savita was comparatively better after her mastectomy. Her PET scans showed no sarcomas or leukemias, although she was still a bit apprehensive about undergoing the same process repeatedly. Since genetic testing for Li-Fraumeni syndrome might have a psychological impact on patients, a weekly psychiatric consultation for Savita was also arranged. Moreover, the genetic pattern of Li-Fraumeni syndrome is autosomal dominant; hence Savita's daughters were under active surveillance, including whole-body MRI scans, genetic counseling, and psychological monitoring. They were kept on metformin, a drug that has been preclinically shown to prevent the development of pre-cancerous lesions (Li & Fraumeni, 1969).

Conclusion: This case therefore emphasizes the need for proper genetic testing and the accurate interpretation of test results. The input of the genetic counselor was crucial in assessing the family history of Savita's mother and sister. Proper testing eventually led to an accurate diagnosis for the family as well as each member (Williams et al., 2008).

9.5.2 Small Cell Lung Carcinoma

With its burden being approximately 14% of all lung cancer cases, small cell carcinoma of the lung is one of the most common carcinomas in the world. The lungs, vital organs for respiration, reside within the mediastinum and possess a cone-like shape. Each lung consists of an apex, base, three surfaces, and three borders. It is important to note that the left lung is somewhat smaller than the right lung, a difference likely attributed to the area occupied by the heart. These extraordinary structures arise from a protrusion of the primitive foregut during the fourth week of intrauterine development, progressing into a configuration of two lobes that ultimately converge to form the lungs as we recognize them in contemporary anatomy (Kumar et al., 2023).

The right lung is divided into three distinct lobes—superior, middle, and inferior—while the left lung features two lobes, superior and inferior, separated by a similarly oriented oblique fissure. The bronchial tree is a branching system of tubes that provides air to the alveoli in the lungs, starting from the trachea and ending at the alveolar sacs.

With the presenting symptoms commonly being commonly hemoptysis, dyspnea, dry cough, and weight loss, lung cancers can be broadly classified into the following categories (Kumar et al., 2023) illustrated in Figure 9.6.

Lung cancers are often present with a history of nodule formation. Any nodule that has been present for more than two years with the presence of calcification of fat is assumed to be benign. Features suggestive of malignancy include greater than 3 cm or a spiculated appearance, particularly with a smoking history. Computed tomography with intravenous contrast provides information regarding the vascularity of the lesion, with the malignant tumors tending to show the greatest contrast enhancement. CT may also depict additional nodules or hilar and mediastinal lymphadenopathy. The latter is a characteristic feature in the staging of primary bronchial carcinoma.

The gold standard for the detection of lung cancer is percutaneous needle biopsy under CT guidance, which has proven to be the most effective procedure for the diagnosis of lung cancers or nodules. However, if the lesion has a higher probability of malignancy in an immunocompetent patient with less serious comorbidities, the best option might be to proceed to resection.

9.5.2.1 Case Scenario

Mukesh, a 60-year-old, retired engineer and also an avid hiker, experiences a lack of sweating and micturition while on a hike. Attributing the cause to be the hot, humid Indian summer, he didn't think too much of it. After coming back from the trip, he started to experience shortness of breath and a dry cough. Thinking it to be a case of aggravated common cold or mild pneumonia, he took some over-the-counter drugs. His symptoms were relieved to an extent, but he continued to cough occasionally over the day.

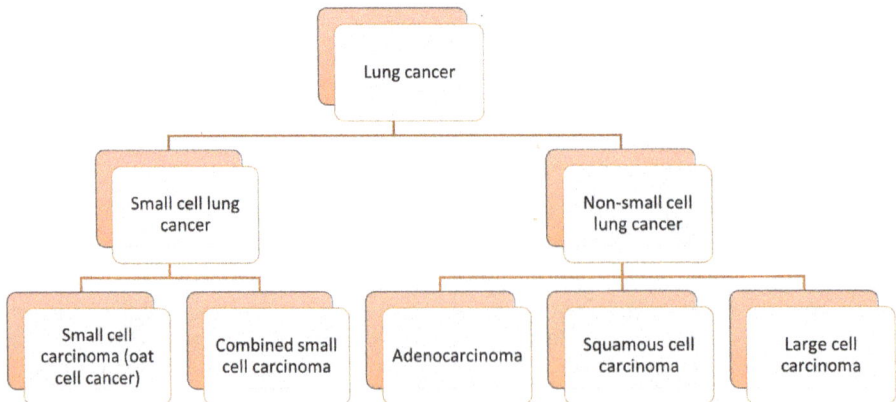

Figure 9.6 Classification of lung cancer.

A few days later, while expressing his concerns about the decreased frequency of micturition to a friend, he was advised to undergo some prostate testing due to the increasing trend of prostatic hyperplasia in the elderly male population. After completing his tests, his doctor advised him to do a serum osmolality and serum sodium test since his prostate revealed no abnormality. His urinalysis revealed highly concentrated urine with high fractional excretion of sodium for serum sodium. His effective serum osmolality was 230 mOsm/kg of water with normal adrenal and thyroid function. The doctor diagnosed him with SIADH (Syndrome of Inappropriate Anti-Diuretic Hormone) and an elevated plasma AVP confirmed the diagnosis. Since SIADH often presents as a paraneoplastic syndrome, the doctor advised Mukesh to undergo a chest CT scan.

Reluctantly, Mukesh complied with the CT despite his initial hesitation and was shocked to learn that his symptoms were not due to the hot weather or cold, but rather because of a pulmonary tumor. After his surgical resection, it was revealed that he was suffering from small cell carcinoma of the lung. When he arrived at the hospital with his family for genetic counseling, Mukesh revealed that he had been an avid smoker for the past 30 years with an estimated 4-pack year history. When it came to familial history, Mukesh had two cancer-free siblings. His father died when he was three years old due to asthma. The genetic counselor discussed with Mukesh the potential for an inherited predisposition to lung carcinoma. She suggested testing for EGFR and ERBB2 as part of a clinical research study.

Mukesh and his wife made appropriate inquiries about whether this test might provide more treatment possibilities and a better prognosis than what they had at that point, which was quite evidently their biggest concern. The counselor emphasized that the detection of an EGFR pathogenic variant may provide him with some additional treatment options, but it is important to appreciate that this is not inevitably the case. She highlighted that a high proportion of the clients who undertake genetic testing receive adverse results, which are irrelevant to their treatment program. The counselor continued to specify the difference between the blood genotyping test and the ongoing tumor genotypic test.

With a patient who is fairly insistent on choices regarding treatment at this time, the counselor explained that there was no need to decide on genetic testing at that moment.

Mukesh expressed that he did not want to waste any time and that he was keen on accumulating as much information as possible, regardless of the minimal likelihood that it might lead to more treatment alternatives. Consequently, he participated in the genetic testing study.

The patient had a germline pathogenic variant of the EGFR gene identified in both him and a specimen taken from his lung tumor. He expressed an interest in this particular variant for the fear of having potentially passed this on to his 14-year-old son. He had the counseling session discuss at length with the patient reasons for delaying the genetic test for his son until his older (Kumar et al., 2023).

During subsequent visits, the sister of the patient was present and indicated interest in undergoing genetic testing. Given the strong family history of lung cancer on the patient's mother's side, the counselor raised the issue of other relatives who may be at risk of carrying the EGFR pathogenic variant. The patient had no objections to sharing his results with other family members.

9.5.2.2 Follow-up

On follow-up, he expressed relief and thankfulness that he had passed the 1-year mark since the diagnosis was having an adequate response to treatment and remained optimistic despite the low survival rate (Schneider et al., 2023). Mukesh and his wife have decided to wait until their son is older before sharing the possibility of him being a carrier.

9.5.2.3 Discussion

Counseling individuals who have recently been diagnosed with cancer can be a challenging task, as their primary focus during this time is on making decisions regarding their active treatment. Therefore, it may prove challenging to navigate questions about treatment. With the increasing prevalence of tumor genetic testing, patients may experience confusion regarding the distinctions between somatic and germline testing in terms of their objectives and findings. For individuals afflicted with cancers associated with unfavorable prognoses, there can be a drive to explore every available test or study that may offer improved treatment alternatives. This quest for information may result in the development of unrealistic expectations on genetic testing.

9.5.3 Leukemia

Childhood leukemia stands as the most prevalent form of pediatric cancer, representing over one-third of all new cancer diagnoses among children and adolescents. In cases of acute leukemia, there is an unchecked proliferation of primitive stem cells, resulting in an overwhelming accumulation of blast cells within the bone marrow. This encroachment diminishes the space available for normal hematopoietic cells, leading to a spectrum of clinical manifestations associated with bone marrow failure, including anemia, increased susceptibility to bleeding, and heightened risk of infections. ALL (Acute Lymphoid leukemia) is usually depicted as anemia and thrombocytopenia whereas the leukocyte count varies from as low as 1×10^9/L to as high as 500×10^9/L or more. The diagnosis is mostly confirmed by the presence of blast cells. The marrow is typically hypercellular, with the replacement of normal elements by leukemic blast cells in varying degrees (Kumar et al., 2023). The risk factors for ALL can be categorized as:

A Environmental (ionizing radiation)

B. Inherited Syndromes

    i. Bloom syndrome

    ii. Ataxia telangiectasia

    iii. Down's syndrome

    iv. Fanconi's anemia

    v. Xeroderma pigmentosa

    vi. Rothmund-Thomson syndrome

    vii. Tuberous sclerosis complex

    viii. Juvenile polyposis

    ix. Leukemia, familial

    x. Li-Fraumeni syndrome

    xi. Blackfan diamond

    xii. Hereditary retinoblastoma

    xiii. Rhabdoid tumor syndrome

    xiv. Schwachman-Diamond syndrome

    xv. Neuroblastoma, familial

    xvi. WT1-related syndromes

Prognostically, ALL can be categorized on the following criteria based on the survival rate and outcomes, as outlined in the Table 9.6.

Table 9.6: Good and Bad Prognosis in ALL

	Good Prognosis	Bad Prognosis
Race	White	Black
Age	2-9 years	<1 or >10 years
Sex	Female	Male
CNS	-	+++
HSM LN	-	+++
Mediastinal mass	-	+++
Type	L1	L2, L3
Cytogenetics	Hyperdiploidy	Hypodiploidy
Immunophenotype	B cell, early pre B cell	T cell
Testicular involvement	Absent	Present
Translocation	T (12;21)	T (9,22)

Source: From Kumar et al. (2023). With permission.

9.5.3.1 Case Scenario

Saman, a lively two-year-old boy, was diagnosed with Beckwith-Wiedemann syndrome (BWS) shortly after birth. His parents, Sama and Ajay, had learned to navigate the complexities of this rare overgrowth disorder, attending regular medical check-ups and following up on cancer surveillance protocols due to BWS's increased cancer risk. Saman had always been a moderately bigger than other children his age, with a distinctive growth pattern typical of BWS, but he was otherwise full of energy and life (Brioude et al., 2018).

However, during one of his routine visits, his pediatrician noticed some unusual symptoms. Saman had been more fatigue than usual, bruising easily, and occasionally experiencing fevers. His parents initially attributed these signs to normal toddler behavior or minor infections. But after a series of blood tests, their worst fears were realized—Saman was diagnosed with acute lymphoblastic leukemia (ALL).

The counselor starts the session by welcoming the family and expressing empathy for the challenging diagnosis. Acknowledging that the news of leukemia is overwhelming, the counselor creates a supportive environment for the family to ask questions. The counselor begins emphatically,

"I understand this is a difficult time for your family. You've been managing Beckwith-Wiedemann syndrome, and now with the recent diagnosis of leukemia, it's natural to have concerns. My role here is to help you understand how these conditions are connected and to guide you through the genetic aspects of this journey".

"Beckwith-Wiedemann syndrome (BWS) is caused by genetic changes that affect the regulation of growth. Children with BWS have increased risk of a given type of cancer, particularly in early childhood. While acute lymphoblastic leukemia is not the most common cancer associated with BWS, the genetic changes that occur in BWS can make some children more vulnerable to developing cancer, including ALL. Understanding these risks helps us to plan the best treatment and surveillance moving forward".

The counselor goes on,

"BWS is often linked to changes on chromosome 11, specifically in a region that controls growth. These changes are usually sporadic, meaning they occur randomly, but in some cases, they can be inherited. We can perform further genetic testing to determine if your child's condition has an inherited component. This information may also be helpful if you're considering having more children, as it can guide reproductive decisions and risk assessments".

The counselor emphasizes the importance of a multidisciplinary approach to care, involving oncologists, pediatricians, and geneticists, to manage both the leukemia and ongoing surveillance for other potential complications of BWS. The counselor provides reassurance about the treatment options and long-term prognosis.

The pediatric oncologist induces the chemotherapy in Saman by giving him steroids and vincristine. They also give an informed detail to the parents explaining the prolonged harmful outcomes of steroids and vincristine in the long term. High-dose methotrexate was added to the regimen to prevent a central nervous system relapse. At further visits, repeated cycles of the drugs were given.

After three months, Saman was scheduled to meet with the genetic counselor again to discuss whether or not genetic testing should be done. Upon entering the consultation room, the counselor was astonished to see a full entourage of individuals of diverse age ranges, seated and standing in front of her. At the start of the discussion, it came to light that the attendees included both the parents of the child, the maternal grandparents and a family friend in addition to the patient's uncles. Presently, he was an in-patient and undergoing high-dose chemotherapy. The counselor described in detail about the multigene panel test and said how the results will be useful, mainly regarding treatment options and follow-up. She gave an in-depth explanation of the BWS genes and the resultant various linked syndromes. She also discussed the drawbacks and risks of testing, involving the chance of identifying variants of uncertain significance. The parents had a high interest in pursuing testing and described their interest in seeking as much detail as possible about the son's potential cancer risks. The participants gave informed consent for the panel test, and the counsellor coordinated the blood sample collection before her next round of chemotherapy.

The counselor also explained to them about the importance of tumor surveillance which involves monitoring the development and progression of tumors in the body. It is a crucial aspect of cancer management, allowing for early detection and timely intervention to improve patient outcomes. Surveillance methods may include regular imaging scans, blood tests, and physical examinations to track changes in tumor size and behavior. Early detection through surveillance can lead to more effective treatment options and increased chances of successful outcomes for patients with cancer. Perspectives on the screening for malignant tumors in childhood vary according to local, national, and international practices. In the region of North America, it is suggested that proactive tumor screening be conducted when the likelihood of tumor development surpasses 1% (Weksberg et al., 2010). In numerous European nations, proactive tumor screening protocols are usually implemented when the likelihood of tumor formation surpasses 5% and is founded on molecular mechanisms (Weksberg et al., 2010).

Since Sama was 14 weeks pregnant, the family also agreed to perform prenatal testing on the fetus. The counselor explained to them that if a genomic variant linking chromosome 11p15.5 (i.e. a cytogenetically visible duplication, translocation or inversion) or a CDKN1C (Cyclin-dependent kinase (CDK)-inhibitor 1C) pathogenic variant has been detected in the proband, fetal DNA from samples can be obtained for prenatal testing (Weksberg et al., 2010). The fetal DNA can be attained by chorionic villus sampling (CVS) or amniocentesis. The parents were also advised that in case the fetus DNA turns positive for fetal methylation changes, it's their decision if they want to go ahead with the pregnancy because there are certain limitations of parental testing for epigenetic alterations.

After three years of continuous maintenance chemotherapy with 6-mercaptopurine and methotrexate, Saman had no relapse and was declared as cancer free by his oncologist.

9.5.3.2 Discussion

Conversations about genetic testing introduce an additional layer of complexity to an already complicated diagnostic and treatment process (Schneider et al., 2023). The process might be increasingly difficult for parents with young children where grief might be multiplied multifold. Providing genetic testing information to multiple individuals, each with varying levels of understanding about genetics, is also a challenge.

9.6 SOCIAL, ETHICAL, AND CULTURAL IMPLICATIONS OF GENETIC COUNSELLING IN ONCOLOGY IN INDIA

9.6.1 Social Implications (Lolkema, 2013)

i) **Social stigma**: In India, genetic factors are often misunderstood, and families can face social stigma when genetic diseases are often considered a "curse" or the result of past actions called karma in previous life. This can lead to stigmatization of affected people and their families, especially in rural areas. Families affected by genetic conditions may experience social isolation. Due to stigma, some families may hide a member's condition to avoid gossip, further marginalizing the affected individual and limiting their social opportunities.

ii) **Marriage**: As arranged marriages become more common, genetic traits identified through counseling can affect a person's marital life. There is often a great deal of effort to hide genetic disorders for fear of diminishing social status and marriage prospects for the fear of getting ostracized by society.

iii) **Female feticide**: Despite laws prohibiting prenatal sex determination, a significant concern is the misuse of genetic counseling for determining the sex of the fetus. In a patriarchal society, the preference for male children can exacerbate gender bias and lead to female feticide (Chakravarty et al., 2022)

iv) **Discrimination against women**: Women are often blamed as the first and foremost culprit in genetic disorders in children, while it is a fact that both parents contribute equally to a child's genetic makeup. Such situations may even lead to social boycotts or, in extreme cases, domestic violence. In India, where a woman has been held responsible for infertility or genetic issues for centuries, a child born with genetic deformities, regardless of the reason, only adds to existing gender disparities.

v) **Views on the issue of reproduction within religious values**: In a country having different religious beliefs, genetic counseling could be viewed from different ethical viewpoints. Some religious groups may forbid genetic testing, abortion, or medical treatments based on their beliefs concerning the character of life and destiny. For example, the decision to abort a pregnancy for genetic defects might contradict some religious beliefs.

vi) **Ethical Dilemmas**: Genetic counselling raises considerable ethical issues when it comes to selective reproduction, the application of genetic information, and the choice to terminate pregnancies. These dilemmas are deeply subjective and could be influenced by individual religious or cultural beliefs.

vii) **Access to services:** Genetic counselling and testing services are costly and unavailable to most economically disadvantaged groups. It, therefore, widens the gap between those who can afford them and those who cannot have them. This will then worsen existing health inequalities (Revathy & Praba, 2022).

viii) **Healthcare infrastructure:** There is a lack of proper infrastructure to provide genetic counselling and diagnostic services in many regions, mainly rural areas in India. Access is often limited to urban centers, which limits the benefits of these developments to rural communities.

ix) **Family involvement:** In Indian society, family plays a crucial role in decision-making, especially regarding health. Genetic counselling decisions are often made not just by individuals but by entire families, which can complicate decision-making processes. There may be pressure from extended family members to make decisions based on social status, finances, or cultural expectations.

x) **Public policy and regulation**: The Government of India has enacted legislation including the Pre-Conception and Pre-Natal Diagnostic Techniques (PCPNDT) Act with the expressed intent of preventing genetic data abuse, especially as it involves sex-selective abortions. However, enforcing this legislation remains a challenge in other areas. With the expansion of genetic counseling, strong ethical standards need to be established and implemented by India to protect the proper use of genetic information and prevent various forms of misuse. Public policy must promote improved genetic service access and affordability to reach other sections of the public at large.

xi) **Discrimination concerns:** Genetic information acquired from genetic susceptibility testing may have medical, financial, and psychosocial implications for the tested individual and his or her relatives. A common fear for individuals considering hereditary cancer genetic testing is employment and insurance discrimination. However, there is insufficient evidence that employment and insurance discrimination occur as a result of the findings from hereditary cancer genetic testing.

9.6.1.1 Conclusion

The gradual change in society's attitudes toward genetic disorders may be likely once genetic counseling becomes more accepted and accessible. The latest advancements in gene technology may still reduce stigma while leading to more open-minded understandings through education and awareness. Genetic counseling also holds promise for better overall health outcomes for individuals with a genetic disorder. It is essential to ensure the accessibility of these technologies for all individuals to avert the widening of the healthcare divide.

9.6.2 Cultural Implications

Genetic counseling in India carries considerable cultural connotations that should be approached as a double-edged sword. In a country marked by a significant number of religious beliefs, social mores, and culture, the introduction of genetic counseling may evoke complex reactions and emotions from individuals as well as families. Cultural, genetic, and medical interplay may create both challenges and opportunities in the offer of genetic counseling services.

Relating to the perception of society about genetic disorders and disabilities, genetic counseling in India has very important cultural impacts. Societal norms and stigmas prevailing in society about disabilities frequently result in shunning, social seclusion, and denial of health services to individuals who suffer from genetic conditions. Hence, overcoming these cultural barriers is very crucial, in which accurate information, support, and counseling facilitate affected individuals and their families.

The concept of genetic inheritance may also go against the dominant ideas and practices in India. For instance, genetic testing for hereditary disorders may raise ethical questions related to issues such as arranged marriages, family honor, and cultural expectations. Genetic counselors need to navigate these complex cultural landscapes sensitively and with due regard to ensure that their intervention is both effective and culturally appropriate (Lolkema, et al., 2013).

9.6.4 Miscellaneous Issues

Mental illness in India is still a stigmatized issue in 2024, hence the provision of genetic counseling to individuals grappling with psychological illnesses such as bipolar disorder, depression, or schizophrenia, may present nuanced differences compared to counseling sessions experienced for those without such diagnoses.

Many patients with mental health challenges encounter the similar fundamental issues as anyone seeking genetic insights; predominantly when their conditions are effectively managed through treatment, the conventional frameworks of counseling can be seamlessly employed. Nonetheless, it remains paramount to ensure that the patient's psychotherapy or psychiatric team is informed of the genetic testing whenever feasible. In instances, where these professionals are integral to the institution's care framework, obtaining explicit consent from the patient to discuss test results may be rendered unnecessary. Conversely, should these mental health providers operate outside the counselor's established practice, the patient's permission to initiate dialogue with them may be essential (Jain et al., 1998).

In both scenarios, the necessity for communication with the treatment team must be thoroughly explored with the patient, allowing for the possibility that additional time may be warranted during sessions to monitor their responses and relay pertinent information. Should the genetic counselor determine that a patient's mental health issues are inadequately controlled—impairing their capacity to provide informed consent, they are compelled to seek further insights from the patient's care providers before proceeding with genetic testing.

Those who care for individuals with mental health conditions are typically equipped to assist counselors in evaluating a patient's ability to consent. In circumstances where a patient has designated a healthcare proxy, the counselor might have to involve the proxy in sessions or at least apprise them of the concerns surrounding the testing process. It is crucial to differentiate between competency, typically determined through a formal legal process, and decisional ability, which is assessed by the healthcare professionals. The evaluation of decision-making capacity often utilizes various instruments and generally revolves around four key components: reasoning, understanding, appreciation, and expressing a choice.

Some may stand at a precipice of personal crisis, seeking the guiding hand of short-term counseling to navigate through turbulent waters. Others may require a more enduring form of support, addressing the shadows cast by loss, the weight of unaddressed mental health problems, or the pervasive dissatisfaction that colors their existence.

Moreover, cancer genetic counselors are urged to forge partnerships with mental health specialists who can lend their expertise in navigating complex cases, propose approaches for engaging with vulnerable patients, and facilitate the coordination of referrals. Preferably, these mental health practitioners will possess a familiarity with the complexities of acute or chronic ailments and a foundational understanding of hereditary cancer syndromes or, at the very least, a willingness to delve into this critical knowledge.

The specter of second cancer looms large for children with hereditary syndromes, leading parents to grapple with the unsettling realization that even if the current affliction is vanquished, their concerns about their child's future health will persist. Lifelong vigilance may be warranted, not only for early indicators of various cancers but also for non-malignant yet potentially lethal conditions associated with the syndrome. Overwhelmed by a multitude of fears, parents may wrestle with guilt if they suspect they have passed on the deleterious mutation to their child (Kumar et al., 2023).

In light of these profound concerns, it becomes evident that psychological insights regarding the parents of children with hereditary cancer syndromes, as well as the children themselves, are of significant importance and could greatly aid in the planning and organization of their treatment and care. Typically, in cases of pediatric cancer, parents can find solace in the knowledge that their other children are not likely at increased risk. However, the discovery that a cancer-stricken child harbors a genetic mutation that also resides in a parent casts a long shadow, suggesting that each of the parent's children may inherit this perilous mutation, thereby elevating their likelihood of developing cancer. The potential for increased risk may extend to the parent as well, necessitating that extended family members be informed, thus widening the circle of anxiety and trepidation.

In less populous and rural locations, there is still a dearth of genetic counseling and testing services. Certain people or neighborhoods may have disproportionate access, even in major cities. Cancer risk reduction and cancer detection recommendations, as well as genetic screenings, may not be available to people with inadequate or no health insurance. Disturbing disparities in cancer-related morbidity and mortality between urban and rural populations persist in India. While this is a small portion of a much bigger demographic and socioeconomic issue, genetic counselors should push for fair treatment for all patients and steer clear of preferential treatment. In addition to adding fresh, significant perspectives to these difficult conversations, increasing diversity in the genetic counseling field will make patients feel more accepted and involved. Genetic counseling providers must exercise much greater caution in terms of transparency and inclusiveness, given the historical record of eugenics and maltreatment of marginalized communities. Genetic counselors are encouraged to support testing for underprivileged populations in addition to offering patients and families ethical genetic counseling, as the high cost of genetic testing and counseling impedes equal access.

9.6.4.1 *Case Scenario*

Ramesh, a 45-year-old recently diagnosed with Stage 1 colon cancer and found to be HNPCC gene positive, was referred to meet with the genetic counselor. Ramesh underwent a partial colectomy with the tumor genetic analysis revealing an HNPCC variant in 30% of cells analyzed, raising concerns about a possible diagnosis of HNPCC (Hereditary Non-Polyposis Colorectal Cancer) (Li & Fraumeni, 1969).

The counselor patiently explained that ethical guidelines necessitated informed consent and thorough documentation, for should the tests yield positive results, Ramesh would need counsel regarding the myriads of HNPCC-related cancer risks that lay ahead.

Ramesh, a father of two daughters aged 21 and 18, was a high school teacher. His parents had succumbed to asthma-related ailments in their 80s, and the only cancer link in his lineage was a maternal cousin, who had faced breast carcinoma at the tender age of 36. Over the next several days, the counselor worked with the oncology service. He had a lively discussion with the service about the appropriateness of radiation therapy for Ramesh.

She provided valuable information regarding his colon cancer and family medical history, which showed only one instance of early breast cancer in a distant relative. The presentation of the clinical dilemma led to a suggestion by one of the clinicians that Ramesh be tested "outside the record" and by another as to whether he would accept testing if knowledge of the results was limited to the oncology service (Axilbund & Peshkin, 2010).

The geneticist discussed in great detail the implications of the somatic HNPCC variant and raised the possibility of a germline genetic test that could shed light on his future management and, more importantly, the necessary screening of his daughters. However, taking into consideration the gravity of what was being presented to him, Ramesh opted not to pursue the latter because of its very high cost. Ramesh had taken a loan from the bank, as he could not stand the surging cost of the treatment and the counseling.

The genetic counselor and radiation oncologist set up a follow-up appointment with Ramesh in a clinical setting that was filled with unease to discuss some of the intricacies involved in genetic testing: namely, its risks and benefits. The key benefit lay in the potential of the germline test to inform personalized decisions related to radiation therapy. Ramesh showed a more guarded ambivalence, indicating that although he "at some point" might consider the possibility of genetic testing, he felt poorly prepared to pursue that now. With Ramesh's high oncotype score and failure to clearly establish a diagnosis of HNPCC, the oncology conference concluded reluctantly as follows: radiation therapy was advised by the oncologists. Ramesh completed the treatment as prescribed, with no complications, and accepted this part of his health with resolve.

Over a period of three years, Ramesh finally gave in to the idea of germline testing, a decision taken almost solely because his family was persistently troubling him with the urge to clarify the mysteries of hereditary breast cancer in their lives. In this tangled world of genetic investigation, however, HNPCC gene testing-as well as other breast cancer genes-showed no pathogenic variants.

9.6.3 Ethical Implications

Common morality is described as the collective set of ethical norms embraced by all individuals who take morality seriously, irrespective of their cultural, ethnic, or religious backgrounds. While many individuals perceive their ethical beliefs as reflective of common morality, it is often the case that these perspectives are influenced by personal experiences, values, and community standards. Those who are immoral consciously decline all ethical principles, while selectively moral individuals adhere to some, but not all, of these standards. From the principles of common morality, governing bodies derive the rules, rights, and codes of conduct that guide their members and constituents.

Genetic counseling often adopts a directive approach, particularly in developing nations such as India. Here, caregivers and patients especially those from low socioeconomic backgrounds tend to prefer that clinicians take the lead in making decisions, showing little inclination to delve into various treatment options. Some practitioners view genetic counseling as a tool for minimizing birth defects and harmful genetic traits within the population, with the overarching aim of enhancing the quality of life for families affected by such conditions. Many clinicians express a degree of acceptance toward the termination of pregnancies upon discovering genetic disorders through prenatal testing. Implicitly or explicitly, the guidance offered to patients frequently leans toward the option of termination; clinicians may employ negative phrasing to sway the patient's decision without openly advocating for such an outcome.

A genetic counselor can recommend the appropriate tests tailored to one's pregnancy. Notably, 54% of respondents are aware that parental histories such as diabetes, anemia, and asthma are often integral to genetic counseling discussions. While genetic testing is not universally mandated, it becomes paramount in the face of potential genetic disorders, such as Down syndrome, especially if suggested (Verma, 1988). This testing is typically indicated for specific cases or those with familial histories of particular diseases and is conducted at various stages throughout pregnancy.

Counseling becomes essential, particularly when the mother is over 30 and has experienced previous difficulties in her quest for motherhood. While engaging in genetic counseling can greatly mitigate the risks linked to severe genetic conditions, such as sickle cell anemia and cystic fibrosis. When a person faces the emotional challenges of repeated miscarriages or the looming possibility of preterm births, it is essential to seek not only a physician's advice but also the specialized knowledge offered by a genetic counselor. Before conception and throughout the complex process of pregnancy, it is highly recommended that pregnant women consult a private genetic counselor who can explain the basic genetic factors involved. In India, the rates of miscarriage, preterm labor, and abortion are higher than in more developed countries. In addition, many are willing to contact a genetic counselor, knowing that this consultation can greatly reduce the risk of these devastating results.

The personal and family nature of the genetic data makes privacy protection very important. Within the intricate meshwork of close-knit familial relationships, especially as realized in the Indian context, the problem of protection for sensitive information from improper appropriation and use is considerably amplified. Without effective safeguarding provisions, such genetic data becomes a weapon for discrimination not by employers or insurance agents but even within the home circle against people according to their intrinsic vulnerabilities, causing damage to their lives. Unlike the traditional healthcare professional, the genetic counselor handles the role differently, having a special ability to communicate potential consequences with sympathy and understanding.

They can guide through the emotional landscape of choice, thus making the entire process less intimidating by relating to the psychological state of the individual. A genetic counselor should not only be proficient in the nuances of communication but also have an intimate understanding of genetic principles. It is in the context of genetic counseling that individuals may unintentionally disclose their familial histories of disease, weaving aspects of their heritage into a pedigree chart to reveal the probability of heritable, significant disorders. However, a pertinent question comes to mind: is it prudent to entrust this confidential medical information to a genetic counselor given the risk of exploitation that might occur? For a counselor to accurately evaluate these disclosures, a basis of trust must first be established, which ensures that families engage in open dialogue to avoid unwanted repercussions and to promote informed decisions regarding prenatal diagnostics.

With the advancement of genetic testing, the necessity for pre-and post-test counseling is becoming more obvious. Genetic counselors are said to be less clinically engaged than medical geneticists, thus consulting services take on a more informal and comprehensive character. The expertise of genetic counselors is necessary in public health programs, which call for an integrated approach. Such an approach should comprise community education, population screening, genetic counseling, and promotion of early diagnosis that are all directed toward the reduction of the incidence of genetic disorders and chromosomal anomalies.

9.6.3.1 Conflicts

Conflicts of interest (COI) arise when a situation jeopardizes the integrity of professional judgment, indicating that providers' choices or actions could be based on personal interests outside of their most significant duty to their clients or patients (Schneider et al., 2023).

Evident conflict of interest combined with the inherent dangers it begets makes it a vital issue regardless of the mere existence of some actual or other form of damage or injury. There indeed two folds objectives of detection and elimination of the conflict of interest, one being guarding against the dangers it can be used for creating for patients and other researchers going underneath their conduct and ensuring public trust and confidence in the study findings provided by healthcare providers and correctness in conducted research.

These goals are critically important to promote transparency and ensure the integrity of medical practices and research efforts. At the same time, it is important to realize that relationships with COI are essential in the creation and advancement of new products that can help recuperate health. The way ahead urges us to develop a more profound awareness, as many conflicts of interest arise not from intentional wrong doing but rather from simple neglect. It is high time that we strive to remove the negative connotation associated with this term, understanding that it is not inherently a harmful notion. Rather, we ought to advocate for a culture of openness among our colleagues, patients, and other practitioners. We, as guardians of our respective professions, need to enforce policies aimed at not only reducing the incidence of conflicts of interest but also addressing them with expertise and ethical considerations.

Conflict of interest is that insidious presence which sits at the periphery of our professional activities and hence requires careful monitoring and deliberate action to maintain the principles of integrity and transparency in our efforts.

Although we are now living in times much more aware and enlightened concerning many details of what comprises COI, as a sad reality, quite several practitioners had to face the uncongenial endeavor of coming to terms with their wrongdoings and questionable moves.

Therefore, it would be fairly rational to conclude that putting robust frameworks in place focused on professional or peer oversight and accountability is critically important. Situations, where the genetic counselor sits on an advisory board, consults, or even receives honoraria or grants from a profitable organization that develops services or products whose utilization is relevant to his clients, raise ethical dilemmas primarily related to conflicts of interest. Experts work in the labyrinthine web of genetic counseling, where they operate at the intersection of an ethical obligation to a profession and an economic incentive in their practice-an open situation requiring a balanced approach. For them, above everything else, is the protection of the trust of their patients in preserving their health essential pillar of their profession. Although the convergence of interests may produce beneficial partnerships that promote the field and support the well-being of those served, counselors and their professional associates must remain alert to the fact that these interests are not always compatible. To navigate this intricate landscape, they must adopt prudent measures, ensuring that ethical considerations prevail in the pursuit of scientific progress.

9.7 FUTURE SCOPE AND CHALLENGES

Genetic counselors will continue to be crucial providers to guarantee excellent, efficient genetic testing services (Schneider et al., 2023). It is well established that improving early detection involves teaching people about their specific risk factors, customizing screening recommendations based on each person's level of risk, and catering to their psychological needs (Schneider et al., 2023). Furthermore, studies indicate that cancer education initiatives are unlikely to succeed unless they address patients' concerns about the disease (Schneider et al., 2023; Schienda & Stopfer, 2020). As cancer genetic services are increasingly included in oncology care, they are changing. Through innovative service delivery methods, testing to determine cancer risk is now available to a broader range of adult and pediatric patient populations (Schienda et al., 2020). Automated techniques are being developed to offer genetic and genomic information on a large scale (Powers et al., 2019). Clinical-grade chatbots that comply with the Health Insurance Portability and Accountability

Act (HIPAA) are one example (www.cleargenetics.com) (Powers et al., 2019). There is a promise for the responsible delivery of automated techniques under clearly defined clinical scenarios by inclusion and review by experts from the significant medical communities, including genetic counselors (Powers et al., 2019). Another example of an automated method for diagnosing genetic risk is ChatGPT, which correctly responds to most of the questions examined regarding hereditary syndromes, genetic testing, and counseling (Patel et al., 2024). With 88.2% (15/17) and 66.6% (2/3) accurate and thorough responses to questions about Lynch syndrome and hereditary breast and ovarian cancer, respectively, ChatGPT also fared in evaluating particular genetic illnesses (Patel et al., 2024). Although more information from gynecologic oncologists would be required to inform patients about genetic disorders, these findings imply that this potent tool can be used as a patient resource for genetic guidance inquiries (Patel et al., 2024). Numerous researchers are developing integrated hybrid models to offer the best genetic counseling services (Hynes et al., 2020; Yala et al., 2019; Contegiacomo et al., 2004). In one study, Hynes et al. developed a framework for genetic counseling services and discovered that the initial assessment of a group and mini-individual genetic counseling model shows that this method is a preferred approach to care delivery and is very well-liked by both patients and genetic counselors (Hynes et al., 2020). Utilizing individual mini-sessions after group information sessions enabled the provision of quality genetic counseling while cutting down on waiting periods. More extensive organized research studies are required to assess this paradigm in greater detail (Hynes et al., 2020). By taking into account the cumulative effect of multiple genetic variants, polygenic risk scores (PRSs) combined with NGS technology and bioinformatic tools will allow for more refined and nuanced risk assessments, improving surveillance and prevention strategies for at-risk individuals and advancing personalized medicine.

Genetic counseling in the field of oncology, although it has a promising future, is also accompanied by certain challenges that must be overcome. There are, however, ethical considerations, and the protection of personal data is highly critical, especially since sensitive genetic data would be available. In addition, as the number of variants of uncertain significance (VUS) increases, more and more educational and training efforts are needed for counselors to accurately evaluate risk. Furthermore, limited resources and sociocultural differences may constrain the availability of such genetic counseling services in low-resource societies, hence the need for more effort in devising measures that promote the availability of these services and consistent guidelines across various healthcare institutions. Moreover, the barriers limiting family history assessment and cancer risk evaluation in oncology centers on patient, provider, and system factors (Lu et al., 2014). Patients frequently lack some knowledge about the history of their family or refrain from sharing the information (Lu et al., 2014). Providers often do not have adequate means or belief in their ability to assess family structure, and the great majority of electronic health records (EHR) systems are just poorly designed for such information (Lu et al., 2014). Global issues like unclear billing or time constraints also make it difficult for oncologists to be comprehensive (Lu et al., 2014). Additionally, a lack of diversity in public databases and large testing cohorts can result in classification errors. Therefore, it is important to increase minority population representation for precise interpretation and fewer VUS, even though this will require time. When it comes to the danger of pediatric cancer, there are still issues with obtaining informed permission, obtaining data on effective surveillance, prevention techniques, and the psychological and financial effects on children and family members. Increased death rates from a variety of cancers in low-income nations, such as India, highlight the lack of qualified genetic counselors and public awareness of the issue. The Professional Society of Genetic Counselors in Asia was founded in 2015, and its mission was described in a 2017 report on genetic counseling (GC) in ten Pacific countries (Verma et al., 2019). According to the survey, there are less than 100 genetic counselors in India, which is a low number compared to the country's population (Verma et al., 2019). Additionally, the profession of genetic counseling is not well-known (Elackatt N. 2013). Indian genetic counselors frequently balance a variety of duties, such as test selection, clinician support, laboratory work, report preparation, psychosocial support, and administrative duties, which takes them away from their primary duties in genetic counseling, making it even more of a barrier to the widespread use of genetic counseling in oncology treatment (Laurino et al., 2018).

9.8 CONCLUSION

Oncology-related genetic counseling has enormous potential to revolutionize cancer treatment in India and worldwide by facilitating individualized, risk-informed treatment. Early diagnosis, focused prevention, and individualized treatment choices for hereditary malignancies are made possible by the increasing accessibility and integration of genetic testing into clinical practice. To fully realize this potential, though, several structural issues must be resolved. These include extending access to genetic services in both urban and rural regions, hiring more qualified genetic counselors, and raising public awareness of the importance of genetic counseling in cancer prevention and treatment. To further dispel social stigma and false beliefs around genetic testing, a culturally aware strategy is necessary. To guarantee that everyone has fair access to these services, legislators, medical professionals, and academic institutions must work together. India can greatly lower its cancer burden and enhance long-term results for patients and their families by filling these gaps and utilizing the power of genetic counseling.

REFERENCES

Abacan M et al. (2019). The global state of the genetic counseling profession. *Eur J Hum Genet* 27(2):183–197.

Amendola LM et al. (2016). Performance of ACMG-AMP variant-interpretation guidelines among nine laboratories in the clinical sequencing exploratory research consortium. *Am J Hum Genet* 98(6):1067–1076.

American Society of Clinical Oncology (2003). American Society of Clinical Oncology policy statement update: genetic testing for cancer susceptibility. *J Clin Oncol* 21(12):2397–2406.

Angus BJ et al. (2022). Participants aux Davidson's principles and practice of medicine, 23 édition. In Innes JA, ed., *Davidson: L'essentiel de la Médecine*, 23rd edn (pp. ix–xiv). Elsevier. doi:10.1016/b978-2-294-77556-7.09990-2.

Antoniou AC et al. (2008). The BOADICEA model of genetic susceptibility to breast and ovarian cancers: updates and extensions. *Br J Cancer* 98(8):1457–1466.

Asmonga D (2008). Getting to know GINA. An overview of the Genetic Information Nondiscrimination Act. *J AHIMA* 79(7):18–22.

Axilbund JE, Peshkin BN (2010). Hereditary cancer risk. In: Tercyak KP, ed., *Handbook of Genomics and the Family*. Springer:267–291.

Baker DL et al. (1998). *A Guide to Genetic Counseling*. Wiley.

Bennett RL et al. (1995). Recommendations for standardized human pedigree nomenclature. *J Genet Counsel* 4(4):267–279.

Bennett RL et al. (2008). Standardized human pedigree nomenclature: update and assessment of the recommendations of the National Society of Genetic Counselors. *J Genet Counsel* 17:424–433.

Bennett RL et al. (2022). Practice resource-focused revision: Standardized pedigree nomenclature update centered on sex and gender inclusivity: a practice resource of the National Society of genetic counselors. *J Genet Counsel* 31(6):1238–1248.

Biesecker BB (1997). Psychological issues in cancer genetics. *Sem Oncol Nursing* 13/2:129–134.

Biggio Jr, JR., Ralston, SJ. (2017). Counseling about genetic testing and communication of genetic test results. Obstetrics and Gynecology, 129(4): E96–E101.

Brioude F et al. (2018). Expert consensus document: Clinical and molecular diagnosis, screening and management of Beckwith-Wiedemann syndrome: an international consensus statement. *Nature Rev Endocrinol* 14(4):229–249.

Carbine NE et al. (2018). Risk-reducing mastectomy for the prevention of primary breast cancer. *Cochrane Database Syst Rev 4*.

Chakravarty N et al. (2022). Cultural and social bias leading to prenatal sex selection: India perspective. *Front Global Women's Health* 3:903930.

Contegiacomo A et al. (2004). An oncologist-based model of cancer genetic counselling for hereditary breast and ovarian cancer. *Ann Oncol* 15(5):726–732.

Croyle RT et al. (1997). Psychologic aspects of cancer genetic testing: a research update for clinicians. *Cancer* 80(S3):569–575.

Elackatt NJ (2013). Genetic counseling: a transnational perspective. *J Genet Counsel* 22:854–857.

Evans N et al. (2019). How should decision aids be used during counseling to help patients who are 'genetically at risk'? *AMA J Eth* 21(10):E865–E872.

Gail MH et al. (1989). Projecting individualized probabilities of developing breast cancer for white females who are being examined annually. *JNCI* 81(24)L1879–1886.

Garber J et al. (2008). Genetic counseling: an indispensable step in the genetic testing process. *J Oncol Pract* 4(2):96–98.

Garber JE, Offit K. (2005). Hereditary cancer predisposition syndromes. *J Clin Oncol* 23(2):276–292.

Global Hallyu Status 2023. (2023).

Heimler A (1997). An oral history of the National Society of Genetic Counselors. *J Genet Counsel* 6(3):315–336.

Hopwood P (1997). Psychological issues in cancer genetics: current research and future priorities. *Patient Educ Counsel* 32(1–2):19–31.

Hunt Brendish K et al. (2021). Genetic counseling clinical documentation: practice resource of the National Society of Genetic Counselors. *J Genet Counsel* 30(5):1336–1353.

Hynes J et al. (2020). Group plus "mini" individual pre-test genetic counselling sessions for hereditary cancer shorten provider time and improve patient satisfaction. *Heredit Cancer Clin Pract* 18:1–7.

Jain U et al. (1998). Prevalence of fragile X(A) syndrome in mentally retarded children at a genetics referral centre in Delhi, India. *Indian J Med Res* 108:12–16.

Kastrinos F et al. (2017). Development and validation of the PREMM$_5$ model for comprehensive risk assessment of lynch syndrome. *J Clin Oncol* 35(19):2165–2172.

Kim YE et al. (2019). Challenges and considerations in sequence variant interpretation for mendelian disorders. *Ann Lab Med* 39(5):421–429.

Kumar V et al. (2023). *Robbins and Kumar Basic Pathology*, 11th edn, New Delhi, India: Elsevier.

Landau C et al. (2021). Effect of inquiry-based stress reduction on well-being and views on risk-reducing surgery among women with BRCA variants in Israel: a randomized clinical trial. *JAMA Network Open* 4(12):e2139670.

Laurino MY et al. (2018). A report on ten Asia Pacific countries on current status and future directions of the genetic counseling profession: the establishment of the Professional Society of Genetic Counselors in Asia. *J Genet Counsel* 27:21–32.

Li FP, Fraumeni JF (1969). Soft-tissue sarcomas, breast cancer, and other neoplasms: a familial syndrome? *Ann Intern Med* 71:747–752.

Lolkema MP et al. (2013). Ethical, legal, and counseling challenges surrounding the return of genetic results in oncology. *J Clin Oncol 31*(15):1842–1848.

Lu KH et al. (2014). American Society of Clinical Oncology Expert Statement: collection and use of a cancer family history for oncology providers. *J Clin Oncol 32*(8):833–840.

Malhotra H et al. (2020). Genetic counseling, testing, and management of HBOC in India: an expert consensus document from Indian Society of Medical and Pediatric Oncology. *JCO Global Oncol 6*:991–1008.

Mikkelson J, Odunsi K (2019). *HHS Public Access 28*(1):26–33.

Offit K, Thom P (2007). Ethical and legal aspects of cancer genetic testing. *Sem Oncol 34*(5):435–443.

Paluch-Shimon S et al. (2016). Prevention and screening in BRCA mutation carriers and other breast/ovarian hereditary cancer syndromes: ESMO Clinical Practice Guidelines for cancer prevention and screening. *Ann Oncol 27*:v103–v110.

Park K (2007). *Park's Textbook of Preventive and Social Medicine*, 19th edn, M/S Banarsidas Bhanot Publishers, Jabalpur.

Patel JM et al. (2024). ChatGPT accurately performs genetic counseling for gynecologic cancers. *Gynecol Oncol 183*:115–119.

PDQ Cancer Genetics Editorial Board. (2024). Cancer genetics risk assessment and counseling (PDQ®): Health professional version. In PDQ Cancer Information Summaries. National Cancer Institute (US).

Petrucelli N et al. (2022). *BRCA1-and BRCA2-Associated Hereditary Breast and Ovarian Cancer*: Adam MP et al., eds, GeneReviews.

Pilarsk R (2021). How have multigene panels changed the clinical practice of genetic counseling and testing. *J Nat Comp Cancer Net 19*(1):103–108.

Pina-Neto JMD (2008). Genetic counseling. *J Pediat 84*:S20–S26.

Powers J et al. (2019). Genetic counseling and oncology: proposed approaches for collaborative care delivery. *Can J Urol 26*(5 Suppl 2):57–59.

Pradhan S (2010). Indian genetic disease database. *Nucleic Acids Res 39*(suppl 1):D933–D938.

Rantanen E et al. (2008). What is ideal genetic counselling? A survey of current international guidelines. *Eur J Hum Genet 16*(4):445–452.

Revathy KS, Praba, LJ (2022). Familiarity, knowledge, attitude, and willingness towards genetic counselling among the South Indian population. Journal of Public Health and Development, 20(2), 228–239. https://doi.org/10.55131/jphd/2022/200217

Richards S et al. (2015). Standards and guidelines for the interpretation of sequence variants: a joint consensus recommendation of the American College of Medical Genetics and Genomics and the Association for Molecular Pathology. *Genet Med 17*(5):405-423.

Sąsiadek MM et al. (2020). Genetics and oncology (part 1.). Fundamentals of genetic testing-based personalised medicine in oncology. *Nowotwory. J Oncol 70*(4):144–149.

Satam H et al. (2023). Next-generation sequencing technology: current trends and advancements. *Biology 12*(7):997.

Sathishkumar K et al. (2022). Cancer incidence estimates for 2022 & projection for 2025: result from National Cancer Registry Programme, India. *Ind J Med Res 156*(4 & 5):598–607.

Schaaf CP (2021). Genetic counseling and the role of genetic counselors in the United States. Medizinische Genetik, 33(1):29–34.

Schienda J, Stopfer J (2020). Cancer genetic counseling—Current practice and future challenges. *Cold Spring Harbor Perspectives in Medicine*, 10(6): a036541.

Schneider KA et al. (2023). *Counseling About Cancer: Strategies for Genetic Counseling.* John Wiley & Sons.

Shah M et al. (2023). Genetic counselling in India: the state of affairs. *Cancer Res Stat Treat 6*(3):484–485.

Steensma DP (2018). Clinical consequences of clonal hematopoiesis of indeterminate potential. *Hematol 2014, ASH Educ Prog 2018*(1):264–269.

Trepanier A et al. (2004). Genetic cancer risk assessment and counseling: recommendations of the national society of genetic counselors. *J Genet Counsel 13*(2):83–114.

Tyrer J et al. (2004). A breast cancer prediction model incorporating familial and personal risk factors. *Stat Med 23*(7):1111–1130.

Ulhaq E et al. (2023). Narrative review on genetic counseling for hereditary cancers: general considerations. *Cancer Res Stat Treat 6*(2):239–247.

Verma A et al. (2019). Mainstreaming genetic counseling for BRCA testing into oncology clinics–Indian perspective. *Ind J Cancer 56*(Suppl 1):S38–S47.

Verma IC (1988). Genetic causes of mental retardation in India. In M. Niermeijer & E. Hicks (Eds.), *Mental retardation, genetics and ethical considerations: International symposium* (pp. 99–106). D. Reidel Publishing Company.

Verma IC, Bijarnia S. (2002). The burden of genetic disorders in India and a framework for community control. *Commun Genet 5*(3):192–196.

Walsh T et al. (2006). Spectrum of mutations in BRCA1, BRCA2, CHEK2, and TP53 in families at high risk of breast cancer. *JAMA 295*(12):1379–1388.

Walsh T et al. (2010). Detection of inherited mutations for breast and ovarian cancer using genomic capture and massively parallel sequencing. *Proc Nat Acad Sci 107*(28):12629–12633.

Weitzel JN et al. (2018). Somatic TP53 variants frequently confound germ-line testing results. *GenetMed 20*(8):809–816.

Weksberg R et al. (2010). *Beckwith–Wiedemann syndrome. Eur J Hum Genet 18*(1):8–14.

Williams N, O'Connell PR (eds). (2008). *Bailey & Love's Short Practice of Surgery.* CRC Press.

Wong SM et al. (2017). Growing use of contralateral prophylactic mastectomy despite no improvement in long-term survival for invasive breast cancer. *Ann Surg 265*(3):581–589.

Yala A et al. (2019). A deep learning mammography-based model for improved breast cancer risk prediction. *Radiology 292*(1):60–66.

10

Ethical, Legal, and Social Implications of Cancer Genetic Testing

Anmol Bhatia and Parul Sharma

10.1 INTRODUCTION

10.1.1 Overview of Cancer Genetic Testing

Genetic testing is a rapidly advancing method for cancer screening, utilizing sophisticated genomics technology to enhance oncology care. Approximately 5% to 10% of cancers possess a hereditary component (Lu et al., 2014), with specific malignancies such as breast, colorectal, ovarian, prostate, pancreatic, and endometrial cancers occasionally exhibiting familial patterns. Individuals possessing inherited mutations in hereditary cancer genes exhibit a markedly elevated risk of developing such cancers, exemplified by Lynch syndrome, associated with mutations in the MLH1, PMS2, MSH2, MSH6, and EPCAM genes (Esplen et al., 2001). Predictive genetic testing is an essential instrument for identifying individuals at risk, providing advantages to both patients and their relatives (Lu et al., 2014). ASCO (American Society of Clinical Oncology) has underscored that the management of individuals with hereditary cancer predispositions is fundamental to oncology practice, with more than 200 genetic tests currently available to evaluate cancer risk (Robson et al., 2015). A favorable outcome may facilitate risk-reduction strategies, encompassing lifestyle modifications, chemoprophylaxis, and prophylactic surgeries.

Nonetheless, genetic testing is still underutilized, as nearly 50 percent of at-risk individuals do not participate in testing (Gray et al., 2012). Although research shows predominantly favorable attitudes towards genetic testing, numerous individuals exhibit reluctance stemming from psychological, financial, and cultural apprehensions (Henneman et al., 2013; Stanislaw et al., 2016; Grady et al., 2003). The choice of the initial family member for testing introduces complexity, as individuals with cancer may be reluctant to engage (Ropka et al., 2006). Consequently, genetic counselling is advised prior to and following testing to address risks, benefits, and limitations. The economic dimension, quantified by willingness to pay (WTP), aids in evaluating individual valuations of genetic testing and informs cost-benefit analyses to enhance healthcare strategies (Drummond et al., 2015). Notwithstanding the advantages, the substantial expense continues to pose a considerable obstacle to extensive testing, and the influence of out-of-pocket costs on testing practices requires additional investigation (Matro et al., 2014; Allford et al., 2014). No survey has specifically investigated consumer interest; however, a study on breast cancer revealed that 82% of high-risk women accepted genetic counselling, yet only 11% of their relatives opted for testing, even when it was provided at no cost (Olejniczak et al., 2016).

While genetic testing services have expanded into low- and middle-income countries (LMICs) through research initiatives and international partnerships, genetic counseling has not developed at the same pace and remains largely a Western concept (Joseph et al., 2004; Kucheria et al., 2003; Huang et al., 1998; Joseph et al., 2006; Parsam et al., 2009; Ramprasad et al., 2007). The shortage of genetic counsellors globally poses a heavy load on physicians, especially in the LMICs, considering the limited training surrounding medical genetics. Therefore, it makes it hard to provide adequate patient education and support (Wonkam et al., 2011; Dimaras et al., 2010; Hill et al., 2016). The motto of bringing genomics from "lab to village" is falling short in the LMICs due to the lack of responsibility and building of ethical genetic services in a way they deem culturally appropriate (Tindana et al., 2012; de Vries et al., 2011; de Vries et al., 2012a; de Vries et al., 2012a; Jenkins, 1999; Masum et al., 2007). Most literature on genetic services in these regions focuses on capacity building and technical success rather than addressing broader ethical considerations (Wonkam et al., 2010; Horovitz et al., 2013; Nivoloni et al., 2010; Vieira et al., 2013; World Health Organization,2016; Chaabouni et al., 2001). However, experts increasingly recognize the need for an ethically grounded approach to ensure genetic services meet the specific needs of LMIC populations (Kingsmore et al., 2012; Melo & Sequeiros, 2012). A growing body of research is beginning to explore the ethical and sociocultural challenges in genetic services, emphasizing the importance of integrating these considerations into their implementation (Wonkam et al., 2011; Tschudin et al., 2011; Jegede, 2009; Ghosh et al., 2002).

At present, genetic testing is predominantly accessible in specialized clinical environments and limited to particular patient demographics, underscoring the necessity for additional research on

DOI: 10.1201/9781003542162-10

public interest and cost-sharing willingness, which could enhance the efficacy of cancer prevention initiatives.

10.1.2 Comprehension and Understanding of Genetic Testing

Genetic testing for disease susceptibility, especially in conditions such as cancer, has generated significant optimism in public perception (Etchegary, 2014). A Dutch survey indicated that 64% of participants acknowledged the prospective advantages of genetic testing. Nonetheless, in conjunction with this optimism, there is a significant concern among the public about the possible misuse of genetic test results, which may result in discriminatory attitudes towards individuals with genetic predispositions (Henneman et al., 2013).

Despite the optimistic potential of genetic testing for evaluating cancer risk, numerous ethnic minority communities in Europe and the United States face considerable disparities in access to genetic services and representation in research initiatives (Godard et al., 2003). A prior evaluation concentrated on the obstacles encountered by ethnic minorities, including South Asian, White Irish, and African populations, in accessing cancer genetic services. This assessment revealed various challenges, such as insufficient awareness and understanding of available genetic testing services, language obstacles, stigma linked to risk status, fatalistic views on cancer, expectations of adverse emotional reactions, uncertainty about the information presented, and a widespread mistrust concerning data utilization (Allford et al., 2014).

Numerous studies involving populations such as Chinese Australians, Hispanics, and African-Americans have revealed a lack of understanding regarding the importance of genetics in relation to cancer, BRCA mutations, and genetic testing. Generational differences in awareness, knowledge, and beliefs, particularly evident in Chinese Australian and Hispanic communities, may have led to hesitance regarding genetic testing for cancer susceptibility among older generations. Certain Chinese Australian participants observed that traditionalists and older generations often ascribed diseases to misfortune or historical transgressions instead of acknowledging the inheritance of mutated genes (Eisenbruch et al., 2004).

A lack of knowledge about hereditary cancer and insufficient experience with genetic testing may discourage individuals from pursuing such testing. Moreover, varying interpretations of the term "close relatives" may hinder the precise evaluation of cancer risk among Chinese Australian populations. The pronounced focus on familial connections among Hispanic women may affect their perspectives on genetic testing and their understanding of cancer risk. The diverse viewpoints highlight the necessity of recognizing and tackling challenges unique to each ethnic group, requiring customized solutions to alleviate these problems (Miki et al., 1994). Privacy issues and the risk of discrimination arising from the disclosure of genetic data to third parties, including insurers and employers, represent considerable disadvantages of genetic testing. The apprehension that employers or health insurers could access such data has deterred numerous Americans from pursuing genetic testing, with some individuals even abstaining from medical care or insurance claims to safeguard their employment prospects. Surveys conducted in Canada and Europe have revealed similar concerns regarding privacy within the domain of genetic testing (Miki et al., 1994). The apprehension regarding genetic discrimination is justified, as there have been occurrences where genetic information has influenced employment and insurance determinations. Despite the existence of legal safeguards against genetic discrimination in certain nations, the public's perceived risk continues to be substantial. This perception may result in hesitance to engage in genetic testing, consequently restricting the advantages of early detection and preventive strategies for at-risk individuals (Miki et al., 1994).

In conclusion, even though there is a possible potentiality in genetic testing for the evaluation of cancer risk, it is extremely important to address the shortcomings linked with its applications. This encompasses augmenting access to genetic services for ethnic minority populations, advancing public comprehension of genetics, and tackling issues related to privacy and discrimination. Customized strategies that account for cultural and generational disparities are crucial for enhancing the adoption of genetic testing and guaranteeing equitable distribution of its advantages among varied populations (Singh et al., 2023).

10.2 GENETIC TESTING FOR CANCERS AND INHERITED CANCER SYNDROMES

10.2.1 Multiple Endocrine Neoplasma

Multiple endocrine neoplasia (MEN) is a group of hereditary cancer disorders that include thyroid tumors, among other conditions. Medullary thyroid carcinoma (MTC) is a rare malignancy found in about 25% of MEN cases, with MEN2A being the most prevalent subtype. Nearly all MEN2A cases exhibit MTC, along with pheochromocytoma and hyperparathyroidism. The expression of MEN2 shows dominant inheritance, with germline RET mutations identified in 92% of MEN2 cases (Eng et al., 1996).

The M918T mutation within exon 16 accounts for approximately 95% of MEN2B mutations, while the A883F mutation in exon 15 is detected in 5% of cases. Historically, preventive measures included preemptive thyroid removal and continuous monitoring for pheochromocytoma and hyperparathyroidism, with genetic testing recommended before surgery or by age six. After six years of age, individuals with RET mutations should undergo annual testing for pheochromocytoma and hyperparathyroidism and may be considered for thyroidectomy. This proactive approach is crucial because MTC can be aggressive and is often diagnosed at an advanced stage if not detected early (Olschwang et al., 1998).

MEN2 is categorized into subtypes MEN2A, MEN2B, and familial medullary thyroid carcinoma (FMTC), all associated with an elevated risk of medullary thyroid carcinoma (MTC) (Burke et al., 1997).

MEN2A: This is the predominant subtype, linked to medullary thyroid carcinoma (MTC), pheochromocytoma, and hyperparathyroidism. MEN2A frequently entails mutations at codons 634, 609, 611, 618, and 620 of the RET gene. Certain families with MEN2A may also exhibit Hirschsprung disease or cutaneous lichen amyloidosis (Decker et al., 1998; Jung et al., 2010).

MEN2B: This less prevalent subtype is more aggressive, characterized by medullary thyroid carcinoma (MTC) that may manifest in early childhood, pheochromocytoma, neuromas, ocular anomalies, and unique physical traits. MEN2B is predominantly linked to mutations at codons 918 (M918T) and 883 (A883F) of the RET gene (Jasim et al., 2011).

FMTC: This condition is regarded as a variant of MEN2A, distinguished exclusively by medullary thyroid carcinoma (MTC) in the absence of the other symptoms characteristic of MEN2A. FMTC is frequently linked to mutations in multiple codons of the RET gene (Jung et al., 2010).

Genetic testing for MEN2 entails sequencing the RET gene to detect pathogenic variants. This testing is essential for early diagnosis and management, especially for individuals with a familial predisposition to MEN2. Prophylactic thyroidectomy is advised for individuals with MEN2 to avert the onset of medullary thyroid carcinoma (MTC), which is frequently aggressive and may metastasise early. The timing of surgery is contingent upon the particular RET mutation and the familial history of medullary thyroid carcinoma onset (Bussières et al., 2018).

The clinical sensitivity of RET gene sequencing is elevated, identifying pathogenic variants in over 98% of MEN2A and MEN2B instances, and exceeding 95% in FMTC cases. The testing strategy encompasses complete coverage of all coding exons of the RET gene, guaranteeing thorough identification of mutations (Ahmed et al., 2018).

Testing is recommended for individuals exhibiting clinical characteristics indicative of MEN2A, MEN2B, or FMTC, as well as for those with a familial history of these disorders. Early genetic testing can identify carriers of RET mutations, facilitating timely preventive interventions like prophylactic thyroidectomy (Bussières et al., 2018).

Notwithstanding advancements in genetic testing and management, challenges persist, particularly in forecasting the onset of MTC and other MEN2 components, potentially resulting in overtreatment or postponed intervention. Moreover, the rising mobility of populations can disrupt clinical care, complicating the tracking and management of affected families (Dralle et al., 2021).

Prophylactic thyroidectomy is an essential preventive intervention for individuals with MEN2, especially those possessing high-risk RET mutations. This procedure markedly diminishes the likelihood of developing MTC and its related mortality. The choice to undertake prophylactic thyroidectomy is determined by the particular RET mutation, familial history, and clinical characteristics (Jasim et al., 2011; Bussières et al., 2018).

Genetic testing for MEN2 presents psychosocial and ethical implications, especially in asymptomatic individuals. Comprehensive counselling prior to testing is crucial to mitigate potential emotional effects and facilitate informed decision-making. The choice to pursue testing must be made with meticulous evaluation of the advantages and possible disadvantages (Giarelli et al., 2002).

In summary, MEN2 is a multifaceted hereditary syndrome managed via genetic testing and preventive measures such as prophylactic thyroidectomy. Comprehending the particular RET mutations and their consequences is essential for efficient management and minimizing the risk of MTC and other related conditions.

10.2.2 Inherited Cancer Syndromes

Von Hippel-Lindau (VHL) Syndrome: Characterized by renal cell carcinoma, pheochromocytoma, and hemangioblastomas. VHL tumor suppressor gene mutations are associated with autosomal dominant inheritance (Maher ER, 2011), and the risk of renal cell carcinoma and retinal/cerebellar hemangioblastoma increases with age (Hong et al., 2019). The age-dependent penetrance of VHL means that the likelihood of developing these tumors escalates significantly as individuals grow older. Early detection and management are critical to prevent severe outcomes (Hong et al., 2019).

Cowden Syndrome (CS): CS is linked with genetic mutations of the gene PTEN giving rise to the risk of breast, thyroid, and endometrial cancers. CS is also associated with other benign growths and developmental abnormalities. The relationship between CS and the PTEN gene is well established, highlighting the importance of PTEN mutations in the development of these cancers (Cummings et al., 2023; Dragoo et al., 2021).

Li-Fraumeni Syndrome (LFS): LFS is linked with genetic mutations of the gene TP53 and is addressed as an uncommon autosomal dominant cancer syndrome. It is known to further manifest various other types of tumors. LFS is characterized by a high risk of developing multiple cancers, often at a young age, including sarcomas, breast cancer, and brain tumors (Franceschi et al., 2017). The TP53 gene plays a crucial role in DNA repair and cell cycle regulation, and mutations in this gene can lead to uncontrolled cell growth and tumor formation (Light et al., 2023).

Hereditary Nonpolyposis Colon Cancer (HNPCC) Syndrome: Results from mutations in DNA mismatch repair genes like MLH1, MSH2, MSH6, and PMS2, elevating the risk of colorectal and endometrial cancer. HNPCC is also associated with an increased risk of other cancers, such as ovarian, gastric, and small intestine cancers (Silva et al., 2005). The syndrome is characterized by the absence of the typical polyps seen in familial adenomatous polyposis (FAP), but it shares a similar risk of developing colorectal cancer (Silva et al., 2005).

Peutz-Jeghers Syndrome (PJS): Identified by LKB1/STK11 mutations and distinctive hyperpigmented macules. PJS is associated with an increased risk of gastrointestinal polyps and various cancers, including breast, colon, and ovarian cancer. The syndrome is characterized by its unique mucocutaneous melanin deposits, which are often seen in the mouth, lips, and digits (Lim et al., 2003).

Hereditary Melanoma: Frequently linked to CDKN2A mutations, whether or not dysplastic nevi are present. CDKN2A mutations are associated with a high risk of developing melanoma, often at a younger age. This highlights the importance of early detection and preventive measures for individuals with a family history of melanoma (Leachman et al., 2017; Pauley K et al., 2012; Rossi et al., 2019).

In summary, these hereditary cancer syndromes underscore the importance of genetic testing and early intervention to manage cancer risk effectively. Understanding the specific genetic mutations and their implications can help tailor preventive strategies and improve outcomes for affected individuals and their families.

10.2.3 Colorectal Cancer

Proactive genetic testing is advantageous in cases with a significant familial medical history of a particular condition, such as hereditary non-polyposis colon cancer (HNPCC) (Strafford, 2012). This condition is frequently signified by three or more affected relatives, with at least one diagnosis made prior to the age of 50. Routine colonoscopic surveillance in these individuals can substantially diminish the incidence of colorectal cancer (CRC), with studies indicating a 62% reduction compared to those who do not receive such monitoring (Farndon et al., 1986).

Colorectal cancer ranks as the third most prevalent cancer among both males and females in the United States, with around 33% of cases occurring in individuals with a familial history of the disease (Siegel et al., 2020). Multiple genes have been linked to hereditary cancer syndromes that increase susceptibility to colorectal cancer as well as other tumor types (Yurgelun et al., 2017). The attributes of colorectal polyps, encompassing their quantity, dimensions, histological type, and anatomical position, are essential for evaluating colorectal cancer risk (Donis-Keller et al., 1993).

The importance of family history is vital in forecasting CRC risk, as the risk escalates with the number of affected relatives. Adenomatous polyps are the primary precursors to the majority of colorectal cancers, and excising these polyps is a fundamental strategy for mitigating risk in patients with adenomatous polyposis. The conventional management for patients exhibiting discernible polyposis characteristics typically entails surgical procedures, including colectomy or proctocolectomy with ileal J-pouch-anal anastomosis. Individuals diagnosed with attenuated adenomatous polyposis may choose rigorous surveillance via endoscopic polypectomies instead of surgical intervention (Roncucci et al., 2017).

Genetic testing is essential in the clinical management of related individuals, facilitating the identification of hereditary mutations in affected persons to confirm specific syndrome diagnoses. This enables the expansion of genetic testing to family members at risk. The Cancer Genome Atlas has revealed significant genetic heterogeneity in colorectal cancers, with over 80% displaying somatic mutations in the APC gene, while a specific subset demonstrates unique gene mutation profiles (Hinoi et al., 2021).

Although genetic testing is beneficial for validating syndromic diagnoses in non-adenomatous polyposis instances, its clinical applicability is frequently constrained (Thayalasekaran, 2022). Colorectal cancer screening has demonstrated efficacy in reducing morbidity and mortality associated with colorectal cancer (Ladabaum et al., 2020). Optimally, aligning CRC screening with risk levels is desirable; however, the difficulty resides in precisely identifying individuals who would derive the greatest benefit from targeted surveillance. The conventional dependence on clinical history as the foundation for evaluating CRC risk is complicated by discrepancies in clinical characteristics and the probability of disease manifestation (Weitzel et al., 2011).

Advanced parallel next-generation sequencing techniques have the potential to identify novel genes or gene combinations associated with genetic susceptibility, which may enhance targeted and effective colorectal cancer prevention strategies. These methodologies, encompassing whole exome or genome analyses, can yield extensive insights into the genetic framework of CRC, facilitating the identification of novel risk factors and enhancing risk stratification (Fatemi et al., 2023).

In summary, proactive genetic testing and early intervention are essential for managing familial colorectal cancer risk. By comprehending genetic predispositions and employing suitable screening strategies, individuals can markedly diminish their risk of developing colorectal cancer (CRC). The incorporation of advanced genetic technologies into clinical practice is expected to improve the accuracy of colorectal cancer risk assessment and prevention strategies, thereby enhancing outcomes for at-risk individuals.

10.2.4 Breast and Ovarian Cancer

Genetic testing for breast and ovarian cancer, specifically targeting the BRCA1 and BRCA2 genes, holds considerable potential in identifying individuals at increased risk for these conditions. Individuals with genetic mutations in these genes may experience diverse potential outcomes, including the risk of developing breast cancer, ovarian cancer, both, or neither (Gabai-Kapara et al., 2014). The penetrance of BRCA1 and BRCA2 mutations exhibits considerable variability, with breast cancer risk spanning from 36% to 85% and ovarian cancer risk from 10% to 44%, affected by factors including age, environmental influences, and genetic variability (Zhang et al., 2018).

Individuals with BRCA1 or BRCA2 mutations are advised to undergo early mammography screening, generally commencing between the ages of 25 and 35, although the efficacy of early surveillance is still ambiguous (Warner, 2018). Tamoxifen chemoprevention demonstrates potential in mitigating breast cancer risk, yet the evidence remains inconclusive (Alpeza et al., 2025). Oral contraceptives may reduce the risk of ovarian cancer but could elevate the risk of breast cancer (Moorman et al., 2013). Prophylactic oophorectomy and mastectomy effectively diminish cancer risk in specific women (Berek et al., 2010).

Recent advancements in molecular techniques, such as next-generation sequencing, have identified multiple genes associated with susceptibility to breast and ovarian cancer. Genes such as TP53, PTEN, STK11, CDH1, and PALB2 markedly elevate cancer risk, albeit with differing penetrance. Although BRCA1 and BRCA2 are widely acknowledged, recent data underscore the significance of additional genes in comprehensive gene panels for identifying at-risk individuals (Dal Molin, 2022).

Genetic testing is instrumental in detecting circulating tumor DNA (ctDNA), a biomarker for breast cancer, which can assist in diagnosis, staging, and treatment determinations. The convergence of genetic predisposition and precision medicine is illustrated by PARP inhibitors, which are efficacious in treating cancers linked to BRCA1/2 mutations, such as ovarian, breast, prostate, and pancreatic cancers. Next-generation sequencing has identified substantial correlations between genetic predisposition to ovarian, gastrointestinal, and breast cancers, underscoring the critical role of genetic testing in cancer management (Mekonnen et al., 2022).

Figure 10.1 provides a flow for the genetic testing decision-making process for the above given disorders.

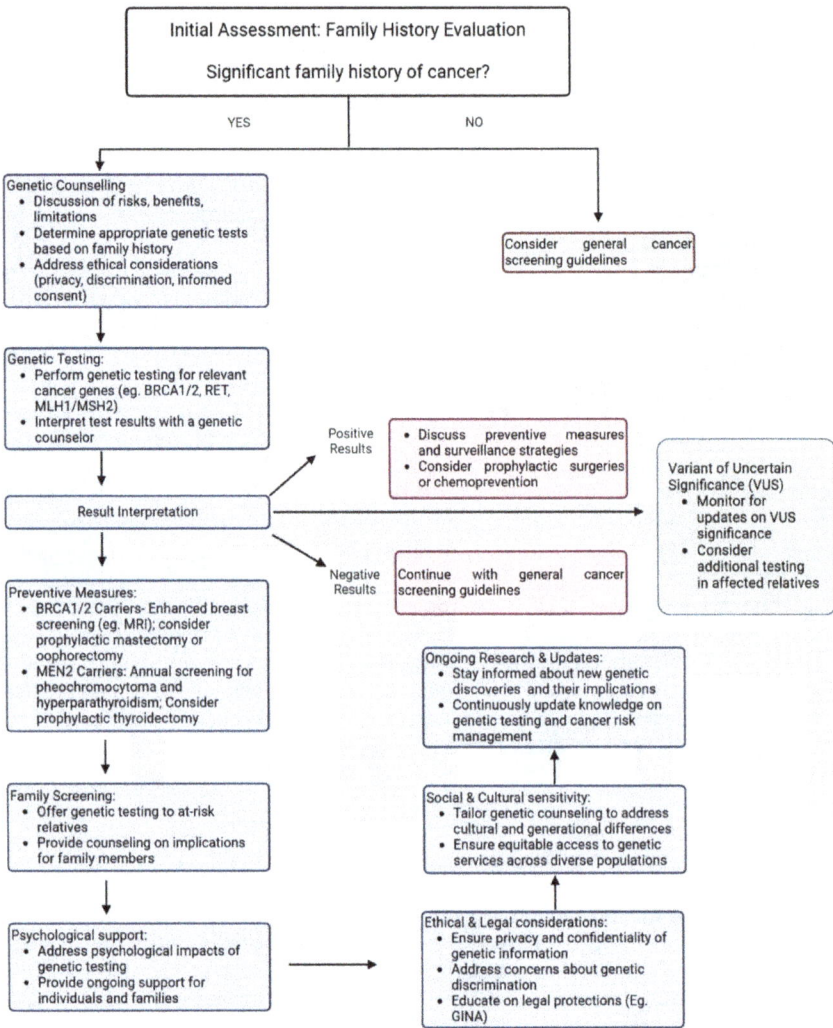

Figure 10.1 Genetic testing decision-making process.

10.3 RISK OF COMMUNICATION

Risk communication is a crucial element of genetic counselling and testing, as it profoundly affects individuals' perceptions and choices concerning genetic testing. Studies indicate that individuals with a low to moderate risk of cancer frequently overestimate their likelihood of developing the disease, particularly if they possess a familial history of it. This overestimation may be intensified by psychological distress and coping strategies, which influence the processing of risk information. Individuals may experience increased anxiety or denial when confronted with potential genetic predispositions, which can skew their perception of actual risk levels (Jamal et al., 2020).

Conventional counselling and educational methods frequently fail to modify individuals' perceptions of their cancer risk, as these perceptions are significantly shaped by emotional influences. Family dynamics significantly influence risk awareness, decisions regarding genetic testing, and resultant outcomes. Effective pretest counselling must thoroughly elucidate the potential risks of genetic testing, encompassing the psychological effects of both positive and negative results, as well as the ramifications for family members. Post-test counselling is crucial, as it entails interpreting genetic test results, evaluating individual and familial risks, and offering feasible risk management strategies (Marteau & Croyle, 1998).

In the realm of cancer genetics, there has been an increase in research regarding risk perception and communication strategies. It is essential to notify carriers of cancer-predisposing mutations regarding screening and risk mitigation alternatives, as inherited mutations are beyond an individual's influence. Familial awareness of a relative's test outcomes can profoundly influence psychological health and risk comprehension. For instance, discovering a family member's genetic mutation may induce heightened anxiety or a sense of fatalism, potentially influencing an individual's choice to pursue testing (Thompson et al., 1992).

Notably, disparities in perceived risk based on gender endure, notwithstanding the gender-neutral characteristics of genetic inheritance. Women, in particular, may be more predisposed to pursue genetic testing due to societal pressures or perceived susceptibility to specific cancers, such as breast cancer. Genetic counselling may not substantially change perceptions of cancer risk or diminish interest in testing, even among individuals with a lower perceived risk threshold. Consequently, delivering thorough information regarding the advantages and disadvantages of testing is imperative, as perceived risk is a pivotal element of genetic counselling (Codori et al., 1999).

The implementation of genetic testing is frequently shaped more by perceived risk than by actual risk, especially regarding colon cancer. Individuals may choose to undergo testing based on their perceived susceptibility, regardless of their actual risk level. Inherited risk is fundamentally familial, underscoring the significance of proficient family risk communication in informing decisions and influencing testing results. Emotions profoundly influence individuals' processing of risk-related information, particularly in the context of serious health threats. For example, the apprehension of losing a family member to cancer may compel individuals to pursue genetic testing, despite their incomplete understanding of the consequences (Leventhal et al., 1983).

Urgent research is required to improve communication methods and resources for genetic testing. This research should concentrate on empirical testing decisions and results rather than mere intentions. Contemporary risk evaluations frequently emphasize lifetime cancer risks; however, transitioning to assessments of immediate relevance may be more beneficial in genetic testing. For instance, comprehending the immediate consequences of a genetic mutation for present health management may be more efficacious in informing decision-making than concentrating exclusively on long-term risks (Leventhal et al., 1983).

Reevaluating counselling strategies is wise, as genetic counselling necessitates a significant time investment. A more efficacious strategy may entail limited pretest counselling succeeded by extensive counselling for individuals who test positive for deleterious mutations. This strategy may enhance resource management efficiency while guaranteeing that individuals requiring comprehensive guidance obtain it. Moreover, integrating novel communication methods, such as interactive tools or tailored risk assessments, may enhance individuals' comprehension and response to genetic risk information (Janis & Mann, 1977).

In summary, effective risk communication in genetic counselling is intricate and shaped by psychological, familial, and societal influences. Improving communication strategies to align with individual needs and risk perceptions is crucial for enhancing genetic testing outcomes and ensuring informed health decisions.

10.4 ETHICAL IMPLICATIONS OF CANCER GENETIC TESTING
10.4.1 Genetic Testing of the Children and Embryos

In the field genetic testing, the principle of autonomy is essential in upholding an individual's right to decide whether to obtain medical information. This principle is especially pertinent in genetic counselling, which prioritizes fully informed decision-making, devoid of coercion, and seeks to educate and empower individuals. Genetic counselling has progressed from the principles of autonomous decision-making, guaranteeing that choices are made with comprehensive understanding and devoid of external coercion.

Challenges emerge when genetic testing pertains to individuals incapable of providing autonomous consent, including children and embryos. Professional guidelines for children aim to balance the preservation of autonomy with the urgency of risk and the accessibility of therapeutic interventions. The American Medical Association (AMA) advocates for genetic testing of early-onset diseases when treatment options exist, but counsels against testing for late-onset conditions unless therapeutic interventions are available. In situations where children are susceptible to early-onset diseases lacking available treatments, the choice to conduct testing is frequently entrusted to the parents' judgement (AMA, Accessed February 20, 2025).

Alternative professional guidelines, including those from the American College of Medical Genetics (ACMG), exhibit greater receptivity towards testing children when the equilibrium of risks and advantages remains ambiguous. These guidelines take into account the psychosocial advantages that may warrant providing tests to capable adolescents (American Society of Human Genetics, 1995). The American Society of Clinical Oncology (ASCO) recommends that decisions regarding testing for potentially affected children should take into account evidence-based risk-reduction strategies and the likelihood of developing a malignancy in childhood.

At the extreme end of this spectrum is the dilemma of genetic testing of embryos, where the definition of "personhood" remains ambiguous. Methods like preimplantation genetic diagnosis (PGD) in in vitro fertilization (IVF) facilitate the identification of single-gene or chromosomal disorders at an early embryonic stage. This technology presents intricate ethical dilemmas, including apprehensions regarding the "slippery slope" towards sexual and trait selection or the testing for multifactorial diseases such as depression or obesity. Professional societies are engaged in deliberations regarding the regulation of preimplantation genetic diagnosis and other assisted reproductive technologies (National Society of Genetic Counselors, 2005).

The AMA Code of Medical Ethics endorses prenatal genetic testing for individuals at heightened risk of foetal genetic disorders, yet cautions that the selection to prevent a genetic disease may not always be suitable, contingent upon factors such as disease severity, likelihood of occurrence, age of onset, and gestational period. Other medical ethics societies have adopted similar stances (AMA, Accessed February 20, 2025).

Ethical concerns encompass issues of equitable access, as these technologies are presently affordable solely to a limited demographic. Due to the lack of long-term outcome data for assisted reproductive technologies, suggested algorithms seek to facilitate patient discussions, considering psychological, ethical, and medical factors (Rhodes, 2006; Cauffman & Steinberg, 2000).

10.4.2 Psychological and Emotional Impact

Empirical research from the United States, Europe, and Australia indicates that genetic testing does not result in significant psychological distress among high-risk individuals; however, it may induce anxiety, concerns regarding cancer, familial discord, and complications in medical decision-making (Thorlacius et al., 1998; Fisher et al., 1998). Although the majority of individuals react favorably, a minority encounters distress that may affect their quality of life. Hereditary cancer risk counselling is essential for identifying families at risk and mitigating cancer-related morbidity and mortality through the recommendation of earlier and more frequent screenings and other risk-reduction strategies. Pre-test counselling is crucial for informed decision-making, and initial testing is typically performed on a family member with a history of a particular cancer type. Individuals who test positive for a mutation are deemed carriers, whereas those with and without a personal history of cancer are categorized as affected and unaffected family members, respectively (Öfverholm, 2024).

While research has predominantly concentrated on potential distress, insufficient attention has been directed towards the positive psychological effects of genetic counselling and test outcomes. A study by Gage et al. emphasized the impact of genetic counselling and a favorable test result on the self-perception of high-risk individuals. Predictive genetic testing should be a fundamental component in managing hereditary cancer risk, as it considerably influences compliance with screening protocols and prophylactic interventions, such as risk-reducing surgeries (Gage et al., 2012). It facilitates the primary prevention of hereditary melanoma, including reducing UV exposure. These findings highlight the significance of genetic counselling and testing for early identification and preventive health strategies. Although research typically discredits the notion that genetic testing induces enduring psychological distress, it concedes that some individuals may be more vulnerable to increased anxiety or melancholy. Early identification of these individuals facilitates targeted interventions. In addition to issues related to anxiety, depression, and cancer-associated stress, studies indicate that genetic counselling offers both advantages and disadvantages. Qualitative data suggest that numerous benefits of inherited risk counselling and testing may not be adequately reflected in standardized psychological evaluations. Comprehending the intricate relationship between positive and negative outcomes, ensuing screening behaviors, and compliance with health strategies is essential for maximizing the advantages of genetic counselling and testing (Tutt et al., 2010).

10.5 LEGAL IMPLICATIONS OF CANCER GENETIC TESTING

10.5.1 Genetic Discrimination

Genetic discrimination, characterized by social stigmatization stemming from hereditary disease risks, can result in negative social consequences, including discrimination against prospective spouses based on their disease risk. Genetic discrimination may lead to financial difficulties, such as when genetic data is utilized by prospective employers in recruitment or advancement choices, or by insurance providers in determining premiums or entirely excluding certain groups from coverage (Hall et al., 2000; Harris et al., 2005; Hall et al., 2005).

While instances of genetic-based insurance discrimination are infrequent, public apprehension regarding such discrimination persists significantly. Initial surveys of medical directors from U.S. life insurance companies revealed that more than 50 percent considered a robust family history of breast cancer adequate grounds to deny all life insurance or significantly raise premiums. In nations such as the United Kingdom, individuals possessing BRCA mutations frequently encounter elevated life insurance premiums (McEwen et al., 1992).

Health insurance is often perceived as a right rather than a commodity, particularly because it is predominantly offered through employment. This viewpoint has prompted arguments against employee discrimination in relation to health insurance as well. Economic rationale exists for health insurers to provide coverage for preventive genetic services without penalties, as the expenses associated with treating diseases often exceed those of enhanced screening or preventive interventions. For example, providing coverage for genetic testing and risk-reducing interventions for individuals with high-risk genetic mutations may ultimately decrease healthcare expenditures by preventing the onset of more severe and expensive conditions (Edwards, 2008).

10.5.2 Intellectual Property and Commercialization

The matter of gene patenting has been a controversial subject in genetics and genomics. In 1991, the U.S. National Institutes of Health (NIH) asserted intellectual property (IP) rights over approximately 3,500 genes derived from fragmentary DNA sequences. By late 2005, roughly 20% of human genes had been patented via over 4,250 distinct patents, with 131 out of 291 cancer-related genes being patented (Futreal et al., 2004; Jensen & Murray, 2005). Advocates of gene patenting contend that it offers essential incentives for investment in novel technologies and promotes the disclosure of innovative inventions. Opponents, however, are concerned that such patents may hinder the advancement of new pharmaceuticals, diagnostic assays, and subsequent research and development.

Concerns have emerged regarding the enforcement of exclusive patents on diagnostic testing by profit-driven entities. Certain academic institutions have indicated that patent holders have improperly claimed exclusivity, resulting in approximately 25% of laboratories discontinuing genetic tests due to patent limitations (Caulfield et al., 2006). The exorbitant expense of patented tests raises concerns, as it may restrict access to genetic testing for individuals in need. The business model of Myriad Genetics for BRCA1 and BRCA2 testing has faced criticism for potentially hindering innovation and escalating costs, which may restrict access to high-quality public genetic testing services (Eccles et al., 2015).

A consortium of researchers in Europe contested existing BRCA patents through the European Patent Convention (EPC) opposition procedure in 2001 and 2002. The Nuffield Council on Bioethics endorsed this dissent (Nuffield Council on Bioethics, 2002). In early 2005, the EPC determined that a company's patent claims for multiple probes identifying BRCA1 should be limited to a single probe. This decision facilitated increased accessibility to genetic testing technologies in Europe (Matthijs, 2006).

Conversely, the BRCA1 and BRCA2 patents were solely possessed in the United States until the Supreme Court determined in 2013 that isolated human genes are not patentable. This decision represented a substantial change, as it facilitated access to genetic testing for these genes and permitted scientists to conduct research without the apprehension of patent infringement. The court determined that artificially engineered DNA molecules, such as cDNA, qualify for patents, whereas naturally occurring isolated DNA segments do not (Mueller J. 2002).

The legal framework regarding gene patents is intricate and dynamic. Judicial bodies have been modifying the criteria for patentability and the rigor of patent enforcement. A rising demand for policy reforms, including compulsory licensing, aims to alleviate the negative impacts of gene patents on public health. The Secretary's Advisory Committee for Genetics Health and Society (SACGHS) has proposed legislation to exempt research and medical diagnosis from patent infringement claims, seeking to reconcile intellectual property incentives with public health requirements (van Zimmeren, 2023).

The NIH has voiced apprehension regarding the influence of gene patents on genetic research and has allocated grants to investigate these effects and offer recommendations to policymakers. The NIH advocates for the unrestricted distribution of research tools whenever feasible, particularly when the likelihood of commercial profit is minimal, while acknowledging the validity of intellectual property protections for innovations linked to valuable products (Mazza & Merrill, 2006).

Gene patents significantly impact personalized medicine, which depends extensively on genetic data to formulate and direct treatments. Although patents on human gene sequences have facilitated the development of novel biologics, their significance in diagnostic testing remains contentious. The intellectual property regulations pertaining to genotype-phenotype associations significantly impact the advancement of personalized medicine. Nonetheless, certain studies indicate that gene patents may obstruct patient access and impede innovation in genetic diagnostics, especially when patents are exclusively licensed to a sole provider (Robertson, 2010)

10.6 SOCIAL IMPLICATIONS OF CANCER GENETIC TESTING
10.6.1 Cultural and Religious Perspectives

There are considerable disparities in access to genetic testing among various socioeconomic and ethnic groups. Research in Europe indicates that upper-class women are disproportionately represented in genetics clinics for breast cancer, whereas lower-class women are underrepresented. This disparity underscores the obstacles encountered by economically disadvantaged groups in obtaining advanced healthcare services (Carstairs & Morris, 1990).

African-American women in the United States encounter distinct obstacles to genetic testing. Although they possess elevated expectations regarding the advantages of BRCA1/2 genetic testing, they frequently lack access to information and understanding of breast cancer genetics. Contributing factors to this disparity encompass awareness of epidemiological data indicating reduced survival rates among African-American cancer patients, potentially fostering fatalistic attitudes towards genetic testing. Education and income are critical factors influencing attitudes, beliefs, and behaviors regarding genetic testing, with extensive studies revealing that African-American participants are considerably less likely to have received genetic counselling (Halbert et al., 2006; Halbert et al., 2005). Despite accounting for factors such as mutation probability, socioeconomic status, cancer risk perceptions, and consultations with primary care physicians, a notable disparity in genetic counselling participation remains among African-Americans. This highlights the intricate interaction of socioeconomic and systemic obstacles that restrict access to genetic services for this demographic.

Access to healthcare constitutes a significant barrier, especially for the working poor and uninsured demographics. In the United States, access to healthcare is frequently contingent upon employment status, resulting in a considerable number of individuals being uninsured at various times. Approximately two-thirds of Hispanics and around one-third of African-Americans experienced periods of being uninsured, in contrast to roughly 20% of European-Americans. The absence of insurance coverage may lead to postponed cancer diagnoses and treatments, intensifying existing health disparities (Doty et al., 2005).

10.6.2 Direct-to-Consumer (DTC) Genetic Testing and Social Risks

Genetic testing may result in psychological distress if not supplemented by adequate genetic counselling or if founded on erroneous test efficacy or interpretation. These issues have reemerged with the proliferation of direct-to-consumer (DTC) genetic testing, enabling individuals to acquire genetic tests independently of healthcare providers. This method has ignited discussions regarding its advantages and disadvantages (Nolan & Ormondroyd, 2023).

Proponents of DTC testing highlight enhanced accessibility to genetic information, which may empower consumers to make informed health choices. Nevertheless, adversaries highlight numerous apprehensions. Consumers may lack a comprehensive understanding of genetic testing complexities, which could result in misinterpretation of results and subsequent errors in health management. In the absence of adequate guidance, individuals may misjudge their risk based on test outcomes, resulting in unwarranted anxiety or misleading reassurance (Nolan & Ormondroyd, 2023).

An illustrative instance of the difficulties linked to DTC testing is a DTC advertising initiative for BRCA testing executed in Atlanta, GA, and Denver, CO, from September 2002 to February 2003. The campaign effectively reached consumers, with advertisements penetrating 90% of households in the targeted markets. It markedly enhanced consumer and provider awareness of BRCA1/2 testing, resulting in an increase in test requests. It was noted that healthcare providers frequently lacked the knowledge to adequately counsel patients regarding genetic testing. In Denver, there was a 300% rise in enquiries from women regarding BRCA testing, yet a 30% decline in referrals of high-risk women during the campaign. This indicates that advertisements may not have effectively communicated the constraints of BRCA testing, possibly resulting in misconceptions regarding the individuals eligible for testing (Jacobellis et al., 2003).

Concerns regarding the quality of DTC testing are substantial. Although fundamental laboratory standards are established under the Clinical Laboratory Improvement Amendments of 1988 (CLIA), there are no explicit requirements for personnel competency assessment or quality control in genetics laboratories. Numerous laboratories voluntarily adhere to industry standards; however, there is a necessity for more rigorous regulation to guarantee uniformity and dependability among all testing facilities (Knowles et al., 2017).

The regulation of DTC testing is presently delegated to individual states, leading to a deficiency in uniformity. Certain states restrict the direct delivery of test results to patients, whereas others lack regulatory statutes on the matter. This variability may result in inconsistent practices and disparate levels of consumer protection. Some companies may offer extensive testing services with expert support, while others provide tests for inadequately validated genomic markers that purport to forecast health tendencies and suggest dietary adjustments or personalized supplements based on genetic profiles (Cernat et al., 2022).

These assessments are occasionally associated with the marketing of products purporting to address conditions identified by the assessments, eliciting ethical concerns regarding the commodification of genetic information. The Federal Trade Commission (FTC) regulates advertising for prescription medications but has not comprehensively addressed direct-to-consumer genetic testing advertising. The absence of regulation exposes consumers to potentially deceptive or unverified assertions regarding the advantages of genetic tests and associated products (Sharkey, 2018).

Moreover, the caliber of DTC testing facilities exhibits significant variability. Certain companies provide comprehensive sequencing services costing more than $3,000, which includes assistance from board-certified genetic specialists. Conversely, other companies offer a variety of tests for both well-established and less established genomic markers, which purportedly forecast potential health predispositions and incorporate dietary adjustments based on genotype. The sale of "customised" supplements designed for weight loss or tailored to an individual's genetic profile is prevalent, further obscuring the distinction between genetic testing and commercial product sales (Wasson et al., 2006).

In conclusion, although DTC genetic testing enhances access to genetic information, it presents considerable challenges concerning consumer education, test interpretation, and quality assurance. Addressing these issues necessitates more extensive regulation and oversight to guarantee that consumers obtain precise and actionable information, and that genetic testing is employed judiciously to enhance health outcomes.

10.7 UNINTENDED CONSEQUENCES IN GENETIC TESTING OF CANCER: Themes in Clinical Case Reports

10.7.1 Wrong Testing Ordered

In many reported cases, the wrong genetic test was ordered, leading to inaccurate medical management recommendations and unnecessary testing. For instance, a 19-year-old woman with a family history of polyposis was tested for an APC gene mutation associated with familial adenomatous polyposis (FAP), but the test was misinterpreted, and she was not referred for further genetic evaluation until a year later. This delay could have significant health implications, as untreated FAP leads to a high risk of colorectal cancer. In fact, 93% of patients with classic FAP develop colorectal cancer by the age of 50 without colectomy, highlighting the urgency of accurate diagnosis and management (Yen et al., 2022).

Another case involved a 63-year-old woman who was tested for BRCA mutations common among individuals of Jewish ancestry, despite not being Jewish herself. The test was negative, but her sister later tested positive for a different BRCA2 mutation. This oversight could have led to missed opportunities for risk management and increased cancer risk for the patient and her family. The failure to identify the correct familial mutation meant that the patient did not receive appropriate counselling or screening recommendations, potentially leading to delayed diagnosis and treatment (Brierley et al., 2012).

In a third case, a 23-year-old woman diagnosed with bilateral breast cancer was referred for genetic counseling. Initially, her physician recommended BRCA testing for surgical decision-making. However, upon taking a detailed family history, the genetic counselor identified a sibling with a childhood brain tumor, suggesting Li-Fraumeni syndrome. Testing revealed a p53 mutation, which significantly altered her management plan, including avoiding chest wall irradiation. This case highlights the importance of comprehensive family histories in guiding genetic testing decisions (Brierley et al., 2012).

Ordering the wrong genetic test can lead to unnecessary expenditure of health care dollars. A patient was charged $4,700 for full sequencing of the MSH2 gene associated with Lynch syndrome, which was not necessary. The appropriate test for the familial mutation would have cost significantly less, around $475. This discrepancy not only wasted resources but also caused distress for the patient, who was denied insurance coverage for the unnecessary test (Brierley et al., 2012).

10.7.2 Results Misinterpreted

Misinterpretation of genetic test results is another common error. In one case, a patient was told she had a normal BRCA test result, but it was later discovered that she carried a deleterious BRCA1 mutation. This misinterpretation delayed her diagnosis and potentially life-saving interventions. The patient had been diagnosed with stage III ovarian cancer and had a strong family history of breast cancer. If her BRCA status had been correctly identified earlier, she might have undergone prophylactic surgery, potentially avoiding advanced cancer (Brierley et al., 2012).

In another case, a patient was incorrectly told she carried a disease-causing MSH6 mutation, leading to unnecessary distress and consideration of prophylactic surgery. The mutation was later found to be of uncertain significance. This misinterpretation highlights the challenges of managing variants of uncertain significance (VUSs), which can cause significant anxiety and lead to unnecessary medical interventions (Brierley et al., 2012).

10.7.3 Inadequate Genetic Counseling

Inadequate genetic counseling can lead to ethical issues, such as testing minors for adult-onset conditions without immediate medical benefit. A case involved a 7-year-old girl who was tested for a BRCA mutation at her parents' request, despite guidelines recommending against such testing in minors. The parents were later informed that this information would also impact whichever parent carried the mutation, raising concerns about the child's future medical management and potential psychosocial impacts (Brierley et al., 2012).

10.8 POTENTIAL FACTORS CONTRIBUTING TO ERRORS

Complexity and Knowledge Gaps: Errors in genetic counseling and testing are often linked to case complexity, time pressures, inadequate experience, insufficient knowledge or training, and poor communication. Many healthcare providers lack the necessary knowledge and training in genetics to provide accurate counseling and testing services. Studies have shown significant deficiencies among nonspecialists in understanding inheritance patterns, risk factors for hereditary cancer syndromes, and gene penetrance (Reason, 1995; Mahlmeister, 2010; Wilson et al., 1999).

Time Pressures: Genetic counseling is a time-consuming process that requires detailed family histories and informed consent discussions. In busy clinical settings, primary care physicians often have insufficient time to provide these services adequately. Professional guidelines suggest that the informed consent process should include discussions of possible test results and their implications for the individual and family members, options for cancer screening and risk reduction, economic considerations, and psychosocial considerations. However, with an average of 20 minutes or less per patient encounter, it is unrealistic to expect primary care physicians to add complex genetic counseling to their workload (Riley et al., 2012; Commission on Cancer, Accessed February 20, 2025).

Ethical and Legal Concerns: Providers may not be aware of current policy guidelines and laws related to genetic testing, such as protections against genetic discrimination (Greendale & Pyeritz, 2001; Brandt et al., 2008; Lowstuter et al., 2008; O'Neill et al., 2010; Laedtke et al., 2012). This lack of awareness can lead to inappropriate testing recommendations and failure to inform patients about their rights. For example, a survey found that more than half of family physicians were unaware of the Genetic Information Nondiscrimination Act (GINA), which provides protections against genetic discrimination by health insurers and employers (Laedtke et al., 2012).

Economic Implications: Unnecessary genetic testing contributes to healthcare waste. Studies have shown that many physicians order inappropriate testing, leading to increased costs without added benefits. In one survey, physicians were asked to distinguish between clinical scenarios where BRCA testing was warranted and those where it was not (Plon et al., 2011). However, many chose to test in low-risk scenarios, highlighting the need for better education and adherence to guidelines to reduce unnecessary testing costs.

Direct-to-Consumer Marketing: Direct-to-consumer marketing of genetic tests can influence practice patterns, potentially leading to more testing without adequate counselling. This marketing often targets both physicians and consumers, raising concerns about the quality of genetic services provided in non-specialist settings. Companies may provide "genetic counselling education" to office staff, which can be inadequate for ensuring that patients receive comprehensive and accurate genetic information (Ray, 2010).

Technological Advances: Recent advances in genetic testing, such as whole exome and whole genome sequencing, offer benefits but also pose significant challenges in interpreting complex genetic data. These tests generate vast amounts of information, much of which is of uncertain clinical significance, creating ethical and legal dilemmas regarding informed consent and data management. The interpretation of how these genetic changes impact health is likely to be far more complex, involving weaker associations, lower-penetrance mutations, and interactions between multiple genes and the environment (Li, 2011; Gonzaga-Jauregui et al., 2012).

In conclusion, errors in genetic counselling and testing can have major medical, legal, financial, and ethical implications. As genetic testing becomes more complex, it is crucial to ensure that healthcare providers have the necessary knowledge, training, and resources to provide accurate and comprehensive genetic services. This includes addressing knowledge gaps, managing time pressures, and staying updated on ethical and legal guidelines. Additionally, there is a need for robust systems to manage and interpret complex genetic data, ensuring that patients receive accurate and actionable information to guide their health decisions. Table 10.1 summarizes key issues, implications, and possible solutions for the Ethical, Legal, and Social Implications of Cancer Genetic Testing.

Table 10.1: Ethical, Legal, and Social Implications of Cancer Genetic Testing

Category	Key Issues	Implications	Possible Solutions
Ethical	Privacy concerns	Risk of misuse of genetic data by insurers, employers, or third parties	Strengthening data protection laws (e.g., GINA)
	Informed consent	Patients may not fully understand the risks, benefits, or limitations of genetic testing	Comprehensive genetic counseling and standardized consent procedures
	Psychological Impact	Anxiety, fear, or fatalism after receiving test results	Pre- and post-test counseling, emotional support services
	Testing in minors and embryos	Autonomy concerns and ethical dilemmas in predictive testing for late-onset conditions	Restrict testing to conditions with immediate medical benefits
Legal	Genetic discrimination	Potential bias in employment and insurance	Enforceable anti-discrimination laws (e.g., GINA)
	Gene patenting	High costs and limited access to patented genetic tests (e.g., BRCA1/2 patents)	Patent law reforms to balance innovation and accessibility
Social	Disparities in access	Unequal availability of genetic testing, particularly in LMICs	Expanding funding, training genetic counselors, and improving healthcare infrastructure
	Cultural and religious factors	Stigma and fatalistic beliefs affecting genetic testing decisions	Culturally sensitive education programs and community engagement
Clinical	Misinterpretation of results	Variants of Uncertain Significance (VUS) may lead to unnecessary anxiety or false reassurance	Improving genetic literacy among healthcare providers
	Direct-to-consumer (DTC) testing	Lack of counseling and misinterpretation of test results	Regulatory oversight and consumer education
	Wrong tests ordered	Unnecessary financial burden and incorrect medical decisions	Clinical decision-support systems and provider training

10.9 OBSTACLES AND CONSTRAINTS OF GENETIC TESTING

In genetic testing, predictive genetic testing primarily illuminates the potential for future health conditions but does not definitively determine their manifestation. The level of uncertainty associated with these findings remains substantial, even in cases where the identified risk is notably high, such as a positive test for Huntington's disease. This unpredictability extends to not only whether the specific ailment will indeed develop but also to the timing and severity of its onset. For instance, while a genetic test might indicate a high risk of developing a particular disease, it cannot predict with certainty whether the disease will occur or when it might manifest (Parthasarathy, 2023).

Predictive genetic testing diverges from traditional diagnostic tests in its immediate impact on not only the individual but also their family members. The motivation for undergoing such testing often arises from concerns about the health of relatives. For example, individuals may seek genetic testing if they have a family history of a specific condition, such as breast cancer, to understand their own risk and potentially inform their relatives about their risk as well (Lerman et al., 1996).

However, the utility of predictive genetic testing can diminish when medical advances render previously menacing conditions, such as breast or colon cancer, increasingly treatable through less-invasive methods. For instance, improvements in cancer screening and treatment have made early detection and management of these diseases more effective, potentially reducing the need for comprehensive predictive genetic testing. Additionally, the widespread availability of efficient screening techniques across the general population may diminish the necessity for predictive genetic testing, especially if these screenings are accessible and effective (Dorval et al., 2000).

Conversely, the appeal of predictive genetic testing rises as the costs associated with screening increase, particularly when more expensive yet superior techniques, like magnetic resonance imaging (MRI), outweigh relatively affordable alternatives such as mammography. Individuals' suitability for predictive genetic testing is significantly influenced by their personal experiences and family medical history. Various factors can either enhance or diminish the utility of such testing. Conditions characterized by high morbidity and mortality rates, therapies that are effective but not curative, and genetic testing with a high predictive value (high penetrance) are associated with increased utility (Esplen et al., 2009).

In contrast, diseases with lower morbidity and mortality rates, treatments that are both effective and well-tolerated, and genetic tests with lower predictive accuracy (low penetrance) tend to reduce utility. The complexity and cost of screening techniques further influence the utility, with more expensive and cumbersome methods diminishing it, while affordable and efficient approaches enhance it. The value of predictive genetic testing is also affected by the affordability and consequences of preventative actions, with expensive or detrimental measures diminishing its value, while straightforward, effective, and widely accepted preventive measures can enhance the overall usefulness of predictive genetic testing (Marzuillo et al., 2014).

Interpreting the implications of positive or negative test results can be challenging. A negative test result often provides reassurance, particularly when the family's predisposing mutation is already identified. For example, if a family member has a known mutation for a specific condition, a negative test result can alleviate concerns about inheriting that mutation. In the domain of cancer genetic testing, with a specific focus on breast cancer, the overarching objectives revolve around enhancing patient and public awareness. Augmenting comprehension is vital to align the burgeoning demand with genuine necessities (National Cancer Institute, 2024b).

The field of genetic testing for cancer is undergoing a remarkable transformation, driven by several influential factors. An increasing number of laboratories are now offering cancer genetic testing services, reflecting the surging interest in personalized genetic insights concerning cancer risk. In response to this heightened demand, the introduction of multiple testing panels, each encompassing a distinct array of genes, signifies a dedicated pursuit to comprehensively investigate genetic risk factors. However, this expansion brings complexities into play, as it entails the management and interpretation of additional genes, compounded by the unforeseen genetic revelations that carry clinical implications (Serani, 2024).

Variants of unknown significance (VUSs), representing genetic alterations with poorly understood clinical implications, are being uncovered concurrently. The accumulation of these VUSs augments the complexity of the genetic data that is already available. This progression indicates a societal inclination towards comprehending genetic makeup and its implications, aligned with the growing public interest in genetic testing. Within this evolving landscape, genetic counseling assumes a broader scope, with genetic counselors adeptly navigating a rapidly expanding genetic

Table 10.2: Advantages and Challenges of Cancer Genetic Testing

Aspect	Advantages	Challenges	Potential Solutions
Early Detection & Prevention	Identifies individuals at high risk for hereditary cancers	Limited awareness and accessibility, especially in LMICs	Public health campaigns and subsidized testing programs
Personalized Medicine	Enables targeted therapies (e.g., PARP inhibitors for BRCA mutations)	High costs of targeted treatments	Insurance coverage and government funding for precision medicine
Family Risk Assessment	Helps relatives make informed healthcare decisions	Psychological distress in families	Genetic counseling for affected families
Ethical Considerations	Empowers individuals with knowledge about their genetic risks	Raises concerns about genetic privacy and discrimination	Stronger legal frameworks to prevent misuse of genetic data
Legal & Policy Framework	Laws like GINA protect against genetic discrimination	Loopholes in laws may still allow indirect discrimination	Stricter enforcement and expanded legal protections
Social & Cultural Factors	Can lead to early interventions and preventive strategies	Cultural stigma and fear of testing results	Culturally sensitive education and awareness program
Direct-to-Consumer (DTC) Testing	Increased accessibility to genetic testing	Lack of regulation, potential misinterpretation of results	Stronger oversight and mandatory genetic counseling for consumers
Variants of Uncertain Significance (VUS)	Continuous research helps improve understanding of genetic variants	VUS can cause anxiety and unnecessary medical interventions	Improved risk communication and physician training

terrain, handling both validated results and the uncertainties introduced by the discovery of VUSs (Burke et al., 2022).

There is also a discernible trend towards proactive identification of risks within larger population groups aimed at enabling early interventions and risk management through genetic marker-based population screening. This approach is particularly relevant for conditions where early detection and intervention can significantly improve outcomes. Evidently, the evolving landscape of cancer genetic testing underscores the imperative need for robust clinical decision-support (CDS) mechanisms. Such mechanisms are indispensable for translating intricate genetic data into actionable insights that healthcare professionals can effectively utilize, thereby underscoring the dynamic interplay between cutting-edge genetics and judicious medical decision-making (Fiol et al., 2020; Sebastian et al., 2021).

Table 10.2 summarizes the advantages, challenges, and potential solutions to the aspects linked to the Cancer Genetic testing.

10.10 CONCLUSION

Cancer genetic testing plays a crucial role in identifying individuals at an increased risk of hereditary cancers, enabling early detection, prevention, and personalized treatment. With technological advancements, genetic testing has expanded globally, yet significant ethical, legal, and social challenges remain. Ethical concerns include privacy risks, genetic discrimination, and informed consent, particularly in testing children and embryos (McLean et al., 2013). Social disparities, such as limited access in low- and middle-income countries and the underrepresentation of ethnic minorities in genetic research, further complicate its widespread adoption. Additionally, psychological impacts, including anxiety and familial distress, highlight the necessity for adequate genetic counselling (Hanson et al., 2023).

Legally, genetic discrimination remains a critical issue, with concerns about insurance and employment biases despite protective legislations like GINA (Genetic Information Nondiscrimination Act). Intellectual property rights, particularly gene patenting, have influenced the cost and accessibility of genetic tests, as seen in the BRCA1/2 legal battles. The rise of direct-to-consumer (DTC) genetic testing has further raised concerns about misinterpretation of results, lack of counseling, and quality control (National Cancer Institute, 2024a).

From a clinical perspective, challenges persist in misordered tests, misinterpretation of results, and inadequate genetic counseling, leading to incorrect risk assessments and unnecessary medical interventions. Variants of Uncertain Significance (VUS) and the growing complexity of genetic findings underscore the need for improved clinical decision support (CDS) systems to guide healthcare providers and patients (National Cancer Institute, 2024b).

Despite these challenges, genetic testing continues to revolutionize oncology, facilitating risk-reducing strategies such as lifestyle modifications, prophylactic surgeries, and targeted therapies. However, its ethical and legal governance, equitable accessibility, and public awareness must evolve alongside technological progress to ensure responsible and effective implementation. Addressing these concerns through policy reforms, interdisciplinary collaboration, and enhanced genetic literacy will be essential in maximizing the benefits of cancer genetic testing while minimizing potential harms.

REFERENCES

Ahmed W, Upasna P, Kim D. Genetics of endocrine tumours. In: Watkinson JC, Clarke RW, eds. *Scott-Brown's Otorhinolaryngology and Head and Neck Surgery*. 8th ed. Vol 1: Basic Sciences, Endocrine Surgery, Rhinology. CRC Press; 2018:83–91.

Allford A et al. What hinders minority ethnic access to cancer genetics services and what may help? *Eur J Hum Genet* 2014;22(7):866–74.

Alpeza F et al. A scoping review of primary breast cancer risk reduction strategies in East and Southeast Asia. *Cancers* 2025;17(2):168.

American Society of Human Genetics. Board of directors: points to consider: ethical, legal, and psychosocial implications of genetic testing in children and adolescents. *Am J Hum Genet* 1995;57:1233–41.

Berek JS et al. Prophylactic and risk-reducing bilateral salpingo-oophorectomy: recommendations based on risk of ovarian cancer. *Obstet Gynecol* 2010;116(3):733–43.

Brandt R et al. Cancer genetics evaluation: barriers to and improvements for referral. *Genet Test* 2008;12(1):9–12.

Brierley KL et al. Adverse events in cancer genetic testing: medical, ethical, legal, and financial implications. *Cancer J* 2012;18(4):303–9.

Burke W et al. Recommendations for follow-up care of individuals with an inherited predisposition to cancer: II. BRCA1 and BRCA2. *JAMA* 1997;277(12):997–1003.

Burke W et al. The challenge of genetic variants of uncertain clinical significance: a narrative review. *Ann Intern Med* 2022;175(7):994–1000.

Bussières V et al. Prophylactic thyroidectomies in MEN2 syndrome: management and outcomes. *J Pediat Surg* 2018;53(2):283–5.

Carstairs V, Morris R. Deprivation and health in Scotland. *Health Bull* 1990;48(4):162–75.

Cauffman E, Steinberg L, (Im)maturity of judgment in adolescence: why adolescents may be less culpable than adults. *Behav Sci Law* 2000;18:741–60.

Caulfield T et al. Evidence and anecdotes: an analysis of human gene patenting controversies. *Nature Biotechnol* 2006;24(9):1091–4.

Cernat A et al. Considerations for developing regulations for direct-to-consumer genetic testing: a scoping review using the 3-I framework. *J Comm Genet* 2022;13(2):155–70.

Chaabouni H et al. Prenatal diagnosis of chromosome disorders in Tunisian population. *Ann Genet* 2001;44: 99–104.

Codori AM et al. Attitudes toward colon cancer gene testing: factors predicting test uptake. *Cancer Epidemiol Biomark Prevent* 1999;8(suppl 1):345–51.

Cummings S et al. Cancer risk associated with PTEN pathogenic variants identified using multi-gene hereditary cancer panel testing. *JCO Precis Oncol* 2023;7:e2200415.

Dal Molin M. Identification and validation of DNA sequence variants in cancer predisposition genes by next generation sequencing approaches. Doctoral thesis, University of Pavia, 2022.

de Vries J et al. Ethical issues in human genomics research in developing countries. *BMC Med Ethics* 2011;12:5.

de Vries J et al. Ethical, legal and social issues in the context of the planning stages of the Southern African Human Genome Programme. *Med Law* 2012a;31:119–52.

de Vries J et al. Investigating the potential for ethnic group harm in collaborative genomics research in Africa: is ethnic stigmatisation likely? *Soc Sci Med* 2012b;75:1400–7.

Decker RA et al. Hirschsprung disease in MEN 2A: increased spectrum of RET Exon 10 genotypes and strong genotype—phenotype correlation. *Human Mol Genet* 1998;7(1):129–34.

Del Fiol G et al. Standards-based clinical decision support platform to manage patients who meet guideline-based criteria for genetic evaluation of familial cancer. *JCO Clin Cancer Inform* 2020;4:1–9.

Dimaras H et al. Challenging the global retinoblastoma survival disparity through a collaborative research effort. *Br J Ophthalmol* 2010;94:1415–6.

Donis-Keller H et al. Mutations in the RET proto-oncogene are associated with MEN 2A and FMTC. *Hum Molec Genet* 1993;2(7):851–6.

Dorval M et al. Anticipated versus actual emotional reactions to disclosure of results of genetic tests for cancer susceptibility: findings from p53 and BRCA1 testing programs. *J Clin Oncol* 2000;18(10):2135–42.

Doty MM, Holmgren AL. Health care disconnect: gaps in coverage and care for minority adults. *Commonwealth Fund* 2006;21:1–2.

Dragoo DD et al. PTEN hamartoma tumor syndrome/Cowden syndrome: genomics, oncogenesis, and imaging review for associated lesions and malignancy. *Cancers* 2021;13(13):3120.

Dralle H, Machens A. Syndromic medullary thyroid cancer: MEN 2A and MEN 2B. In: Randolph GW, ed, *Surgery of the Thyroid and Parathyroid Glands*, 3rd edn, Elsevier, 2021:235–245.

Drummond MF et al. *Methods for the Economic Evaluation of Health Care Programmes*, 4th edn, Oxford University Press; 2015.

Eccles DM, Mitchell G, Monteiro ANA, Schmutzler R, Couch FJ, Spurdle AB, et al. BRCA1 and BRCA2 genetic testing—pitfalls and recommendations for managing variants of uncertain clinical significance. Ann Oncol 2015;26(10):2057–65.

Edwards A et al. Interventions to improve risk communication in clinical genetics: systematic review. *Patient Educ Counsel* 2008;71(1):4–25.

Eisenbruch M et al. Optimising clinical practice in cancer genetics with cultural competence: lessons to be learned from ethnographic research with Chinese-Australians. *Soc Sci Med* 2004;59(2):235–48.

Eng C et al. The relationship between specific RET proto-oncogene mutations and disease phenotype in multiple endocrine neoplasia type 2: International RET Mutation Consortium analysis. *JAMA* 1996;276(19):1575–9.

Esplen MJ et al. Motivations and psychosocial impact of genetic testing for HNPCC. *Am J Med Genet* 2001;103(1):9–15.

Esplen MJ et al. The BRCA Self-Concept Scale: a new instrument to measure self-concept in BRCA1/2 mutation carriers. *Psycho-Oncol* 2009;18(11):1216–29.

Etchegary H. Public attitudes toward genetic risk testing and its role in healthcare. *Pers Med* 2014;11(5):509–22.

Farndon JR et al. Familial medullary thyroid carcinoma without associated endocrinopathies: a distinct clinical entity. *Br J Surg* 1986;73(4):278–81.

Fatemi N et al. Whole exome sequencing identifies MAP3K1, MSH2, and MLH1 as potential cancer-predisposing genes in familial early-onset colorectal cancer. *Kaohsiung J Med Sci* 2023;39(9):896–903.

Fisher B et al. Tamoxifen for prevention of breast cancer: report of the National Surgical Adjuvant Breast and Bowel Project P-1 Study. *JNCI* 1998;90(18):1371–88.

Franceschi S et al. Whole-exome analysis of a Li–Fraumeni family trio with a novel TP53 PRD mutation and anticipation profile. *Carcinogen* 2017;38(9):938–43.

Futreal PA et al. A census of human cancer genes. *Nature Rev Cancer* 2004;4(3):177–83.

Gabai-Kapara E et al. Population-based screening for breast and ovarian cancer risk due to BRCA1 and BRCA2. *Proc Nat Acad Sci* 2014;111(39):14205–10.

Gage M et al. Translational advances regarding hereditary breast cancer syndromes. *J Surg Oncol* 2012;105(5):444–51.

Ghosh K et al. Carrier detection and prenatal diagnosis in haemophilia in India: realities and challenges. *Haemophil* 2002;8:51–5.

Giarelli E. Multiple endocrine neoplasia type 2a (MEN2a): a call for psycho-social research. Psycho-Oncology: Journal of the Psychological, Social and Behavioral Dimensions of Cancer 2002;11(1):59–73.

Godard B et al. Provision of genetic services in Europe: current practices and issues. *Eur J Hum Genet* 2003;11(2):S13–48.

Gonzaga-Jauregui C et al. Human genome sequencing in health and disease. *Ann Rev Med* 2012;63(1):35–61.

Grady WM. Genetic testing for high-risk colon cancer patients. *Gastroenterol* 2003;124(6):1574–94.

Gray SW et al. Attitudes of patients with cancer about personalized medicine and somatic genetic testing. *J Oncol Pract* 2012;8(6):329–35.

Greendale K, Pyeritz RE. Empowering primary care health professionals in medical genetics: how soon? How fast? How far? *Am J Med Genet* 2001;106(3):223–32.

Halbert CH et al. Low rates of acceptance of BRCA1 and BRCA2 test results among African American women at increased risk for hereditary breast-ovarian cancer. *Genet Med* 2006;8(9):576–82.

Halbert CH et al. Genetic testing for inherited breast cancer risk in African Americans. *Cancer Investig* 2005;23(4):285–95.

Hall MA et al. Concerns in a primary care population about genetic discrimination by insurers. *Genet Med* 2005;7(5):311–6.

Hall MA, Rich SS. Laws restricting health insurers' use of genetic information: impact on genetic discrimination. *Am J Hum Genet* 2000;66(1):293–307.

Hanson EN et al. Psychosocial factors impacting barriers and motivators to cancer genetic testing. *Cancer Med* 2023;12(8):9945–55.

Harris M et al. Controversies and ethical issues in cancer-genetics clinics. *Lancet Oncol* 2005;6(5):301–10.

Henneman L et al. Public attitudes towards genetic testing revisited: comparing opinions between 2002 and 2010. *Eur J Hum Genet* 2013;21(8):793–9.

Hill JA et al. Achieving optimal cancer outcomes in East Africa through multidisciplinary partnership: a case study of the Kenyan National Retinoblastoma Strategy group. *Global Health* 2016;12:23.

Hinoi T. Cancer genomic profiling in colorectal cancer: current challenges in subtyping colorectal cancers based on somatic and germline variants. *J Anus Rect Colon* 2021;5(3):213–28.

Hong B et al. Frequent mutations of VHL Gene and the clinical phenotypes in the Largest Chinese Cohort with Von Hippel–Lindau Disease. *Front Genet* 2019;10:867.

Horovitz DDG et al. Genetic services and testing in Brazil. *J Community Genet* 2013;4:355–75.

Huang Q et al. Gene diagnosis and genetic counselling of Rb gene mutations in retinoblastoma patients and their family members. *Zhonghua Yi Xue Yi Chuan Xue Za Zhi* 1998;15:65–8.

Jacobellis J, Martin L, Engel J, VanEenwyk J, Bradley L, Kassim S, et al. Genetic testing for breast and ovarian cancer susceptibility: evaluating direct-to-consumer marketing—Atlanta, Denver, Raleigh-Durham, and Seattle, 2003. Morbidity and Mortality Weekly Report. 2004;53(27):603–606.

Jamal L et al. An ethical framework for genetic counseling in the genomic era. *J Genet Counsel* 2020;29(5):718–27.

Janis IL, Mann L. *Decision Making: A Psychological Analysis of Conflict, Choice, and Commitment*. Free Press; 1977.

Jasim S et al. Multiple endocrine neoplasia type 2B with a RET proto-oncogene A883F mutation displays a more indolent form of medullary thyroid carcinoma compared with a RET M918T mutation. *Thyroid* 2011;21(2):189–92.

Jegede AS. Culture and genetic screening in Africa. *Dev World Bioeth* 2009;9:128–37.

Jenkins T. Ethics and the Human Genome Diversity Project: an African perspective. *Polit Life Sci* 1999;18:308–11.

Jensen K, Murray F. Intellectual property landscape of the human genome. *Science* 2005;310(5746):239–40.

Joseph B et al. Retinoblastoma: a diagnostic model for India. *Asian Pac J Cancer Prev* 2006;7:485–8.

Joseph B et al. Retinoblastoma: genetic testing versus conventional clinical screening in India. *J Mol Diagn* 2004;8:237–43.

Jung J et al. A Korean family of familial medullary thyroid cancer with Cys618Ser RET germline mutation. *J Korean Med Sci* 2010;25(2):226.

Kingsmore SF et al. Next-generation community genetics for low- and middle-income countries. *Genome Med* 2012;4:25.

Knowles L et al. Paving the road to personalized medicine: recommendations on regulatory, intellectual property and reimbursement challenges. *J Law Biosci* 2017;4(3):453–506.

Kucheria K et al. Human molecular cytogenetics: diagnosis, prognosis, and disease management. *Teratog Carcinog Mutagen* 2003:225–33.

Ladabaum U et al. Strategies for colorectal cancer screening. *Gastroenterol* 2020;158(2):418–32.

Laedtke AL et al. Family physicians' awareness and knowledge of the Genetic Information Non-Discrimination Act (GINA). *J Genet Counsel* 2012;21(2):345–52.

Leachman, S. A., Lucero, O. M., Sampson, J. E., Cassidy, P., Bruno, W., Queirolo, P., & Ghiorzo, P. (2017). Identification, genetic testing, and management of hereditary melanoma. Cancer and Metastasis Reviews, 36(1), 77–90.

Lerman C et al. BRCA1 testing in families with hereditary breast-ovarian cancer: a prospective study of patient decision making and outcomes. *JAMA* 1996;275(24):1885–92.

Leventhal H et al. The impact of communications on the self-regulation of health beliefs, decisions, and behavior. *Health Educ Q* 1983;10(1):3–29.

Li C. Personalized medicine–the promised land: are we there yet? *Clin Genet* 2011;79(5):403–12.

Light N et al. Germline TP53 mutations undergo copy number gain years prior to tumor diagnosis. *Nature Communicat* 2023;14(1):77.

Lim W et al. Further observations on LKB1/STK11 status and cancer risk in Peutz–Jeghers syndrome. *Br J Cancer* 2003;89(2):308–13.

Lowstuter KJ et al. Influence of genetic discrimination perceptions and knowledge on cancer genetics referral practice among clinicians. *Genet Med* 2008;10(9):691–8.

Lu KH et al. American Society of Clinical Oncology Expert Statement: collection and use of a cancer family history for oncology providers. *J Clin Oncol* 2014;32(8):833–40.

Maher ER. von Hippel-Lindau disease. *Curr Molec Med* 2010;4(8):833-42.

Mahlmeister LR. Human factors and error in perinatal care: the interplay between nurses, machines, and the work environment. *J Perinat Neonat Nursing* 2010;24(1):12-21.

Marteau TM, Croyle RT. The new genetics: psychological responses to genetic testing. *BMJ* 1998;316(7132):693–6.

Marzuillo C et al. Predictive genetic testing for complex diseases: a public health perspective. *QJM* 2014;107(2):93–7.

Masum H, Singer PA. A visual dashboard for moving health technologies from 'lab to village'. *J Med Internet Res* 2007;9:e32.

Matro JM et al. Cost sharing and hereditary cancer risk: predictors of willingness-to-pay for genetic testing. *J Genet Counsel* 2014;23(6):1002–11.

Matthijs G. The European opposition against the BRCA gene patents. *Famil Cancer* 2006;5:95–102.

Mazza AM, Merrill SA, eds. *Reaping the Benefits of Genomic and Proteomic Research: Intellectual Property Rights, Innovation, and Public Health.* National Academies Press; 2006.

McEwen JE et al. A survey of state insurance commissioners concerning genetic testing and life insurance. *Am J Hum Genet* 1992;51(4):785.

McLean N et al. Ethical dilemmas associated with genetic testing: which are most commonly seen and how are they managed? *Genet Med* 2013;15(5):345–53.

Mekonnen N et al. Homologous recombination deficiency in ovarian, breast, colorectal, pancreatic, non-small cell lung and prostate cancers, and the mechanisms of resistance to PARP inhibitors. *Front Oncol* 2022;12:880643.

Melo DG, Sequeiros J. The challenges of incorporating genetic testing in the Unified National Health System in Brazil. *Genet Test Mol Biomarkers* 2012;16:651–5.

Miki Y et al. A strong candidate for the breast and ovarian cancer susceptibility gene BRCA1. *Science* 1994;266(5182):66–71.

Moorman PG et al. Oral contraceptives and risk of ovarian cancer and breast cancer among high-risk women: a systematic review and meta-analysis. *J Clin Oncol* 2013;31(33):4188–98.

Mueller, J. M. (2002). Public Access versus Proprietary Rights in Genomic Information: What Is the Proper Role of Intellectual Property Rights. J. Health Care L. & Pol'y, 6, 222.

National Cancer Institute. BRCA gene changes: cancer risk and genetic testing [Internet]. Bethesda, MD: National Cancer Institute; 2024. Updated July 19, 2024. Available from: https://www.cancer.gov/about-cancer/causes-prevention/genetics/brca-fact-sheet

National Cancer Institute. The genetics of cancer, 2024b: www.cancer.gov/about-cancer/causes-prevention/genetics#should-i-get-genetic-testing-for-cancer-risk (accessed February 2025).

National Society of Genetic Counselors. Position statement: prenatal and childhood testing for adult-onset disorders, 2005: www.nsgc.org/about/Prenatal_two (accessed February 2025).

Nivoloni K et al. Newborn hearing screening and genetic testing in 8974 Brazilian neonates. *Int J Pediatr Otorhinolaryngol* 2010;74:926–9.

Nolan JJ, Ormondroyd E. Direct-to-consumer genetic tests providing health risk information: a systematic review of consequences for consumers and health services. *Clin Genet* 2023;104(1):3–21.

Nuffield Council on Bioethics. The ethics of patenting DNA: a discussion paper, 2002: www.nuffieldbioethics.org/publication/the-ethics-of-patenting-dna-a-discussion-paper/ (accessed February 2025).

O'Neill SC et al. Primary care providers' willingness to recommend BRCA1/2 testing to adolescents. *Famil Cancer* 2010;9:43–50.

Öfverholm A. *Cancer genetic risk assessment: Studies on genetic testing, genetic counselling and risk management.* Doctoral thesis, Gothenburg University, 2024.

Olejniczak D et al. Acceptance of, inclination for, and barriers in genetic testing for gene mutations that increase the risk of breast and ovarian cancers among female residents of Warsaw. *Contemp Oncol/Współczesna Onkologia* 2016;20(1):80–5.

Olschwang S et al. Germline mutation profile of the VHL gene in von Hippel-Lindau disease and in sporadic hemangioblastoma. *Hum Mutat* 1998;12(6):424–30.

Parsam V et al. A comprehensive, sensitive and economical approach for the detection of mutations in the RB1 gene in retinoblastoma. *J Genet* 2009;88:517–27.

Parthasarathy S. Breast cancer (BC) and the role of circulating tumor DNA. *Int J Trends OncoSci* 2023;1:33–7.

Pauley K et al. Considerations for germline testing in melanoma: updates in behavioral change and pancreatic surveillance for carriers of CDKN2A pathogenic variants. *Front Oncol* 2022;12:837057.

Plon SE et al. Genetic testing and cancer risk management recommendations by physicians for at-risk relatives. *Genet Med* 2011;13(2):148–54.

Ramprasad V et al. Retinoblastoma in India: microsatellite analysis and its application in genetic counseling. *Mol Diagn Ther* 2007;11:63–70.

Ray T. Myriad defends policy of urging docs to genetically counsel BRCAnalysis customers. Pharmacogenomics Reporter, 2010: www.genomeweb.com/dxpgx/myriad-defends-policy-urging-docs-genetically-counsel-bracanalysis-customers (accessed February 2025).

Reason J. Understanding adverse events: human factors. *BMJ Qual Safe* 1995;4(2):80–9.

Rhodes R. Why test children for adult-onset genetic diseases? *Mt Sinai J Med* 2006;73:609–16.

Riley BD et al. Essential elements of genetic cancer risk assessment, counseling, and testing: updated recommendations of the National Society of Genetic Counselors. *J Genet Counsel* 2012;21:151–61.

Robertson AS. The role of DNA patents in genetic test innovation and access. *Nw J Tech Intell Prop* 2010;9:377.

Robson ME et al. American Society of Clinical Oncology policy statement update: genetic and genomic testing for cancer susceptibility. *J Clin Oncol* 2015;33(31):3660-7.

Roncucci L et al. Attenuated adenomatous polyposis of the large bowel: present and future. *World J Gastroenterol* 2017;23(23):4135.

Ropka ME et al. Uptake rates for breast cancer genetic testing: a systematic review. *Cancer Epidemiol Biomark Prevent* 2006;15(5):840–55.

Rossi M et al. Familial melanoma: diagnostic and management implications. *Dermatol Pract Concept* 2019;9(1):10.

Sebastian A et al. Effect of genetics clinical decision support tools on health-care providers' decision making: a mixed-methods systematic review. *Genet Med* 2021;23(4):593-602.

Serani S. Evolving landscape of genetic testing in oncology, targeted oncology, 2024: www.targetedonc.com/view/evolving-landscape-of-genetic-testing-in-oncology (accessed February 2025).

Sharkey CM. Direct-to-consumer genetic testing: the FDA's dual role as safety and health information regulator. *DePaul L Rev* 2018;68:343.

Siegel RL et al. Colorectal cancer statistics, 2020. *CA* 2020;70(3):145–64.

Silva RV et al. Hereditary nonpolyposis colorectal cancer identification and surveillance of high-risk families. *Clinics* 2005;60:251–6.

Singh DN, Daripelli S, Elamin Bushara MO, Polevoy GG, Prasanna M. Genetic testing for successful cancer treatment. Cureus. 2023;15(12):e49889. doi:10.7759/cureus.49889

Stanislaw C et al. Genetic evaluation and testing for hereditary forms of cancer in the era of next-generation sequencing. *Cancer Biol Med* 2016;13:55–67.

Strafford JC. Genetic testing for lynch syndrome, an inherited cancer of the bowel, endometrium, and ovary. *Rev Obstet Gynecol* 2012;5(1):42.

Thayalasekaran S. *Endoscopic techniques for the detection, characterisation and treatment of gastrointestinal neoplasia*. Doctoral dissertation, University of Portsmouth, 2022.

Thompson RJ et al. Stress, coping, and family functioning in the psychological adjustment of mothers of children and adolescents with cystic fibrosis. *J Pediat Psychol* 1992;17(5):573–85.

Thorlacius S et al. Population-based study of risk of breast cancer in carriers of BRCA2 mutation. *Lancet* 1998;352(9137):1337–9.

Tindana P et al. Seeking consent to genetic and genomic research in a rural Ghanaian setting: a qualitative study of the MalariaGEN experience. *BMC Med Eth* 2012;13:1–2.

Tschudin S et al. Prenatal counseling–implications of the cultural background of pregnant women on information processing, emotional response and acceptance. *Eur J Ultrasound* 2011;32:e100–107.

Tutt A et al. Oral poly (ADP-ribose) polymerase inhibitor olaparib in patients with BRCA1 or BRCA2 mutations and advanced breast cancer: a proof-of-concept trial. *Lancet* 2010;376(9737):235–44.

van Zimmeren E. Legal empirical studies of patenting and patent licensing practices. In: Derclayre E, ed, *Research Handbook on Empirical Studies in Intellectual Property Law*. Edward Elgar Publishing, 2023:27–46.

Vieira TP et al. Genetics and public health: the experience of a reference center for diagnosis of 22q11.2 deletion in Brazil and suggestions for implementing genetic testing. *J Community Genet* 2013;4:99–106.

Warner E. Screening BRCA1 and BRCA2 mutation carriers for breast cancer. *Cancers* 2018;10(12):477.

Wasson K et al. Direct-to-consumer online genetic testing and the four principles: an analysis of the ethical issues. *Eth Med* 2006;22(2):83.

Weitzel JN et al. Genetics, genomics, and cancer risk assessment: state of the art and future directions in the era of personalized medicine. *CA* 2011;61(5):327–59.

Wilson RM et al. An analysis of the causes of adverse events from the Quality in Australian Health Care Study. *Med J Austral* 1999;170(9):411–5.

Wonkam A et al. Acceptability of prenatal diagnosis by a sample of parents of sickle cell anemia patients in Cameroon (sub-Saharan Africa). *J Genet Couns* 2011;20:476–85.

Wonkam A et al. Capacity-building in human genetics for developing countries: initiatives and perspectives in sub Saharan Africa. *Public Health Genom* 2010;13:492–4.

Yen T et al. APC-associated polyposis conditions. In: Adam MP et al., eds, *GeneReviews*, 2022: www.ncbi.nlm.nih.gov/books/NBK1345/ (accessed February 2025).

Yurgelun MB et al. Cancer susceptibility gene mutations in individuals with colorectal cancer. *J Clin Oncol* 2017;35(10):1086–95.

Zhang L et al. Breast and ovarian cancer penetrance of BRCA1/2 mutations among Hong Kong women. *Oncotarget* 2018;9(38):25025.

11

Implementing Cancer Genetic Testing in Clinical Practice

Changanamkandath Rajesh, Harsimran Kaur, and Preeti Rajesh

11.1 INTRODUCTION

Cancer diagnosis at an early stage is the best and most effective method to prevent death from cancer. Early diagnosis, and more importantly, methods that can be used in prognosis or early diagnosis, will help us manage disease treatment options more effectively. Multiple tests currently in use for diagnosis, however, are not effective in deducing the disease, especially at or near its onset. As discussed extensively in this book, physicians look to use traditional tests that include imaging techniques, tumor marker detection, endoscopy, and more recently, genetic tests, only once a patient is already diagnosed from the expected symptoms of cancer. The tests determine whether the symptoms are actually cancer or just other infections or disease conditions that are mimicking cancer. The advent of more advanced technologies, which lower the cost and the time taken, with the ability to predict as well as detect cancer at multiple stages, underscores the significance genetic testing is providing in cancer diagnosis.

The cancer diagnostic tests have shown drastic improvements, especially with advanced imaging techniques such as Positron Emission Tomography (PET), X-Ray Computed Tomography (CT), and Magnetic Resonance Spectroscopy (MRS), and more recently, molecular techniques (Pulumati et al., 2023). These advances have not only helped early detection but also provided better therapeutic management. These diagnostic techniques have several advantages, including better accessibility and non-invasiveness, as well as providing a more clearly understood diagnosis to the general public and clinicians who are not well-versed with the "ATGC" code of human genes. The intricacies associated with genetic diversity and the inability, in many cases to give a foolproof prediction have resulted in inability of clinicians to move on from the current diagnostic methods in a more confident manner. However, the ability to generate more genetic markers that can be used to determine predisposition to cancer can promote the replacement of existing clinical strategies for diagnosis with genetic testing. The overall complexity of cancer prognosis, coupled with a more expanded genetic testing strategy that can be associated with cancer therapy, will enhance the use of these technologies in clinical practice.

This chapter will summarize the tests already in use for cancer diagnosis presently, as discussed throughout the book, in the first part, along with the advances and limitations of these strategies. It will then go on to discuss the need to develop more advanced clinical practices to actually look beyond just the diagnosis of cancer once it has already reached stages where intervention is not easy. The advances in genetic testing strategies, especially with the advent of Next Generation Sequencing (NGS) technologies and other more recent techniques, will be discussed for their large-scale and cost-effective methods in predicting the disease. The ability to provide physicians with sufficient reliable data to make informed decisions regarding potential personalized treatment decisions that will enhance treatment efficacy will be discussed. The chapter will also list those genetic tests which will effectively popularize these genetic tests among physicians, in addition to their prognostic values, so that the tests can be made available for general public usage.

11.2 CLINICAL PRACTICES IN CANCER DIAGNOSIS

Traditional clinical practices involve several screening tests on diagnosis of symptoms of cancer to find out if the symptoms seen are a result of cancer. This cannot be done using any single diagnostic test but using a series of tests that involve biochemical laboratory tests, imaging tests (scans), and other more advanced tests. The diagnostic approach by clinicians always starts with physical evaluation for symptoms, followed by a series of laboratory tests. In the final chapter we discuss the different technological advances that have evolved with time starting from imaging techniques, biomarker identifications and more recently by usage of artificial intelligence. Each of these techniques in combination should provide screening, estimate the stage of cancer and be able to suggest a method of therapeutic strategy as well as be able to follow the therapeutic response.

11.2.1 Diagnostic Imaging Techniques

Imaging techniques used in diagnosis uses a variety of imaging tools other than light. These sensitive tools will give a clear picture of the tumor and are generally used as a most convincing tool in diagnosis. The various imaging techniques are as follows

11.2.1.1 Positron Emission Tomography (PET)

One of the most widely used tools in the diagnosis of several types of tumors, PET generates an image of the tumor tissue by capturing the gamma radiations emitted from tissues in response to positrons from the cyclotron device used for imaging. The PET scanner detects the region of blood flow within the areas of tumor giving it both diagnostic as well as provide an idea into therapeutic potential due to the anatomical information. These also identify cancerous lesions as well as lymph node metastasis missed via conventional imaging. However, the technique has a major limitation of introduction of intravenous administration of radioactive compounds used in detection that will lead to radiation exposure (Frangioni, 2008; Lopci et al., 2010). Advances in software and hardware of PET imaging devises have made it better suited for early detection of cancer.

11.2.1.2 X-Ray Computed Tomography (CT)

Computed Tomography uses a series of X-Ray images taken from multiple angles to construct three dimensional image of the tumor tissue along with the surrounding blood vessels and tissues. The digitally recreated radiographs provide a very accurate information of the spatial information of the tumors. The lack of functional information and sub-optimal imaging does pose challenges in its use in tumor imaging, although recent advances in instrumentation in speed, dual energy, lower voltage use, etc have improved its use as in tumor imaging especially for screening in cases of colon, lung, head and neck and breast cancers, Use of CT along with PET is also a useful combination tool to precisely detect the tumor image efficiently especially in cases of metastasis (Zhou et al., 2021; Wang et al., 2021).

11.2.1.3 Magnetic Resonance Imaging (MRI)

MRI involves the use of magnetic field and radiowaves that are used to produce images of the tumors as well as the surrounding tissues and organs. The principle uses the change in frequency of charged particles on application of magnetic fields to provide the composition and images of the tissues. Used primarily for detection of brain cancers it is also used in several soft tissue sarcomas in addition to spinal cord prostatic, bladder, uterine, and ovarian tumors. Its primary advantage is in the lack of ionizing radiation exposure and lower chances of allergic reaction compared to CT and X-Rays where allergic contrasting agents might be used. Advanced MRI techniques as hyperpolarized MRI can be used to detect and characterize types of cancers (Haris et al., 2015).

11.2.1.4 Magnetic Resonance Spectroscopy

MRS is different from MRI in the use of signals for imaging being used from compounds as Carbon, hydrogen, creatinine, lactate and N-acetyleaspartate etc. The magnetic fields therefore used in MRS is much stronger therefore making it possible to construct images of metabolic activity as well as the vascular movement. The ability to detect metabolic changes with respect to changes in ratio of metabolites in tumors the method can be extrapolated in differentiating tumor recurrence nectrosis as well as the proliferative potential and aggressiveness of tumor. Limitations of this technique include the cost and time taken for tests in addition to the inability to derive anatomical information using these techniques (Verma et al., 2016).

11.2.2 Molecular Diagnostic Advances

Although the imaging techniques have been the potential go to method for cancer detection by clinicians as it provides a clear image and actionable target for them, the advent of molecular biology and advances in healthcare biotechnology has now shifted the field to molecular diagnosis to be able to conclusively state the cancer type, stage and targeting strategy. The broad molecular diagnostic techniques are gaining popularity in diagnosis of cancer.

11.2.2.1 Flow Cytometry for Biomarkers

Flow cytometry has been a technique that has been used to analyze single cells of a large population of cells using markers both on surface or intracellular along with analysis involving variations in the cell size, morphology and DNA ploidy. Use of fluorescently labeled antibodies have been used for multiple hematological malignancies as Hairy cell Leukemia using BRAF V600E specific antibody or detecting clonality of B and T cells in Acute Lymphoblastic Leukemia (ALL). Panel of markers have also been used for detection in Chronic Lymphocytic Leukemia (CLL) (Ahmad et al., 2022).

11.2.2.2 Synthetic Biosensors and Biomarker Analysis

More recent advances in cancer diagnosis has evolved from advances in synthetic biology and cell engineering due to identify biomarkers arising out of changes in cellular make up in early stage of cancer. These markers can be tracked and detected in cancer pathways by using biosensors placed within the body so that their quantification can result in ability to diagnose the tumors early in their onset. These biomarkers once identified and if released into blood or other body fluids can also be identified by routinely available test strategies (Li et al., 2022).

Use of extracellular vesicles as exosomes as stable biomarkers that are found in body fluids and are associated with the cells of their origin is now tried. They can be analyzed for altered protein or genotypic changes of cells of origin (Soung et al., 2017). Use of nanoparticles as biosensors are gaining high amount of traction mainly due to their small size, biosafety and better loading characteristics. The use of quantum dots, gold, silver, or graphene, known for better penetration in combination with specific biological molecules as targeting peptides or antibodies have found its place in imaging as well as therapeutic advances in the field (Zhang et al., 2020; Chhabra et al., 2018).

11.2.2.3 Fluorescence in Situ Hybridization (FISH)

FISH analysis to detect the chromosomal changes have now replaced the classical cytogenetic testing that have been in use from early times of cancer detection in the 20th century. The technique uses fluorescent probes specific to individual chromosomes that can identify chromosomal abnormalities as aneuploidy, rearrangements, deletions etc. The use of variations of probes and reporters there are multiple variations of FISH are in use that include Multiplex FISH (MFISH), Spectral Karyotyping (SKY), COmBined RAtio Labeling (COBRA) etc. (Speicher et al., 1996; Schröck et al., 1996). The use of FISH patterns of normal and cancerous cells can be used to identify variations in chromosome numbers, structures or any variations of loci by Comparative Genomic Hybridization (CGH) which can give extensive differential pattern of cancerous cells. A combination of FISH and immunocytochemistry can provide additional details on the gene activity at DNA and mRNA level as well (Tanke et al., 1999).

11.2.2.4 Volatile Organic Compound (VOC) Analysis

VOC analysis aims at early detection of lung cancer by attempting to identify the molecular biomarker compounds exhaled from breath of lung cancer patients. Investigation has led to identification of over 1000 volatile compounds depending on various patient conditions both physiological or disease related including ethanol. toluene, benzene, styrene, ethylbenzene, pentanal etc. The studies are underway to generate a consistent molecular signatures that can identify patterns of lung cancer by using patient sample analyzed using Mass Spectrometry (Jia et al., 2019)

11.2.2.5 Liquid Biopsy

Liquid biopsy is an important novel concept of cancer diagnosis that uses body fluids as blood, saliva and urine in monitoring the progress of tumor. The key target in this diagnostic technique is the circulating tumor cells (CTCs), circulating tumor DNA (ctDNA), the cell free circulating miRNA (ctmiRNA) or extracellular vescicles (EVs) present in the bodily fluids. This study has not only resulted in diagnosis at an early stage of cancer but also can be extended to prognosis as well as in response to therapy. This analysis can determine the possibility of recurrence of cancer after therapeutic intervention and predict the disease free survival of the patient after therapy.

11.2.2.6 Immunohistochemistry and Microarray Based Diagnosis

Immunohistochemistry refers to technique of using antibodies against specific tumor antigens and measuring their changes in expression in cancerous cells. The antibodies are fluorescently labeled and used on tissues to differentiate the cancerous cells where the expression difference is observed clearly. The technology can be used to differentiate the different forms of cancer using targeted antigens to specific cells e.g. in identifying the "Cluster of Differentiation (CD)" markers within lymphomas (Goyal et al., 1996). It is also useful in prognostic indication as well, as in Her2/neu protein, estrogen and progesterone specific breast cancer prognosis.

Hybridization based molecular diagnostic methods are also being used in cancer diagnosis using the technique of microarrays. The technique can detect DNA, RNA and proteins differentially in cancer and normal cells respectively. It can be used to detect and quantify the expression using specific predetermined probes for the biomarkers in several genes. The assay is a high-throughput strategy that can be used to scan and analysis several genes and markers at one go. There are cDNA microarray panels that include over 1000s of genes for multiple cancer types that can be diagnosed. However, the use of microarrays has not gained popularity due to lack of specific tumor markers that are useful in using such expensive technique.

11.2.3 Limitations in Existing Cancer Diagnosis

The traditional cancer diagnostic strategies are convenient for usage due to their cost effectiveness and have been effective in prevention, identification and treatment of multiple cancers. The challenge in all these diagnostic techniques is the ability to provide timely and accurate diagnosis with a possibility or suggestion of intervention at the right time. The current cancer diagnostic processes involve multiple steps of imaging and tumor excision followed by biopsy. Although imaging techniques have been a very effective tool in detecting and identifying cancer for a long time, they stay largely ineffective as a screening tool in case of large populations. These technologies in spite of all advances still miss several smaller lesions and detection is mostly done at relatively advanced stages. Achieving these goals require more advanced for identifying individual's propensity to cancer either prior to the onset or very early in the onset.

The field of molecular imaging and the advances discussed above has been part of evolving field of precision medicine, that should help in early diagnosis as well as individual specific treatment at the exact time. However, cancer is a genetic disease that arises due to accumulation of mutations, genome instability and alteration of proteins in the cells. Therefore, any test that does not evaluate these and other molecular signals cannot successfully be a tool that can detect early diagnosis or used as a tools for assessing the therapeutic efficiency. The use of the current diagnostic imaging techniques although cannot be replaced anytime in the near future due to the obvious advantages, the molecular techniques will need to complement the existing techniques for effective tackling of the cancer load especially in screening processes. The era of precision medicine that includes all the omics technology genomics, transcriptomics, proteomics, meatabolomics in complementation with molecular imaging is the need of the hour to transition towards predictive, preventive, and proactive measures to disease diagnosis rather than the current reactive strategy.

11.3 GENETIC TESTING FOR CANCER DIAGNOSIS AND PROGNOSIS

As discussed throughout the book the role of genetic tests has been increasing significantly in oncology, be it genetic profiling of somatic mutations or for informed preference of molecular targets in therapy. The tests that provide information on the inherited or germline or constitutive mutations that has helped in giving a choice of therapeutic agent as well as somatic variations will be the way forward in the diagnosis as well as in predicting the occurrence or recurrence of the tumors. An array of techniques from karyotyping, FISH, *in situ* hybridization, Real Time PCR, Sequencing and microarray all provide a range of diagnostic methods that can work as high-throughput genome-wide screens or in specific targeted tests for therapy or diagnosis (Gully et al., 2010). The advent of next generation sequencing technology and the advances in the field has revolutionized the field of molecular diagnosis due to massive advantage it offers in screening and making it cost effective in analysing more and identifying most markers in a sample (Serratì et al., 2016). This high-throughput method that can provide massive parallel sequencing in reduced time span can identify several genomic alterations at genomic and transcript level including Copy number variations (CNVs), Single nucleotide variations/polymorphisms (SNPs), Insertions and Deletions (INDELs) as well as fusion transcripts in single cycle that used to take several different tests previously. Although its usage in clinical set-up is still limited due to the lack of understanding and the ability to streamline and analyze the huge amount of data in a more simplified and clinician friendly way. The advent of gene panels specific to each cancer type has started giving more access to relevant small panel tests, so that molecular technology is now gaining more acceptability worldwide.

11.3.1 Genetic Testing for Hereditory Cancers

Hereditary cancers account for around 10% of all cancers. The identification of these genetic variations as genetic markers can be used to diagnose cancer early or before its onset in addition to suggesting therapeutic strategy. Most significantly they can be used in management of cancer by preventive testing programs as well as screening the family for effective prognosis (Garutti et al., 2023). The American College of Medical Genetics and Genomics with the Association for Molecular Pathology have developed a method of classifying these genetic variations into Pathogenic (P), Likely pathogenic (LP), Uncertain significance (VUS), Likely benign (LB), and Benign (B) that gives clinicians a clear indication to determine the significance in each identified variation (Richards et al., 2015). The list of the genes associated with germline mutations are indicated in Figure 11.1 and the details listed in Table 11.1 with the potential significance of these in terms of prognostic, diagnostic and therapeutic potential.

There are several known hereditary signature variations associated with different cancer types, the most significant one being the hereditary association of *Trp53, BRCA1/BRCA2, STK11, PALB2, ATM*, etc., in breast, ovarian, pancreatic, and prostate cancers. Similar hereditary cancer associations can be attributed to *MEN2A/2B* for thyroid cancer, etc., as has been discussed in detail throughout this book. The increase in similar genetic dispositions associated with various cancers has made it significant to have a global attribution to these associations via large-scale genome-wide association studies (GWAS) to develop a more definite relationship between the genotype and clinical manifestation. Recent advances in diagnostic technologies have resulted in the development of specific panels, as shown in Table 11.1, that can be used to screen larger cohorts of the population for their association with different markers. Such large-scale studies, though significant in discovering novel markers, mean that the analysis of individual characterized polymorphisms can be utilized for personalized management of disease (Garutti et al., 2023). The use of AI to combine these genetic markers with clinical markers can give even higher impetus to the field of cancer diagnosis and prognosis.

11.3.2 Genetic Testing for Somatic Variation Diagnosis

The somatic variations associated with tumor samples and identification of genetic variations in those generally define cancer diagnosis and targeted therapy that can be administered. Identification of these variations, the significant cancer-causing ones, also known as "Driver Mutations" along with a few benign "Passengers" is a more targeted approach in cancer diagnosis. Several cancer diagnosis studies have identified a whole catalog of mutations that are associated with predicted diagnostic, prognostic, as well as therapeutic values (Watson et al., 2013; Pleasance et al., 2010). The origin of cancer is predicted to be from a small subset of clones that have

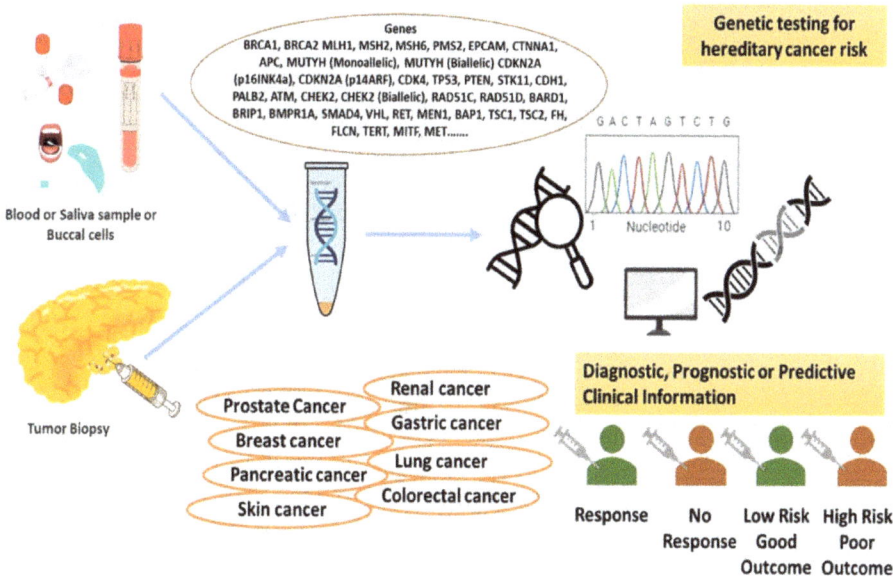

Figure 11.1 The common genetic tests associated with hereditary cancer risk. The figure summarizes the various genes that are used for diagnostic, prognostic, and predictive clinical information in a variety of cancer types as a result of genetic analysis. Therapeutic use of these genetic alterations can be classified into no response to risk and treatment outcomes as outlined in Table 11.1.

Table 11.1: Germline Genetic Testing for Hereditary Cancer Risk

Cancer Type	Test/Panel Name	Genes Included	Company	Clinical Utility
Breast	BRACAnalysis CDx	Germline BRCA1/2 pathogenic variants	Myriad Genetics	Identifies mutations linked to increased cancer risk; guides prevention, surveillance, and treatment options including recommending an appropriate PARP inhibitor.
Hereditary Breast Cancer	Breast Cancer Comprehensive Panel	ABRAXAS1, AKT1, ATM, BARD1, BLM, BRCA1, BRCA2, BRIP1, CDH1, CHEK2, CTNNA1, DICER1, EPCAM, FANCC, FANCM, MLH1, MRE11, MSH2, MSH6, MUTYH, NBN, NF1, NTHL1, PALB2, PIK3CA, PMS2, PTEN, RAD50, RAD51C, RAD51D, RECQL, SDHB, SDHD, SMARCA4, STK11, TP53, XRCC2 (37 genes)	Fulgent Genetics	Confirming the presence of a germline pathogenic variant linked to breast cancer. Recommended for a patient or a family member diagnosed with breast cancer before age 50, triple-negative breast cancer, male breast cancer, or if there have been multiple cases of cancer in a single individual. This test is designed to detect individuals with a germline pathogenic variant and is not validated to detect mosaicism below the level of 20%.
Hereditary Breast and Ovarian cancer syndrome and Lynch syndrome	Hereditary Breast and Gynecological Cancer Panel	ATM, BARD1, BLM, BRCA1, BRCA2, BRIP1 CDH1, CHEK2, DICER1, EPCAM, FANCM, MLH1, MRE11A, MSH2, MSH6, NBN, NF1, PALB2, PMS2, PTEN, RAD50, RAD51C, RAD51D, RECQL, SMARCA4, STK11, TP53 XRCC2 (28 genes)	Blueprint Genetics	Identification of the variants that could potentially explain the patient's phenotype, guided patient management and family member risk stratification.
Gastrointestinal cancer	ColoNext ®	APC, AXIN2, BMPR1A, CDH1, EPCAM, GREM1, MBD4, MLH1, MSH2, MSH3, MSH6, MUTYH, NTHL1, PMS2, POLD1, POLE, PTEN, SMAD4, STK11, TP53	Ambry Genetics	Inherited risk for colorectal cancer, gastric cancer, &/or polyposis based on personal &/or family history; informs prophylactic and management decisions.
Prostate Cancer	Prostate Cancer Panel	ATM, BRCA1, BRCA2, BRIP1, CHEK2, EPCAM, HOXB13, MLH1, MSH2, MSH6, NBN, PALB2, PMS2, RAD51C, RAD51D, TP53	Prevention Genetics	Evaluates genetic risk factors for aggressive prostate cancer; informs personalized management.
Pancreatic Cancer	Invitae Hereditary Pancreatic Cancer Panel	APC, ATM, BRCA1, BRCA2, CDKN2A, EPCAM, MEN1, MLH1, MSH2, MSH6, NF1, PALB2, PMS2, STK11, TP53, TSC1, TSC2, VHL	Labcorp and Invitae	Predisposition to adult-onset pancreatic cancer; supports risk assessment and surveillance.
Melanoma	Melanoma Comprehensive Panel	BAP1, BRCA2, CDK4, CDKN2A, CHEK2, MITF, MUTYH, POT1, PTEN, RB1, SLC45A2, TERT, TP53, TYR	Fulgent Genetics	Assesses genetic predisposition to melanoma; aids early detection and prevention strategies.
Colorectal Cancer, Endometrial Cancer, Lynch Syndrome, Ovarian Cancer, Pancreatic Cancer, Paraganglioma, Pheochromocytoma, Renal Cancer, Attenuated Familial Adenomatous Polyposis (AFAP), Thyroid Cancer, Brain Cancer, Breast Cancer	OncoGeneDx Custom Panel	Combination of gene can be selected from a list of 91 genes	GeneDx	Identify the genetic basis of cancer for individuals who have features and/or a family history consistent with one of the hereditary cancer syndromes; Determine appropriate clinical management recommendations based on a molecular diagnosis Identify family members at-risk.
Hereditary Diffuse Gastric Cancer (HDGC)	CDH1 specific site analysis	CDH1	Ambry Genetics	Detects mutations that increase the risk of diffuse gastric cancer; informs consideration of prophylactic surgery, such as gastrectomy, or other risk-reducing measures, as appropriate and Identify at-risk family members

accumulated such somatic changes, and therefore, analysis to identify these mutation subsets is important clinically. The prior technologies, mostly involving Sanger sequencing, PCR hybridization, and cytogenetics, had the limitation of targeting only a limited number of such mutations in a subset of genes that were associated with cancer initiation or progression as oncogenes or tumor suppressors. The emphasis was and is still given to specific mutations that are targetable therapeutically. However, advances in sequencing technologies have vastly increased this landscape, and recent data have seen an explosion in the number of such somatic mutations, expanding the spectrum significantly. There are several test panels and commercial kits that have now come into existence, which has been discussed in detail throughout this book previously and is summarized in Table 11.2.

The early attempts to identify the whole spectrum of aberrations in the protein-coding sequences in colon, breast, and glioblastoma were done by Sanger sequencing and required vast amounts of sequencing (Sjoblom et al., 2006; Parsons et al., 2008). Still these pioneering work provided several novel markers associated with cellular metabolism and DNA modification that formed the basis of similar work.

11.4 GENETIC TESTING AS A TOOL FOR TARGETED THERAPY

The most significant and clinically lucrative application of genetic testing is in revolutionizing the aspects of prevention, therapeutic potential in targeted therapy, as well as the ability to monitor and treat progress. Prevention is achieved by testing for genetic markers that are associated with cancer in healthy individuals or family members, which can provide them with facts in order to make informed decisions to manage the disease by taking preventive strategies in lifestyle. The ever-increasing knowledge of genetic mutations has not only propelled predictive testing but also provided knowledge of genetic predisposition to cancer. This knowledge can help design personalized risk management strategies. Unlike traditional methods these tests can be performed before disease onset or during early stages of disease in high-risk individuals. As summarized in Table 11.1 and Table 11.2 as well as discussed throughout the book, several of the genetic tests available have potential treatment and preventive potential.

Targeted therapy is in use in mostly breast, colorectal, lung, and pancreatic cancers and in hematological malignancies. The common therapeutic agents are monoclonal antibodies and small molecule inhibitors that target several carcinogenic processes such as growth factors, apoptotic pathways, cell signalling, and cell cycle proteins.

11.4.1 Monoclonal Antibody for Targeted Therapy

The first Food and Drug Administration (FDA) approved monoclonal antibody (Mab) for cancer therapy targeted Epidermal Growth Factor Receptor (EGFR) antagonists and Human Epidermal Growth Factor Receptor 2 (HER2) (Sliwkowski & Mellman, 2013). The anti-cancer effect of these antibodies could be by binding to receptors, preventing oncogenesis, or by targeting the cancerous cells with linked toxins or therapeutic agents. They could also activate the immune system to target cancer cells by blocking cytotoxic T lymphocyte antigen (CTLA-4), e.g., Ipilimumab in melanoma, Programmed cell death receptor (PD-1) e.g., Pembrolizumab and Durvaluman in Non-Small Cell Lung Cell carcinoma (NSCLC) or chimeric antigen receptor CT-cells (CAR-T) (Yang, 2015). Other examples of therapeutic monoclonal antibodies include CD19 and CD20 targeting Blinatumomab, Ibritumomab tiuxetan against leukemia and lymphoma, CD30 targeting Brentuximan vedotin in multiple lymphomas, Vascular Endothelial Growth Factor Receptor 2 (VEGFR2) targeting Ramucirumab in hepatocellular Cancinoma (HCC), Vascular Endothelial Growth Factor A (VEGF-A) targeting Bevacizumab in colorectal, breast, NSCLC etc. are few examples that have been discussed extensively previously (Orzetti et al., 2022). These therapeutic drugs have to be administered intravenously as they may be denatured in the GI tract when taken orally. As a passive immunization strategy these therapeutic molecules require frequent or continuous boosters mainly due to short *in vivo* half-life. The cost of these treatments are also quite high.

11.4.2 Small Molecule Inhibitors for Targeted Therapy

Small molecules refer to less than 900 Dalton molecular weight compounds that can penetrate and block the targets mostly components of signalling pathway contributing to carcinogenesis as Cyclin-dependent kinases (CDKs) (e.g., Ribociclib, Palbociclib and Abemaciclib in metastatic breast cancers) and poly (ADP-ribose) polymerases (PARPs) (e.g., Rucaparib, Olaparib, Niraparib in ovarian and peritoneal cancers) and proteasomes (e.g., Carfilzomib, Bortezomib and Ixazomib in Multiple Myeloma). Other targets include EGFR specific Afatinib, Erlotinib, Gefitinib for NSCLS,

Table 11.2: Genetic Testing for Somatic Variations

Cancer Type	Test/Panel Name	Markers/Genes/Assay	Company	Clinical Utility
Non-Small Cell Lung Cancer (NSCLC)	cobas® EGFR Mutation Test v2	EGFR mutations (e.g., Exon 19 deletions, L858R and T790M)	Roche Diagnostics	Identifies EGFR mutations to guide targeted therapy with EGFR inhibitors (e.g., osimertinib).
Solid Tumors, Non-Small Cell Lung Cancer (NSCLC), Melanoma, Colorectal Cancer, Breast Cancer, Ovarian Cancer, Cholangiocarcinoma, Prostate Cancer	FoundationOne CDx	More than 300 genes	Foundation Medicine	Broad genomic profiling to detect actionable alterations for personalized treatment strategies.
Acute myeloid leukemia (AML) and myelodysplastic syndrome (MDS)	Abbott RealTime IDH1	IDH1	Abbott	Identifies patients with an isocitrate dehydrogenase-1 (IDH1) mutation for treatment with TIBSOVO® (ivosidenib) or in identifying AML patients for treatment with REZLIDHIATM (olutasidenib).
Acute myeloid leukemia (AML)	Abbott RealTime IDH2	IDH2	Abbott	Testing acute myeloid leukemia (AML) patients with an isocitrate dehydrogenase-2 (IDH2) mutation for treatment with IDHIFA® (enasidenib).
Synovial sarcoma	MAGE-A4 IHC 1F9 pharmDx	Melanoma-associated antigen 4 (MAGE-A4)	Agilent (Dako)	Evaluates patients with synovial sarcoma for treatment with TECELRA®.
Non-small cell lung cancer (NSCLC)	PD-L1 IHC 22C3 pharmDx	PD-L1 protein expression	Agilent (Dako)	Evaluates PD-L1 status to determine eligibility for treatment with KEYTRUDA® (pembrolizumab), an immune checkpoint inhibitor.
Melanoma	cobas 4800 BRAF V600 Mutation Test	BRAF V600 mutations	Roche Diagnostics	Guides the use of BRAF inhibitors (e.g., vemurafenib, dabrafenib) in melanoma patients.
Colorectal Cancer	Cobas KRAS Mutation Test	KRAS mutations	Roche Diagnostics	Determines KRAS status to predict response to anti-EGFR monoclonal antibodies.
Colorectal/Multiple Tumors	MSI Analysis System v1.2	Microsatellite instability (MSI) markers	Promega	Detects MSI-high status, aiding in immunotherapy decisions across various tumor types.
Ovarian Cancer	Myriad myChoice CDx	BRCA1/2 mutations and Homologous Recombination Deficiency (HRD) score	Myriad Genetics	Homologous recombination deficiency (HRD) test to select ovarian cancer patients who may benefit from PARP inhibitors.
Non-Small Cell Lung Cancer (NSCLC)	Vysis ALK Break Apart FISH Probe Kit	ALK gene rearrangements	Abbott	Detects ALK rearrangements to guide treatment with ALK inhibitors.

BCR-ABL specific Nilotinib, Ponatinib and Dasatnib in Chronic Myeloid leukemia (CML) VEGFR specific Nintedanib in NSCLC etc. These molecules can be administrated orally and are more cost effective than the monoclonal antibody strategies. Their low specificity towards target and the drug-drug interaction is major disadvantage in comparison to the antibodies used for therapy. They also might require a daily dose due to extremely low *in vivo* half-life of just few hours.

The primary goal in this therapeutic strategy is to prevent the collateral damage caused by common chemo-therapeutic and radio-therapeutic methods. This targeted therapy has been made possible mainly due to the advancement in genetic testing and identification of more and more biomarkers. Once identified these targets have added advantage of determining optimal doses, therapeutic efficacy and follow ups. These therapeutic strategies promote the overall and disease free survival and can be used either by themselves or by using in combination with other treatment regimens. Although the classical methods of cancer therapy is still not wholly replaceable, the biomarker identification in coherence with the genetic testing strategies can give clinicians an enhanced therapeutic strategy by combining the existing strategy with these targeted approaches for reduced toxicity.

11.5 CHALLENGES AND LIMITATIONS IN INTEGRATION OF GENETIC TESTING TO CLINICAL PRACTICE

With cancer incidence occurring more and more in low income countries pose a big challenge to bring the high cost molecular diagnostics to general clinician's table. The public in these developing countries where the rates of cancer both in terms of morbidity and mortality rates are much higher would not be able to afford the expensive diagnostic tools especially if it does not provide sufficient advantages that the high cost can justify. The support of large-scale programs like the World Health Organization (WHO)'s global program to prevent Cervical cancer in the early part of this decade with Vaccinations, Screening and treatment support can give an added impetus to the implantation fot the more expensive genetic testing strategies into public usage. The emphasis however if we want to bring these tests accessible to general public is to develop the technologies that are cheaper and be able to have added advantage in providing treatment paths. Another advantage would be to have tests that can either be capable of prognoses or detection right before the onset that can be used as a screening tool especially in more prevalent populations.

11.6 OVERCOMING CHALLENGES IN IMPLEMENTING GENETIC TESTING IN CLINICS

A healthy collaboration between clinicians of various fields with the scientific community as well as genetic councillors would be the first major step in implementation in clinics. The development of an Artificial Intelligence (AI)-based system of integration of these steps for a more practical access to the clinician regarding the molecular interpretations and the options available at the fingertips of the clinician can make the tests more useful. This will give the clinician more confidence in prescribing the tests. The result, interpretation, and actionable data requires exploration of multiple databases and literature which can be automated with available AI tools and algorithms. The integration will help to make the clinicians and the general public aware of the actual advantage of the benefits of genetic testing over the conventional even advanced methods that will have to go hand in hand with the molecular testing strategies.

The studies involving the perceptions of clinical oncologists and geneticists have indicated that in order to bring the genetic tests to general clinical usage the most important parameters were to have the genetic results in therapeutic decisions and to have the ability to order tests directly by having sufficient and clear information and rapid testing panels (Korngiebel, 2019). This emphasizes an urgent need to have geneticists and genetic counsellors actively training and adopting practice guidelines hand in hand with clinicians.

Although the use of information tools to streamline the integration of basic and clinical fields would be a practical solution to the implementation of these diagnostic tools into clinics, the real advantage of these genetic tools in early prognosis and diagnosis as well as in providing personalized targeting options will be the key aspects that drive the popularity of genetic tests. These personalized strategies will improve the therapeutic efficacy by minimising the side effects of traditional therapy. Therefore, although the last few decades have seen a lot of advances to the classic diagnostic techniques that have existed for generations to improve the diagnostic potential, more novel approaches including the genetic tests developed will be the way forward in the future. The molecular diagnosis techniques discussed in this chapter in combination with environmental and lifestyle choices can provide the ideal effective management of cancer diagnosis that forms the backbone of the upcoming field of precision medicine as a variation of personalized medicine

(Hood et al., 2012). One of the most important tools in promoting and popularizing precision medicine are the molecular diagnosis testing including genetic testing. Several multi genetic panels that are now being made available that include Mammaprint™ for 70 breast cancer gene signatures and Oncotype Dx for different types of panels have made assessment of cancer and its relapse potential that makes cancer management possible (Slodkowska & Ross, 2009; Carlson & Roth, 2013). Similar advances are seen by use of next generation sequencing in aberrant expression of long coding RNAs (lncRNAs) in different cancer types as an analysis tool for diagnosis (Huarte, 2015). One of the best preliminary example of application of the technology was seen in a pilot study of clinical oncology where within a month of collection of an advanced stage cancer sample and by making use of a series of high-throughput sequencing data analysis oncologists were able to generate a cancer mutational landscape which could be used for biomarker driven clinical trials (Roychowdhury et al., 2011). In conclusion, the future of cancer diagnosis is in the field of precision medicine which will focus on delivering correct and effective treatment based on molecular tools that will accelerate and improve the management of the disease.

REFERENCES

Ahmad E et al. (2022). Molecular markers in cancer. *Clin Chim Acta 532*:95–114.

Carlson JJ, Roth JA. (2013). The impact of the Oncotype Dx breast cancer assay in clinical practice: a systematic review and meta-analysis. *Breast Cancer Res Treat 141*:13–22.

Chhabra VA et al. (2018). Synthesis and spectroscopic studies of functionalized graphene quantum dots with diverse fluorescence characteristics. *RSC Adv 8*(21):11446–11454.

Frangioni JV (2008). New technologies for human cancer imaging. *J Clin Oncol 26*(24):4012–4021.

Garutti M et al. (2023). Hereditary cancer syndromes: a comprehensive review with a visual tool. *Genes 14*(5):1025.

Goyal RK, et al. (1996). Hodgkin disease after renal transplantation in childhood. *J Pediatr Hematol Oncol 18*(4):392–395.

Gulley ML et al. (2010). Genetic tests to evaluate prognosis and predict therapeutic response in acute myeloid leukemia. *J Molec Diagnost 12*(1):3–16.

Haris M et al. (2015). Molecular magnetic resonance imaging in cancer. *J Translat Med 13*:1–16.

Hood L et al. (2012). Revolutionizing medicine in the 21st century through systems approaches. *Biotechnol J 7*(8):992–1001.

Huarte M. (2015). The emerging role of lncRNAs in cancer. *Nature Med 21*(11):1253–1261.

Jia Z et al. (2019). Critical review of volatile organic compound analysis in breath and in vitro cell culture for detection of lung cancer. *Metabolites 9*(3):52.

Korngiebel DM et al. (2019). Practice implications of expanded genetic testing in oncology. *Cancer Investigat 37*(1):39–45.

Lopci E et al. (2010). Imaging with non-FDG PET tracers: outlook for current clinical applications. *Insights Imaging 1*:373–385.

Li M et al. (2022). Recent progress in biosensors for detection of tumor biomarkers. *Molecules 27*(21):7327.

Orzetti S et al. (2022). Genetic therapy and molecular targeted therapy in oncology: safety, pharmacovigilance, and perspectives for research and clinical practice. *Int J Molec Sci 23*(6):3012.

Parsons DW et al. (2008). An integrated genomic analysis of human glioblastoma multiforme. *Science 321*(5897):1807–1812.

Pleasance ED et al. (2010). A comprehensive catalogue of somatic mutations from a human cancer genome. *Nature 463*(7278):191–196.

Pulumati A et al. (2023). Technological advancements in cancer diagnostics: improvements and limitations. *Cancer Rep 6*(2):e1764.

Richards S et al. (2015). Standards and guidelines for the interpretation of sequence variants: a joint consensus recommendation of the American College of Medical Genetics and Genomics and the Association for Molecular Pathology. *Genet Med 17*(5):405–423.

Roychowdhury S et al. (2011). Personalized oncology through integrative high-throughput sequencing: a pilot study. *Science Translat Med 3*(111):111ra121.

Schröck E et al. (1996). Multicolor spectral karyotyping of human chromosomes. *Science 273*(5274):494–497.

Serratì S et al. (2016). Next-generation sequencing: advances and applications in cancer diagnosis. *OncoTargets Ther 9*:7355–7365.

Sjoblom T et al. (2006). The consensus coding sequences of human breast and colorectal cancers. *Science 314* (5797):268–274.

Sliwkowski MX, Mellman I (2013). Antibody therapeutics in cancer. *Science 341*(6151):1192–1198.

Slodkowska EA, Ross JS (2009). MammaPrint™ 70-gene signature: another milestone in personalized medical care for breast cancer patients. *Expert Rev Molec Diagnost 9*(5):417–422.

Soung YH, et al. (2017). Exosomes in cancer diagnostics. *Cancers 9*(1):8.

Speicher MR et al. (1996). Karyotyping human chromosomes by combinatorial multi-fluor FISH. *Nature Genet 12*(4):368–375.

Tanke HJ et al (1999). New strategy for multi-colour fluorescence in situ hybridisation: COBRA: COmbined Binary RAtio labelling. *Eur J Hum Genet 7*(1):2–11.

Verma A et al. (2016). Magnetic resonance spectroscopy—revisiting the biochemical and molecular milieu of brain tumors. *BBA Clin 5*:170–178.

Wang X et al. (2021). Dual-energy CT quantitative parameters for evaluating immunohistochemical biomarkers of invasive breast cancer. *Cancer Imaging 21*:1–10.

Watson IR et al. (2013). Emerging patterns of somatic mutations in cancer. *Nature Rev Genet 14*(10):703–718.

Yang Y (2015). Cancer immunotherapy: harnessing the immune system to battle cancer. *J Clin Investigat 125*(9):3335–3337.

Zhang Y et al. (2020). Controlled synthesis of Ag2Te@ Ag2S Core–Shell quantum dots with enhanced and tunable fluorescence in the second near-infrared window. *Small 16*(14):2001003.

Zhou Y et al. (2021). Pre-colectomy location and TNM staging of colon cancer by the computed tomography colonography: a diagnostic performance study. *World J Surg Oncol 19*:1–13.

Index

A

Absolute risk, 163
Activated oncogenes, 23
Adenomatous polyposis coli (APC) gene, 72
ADP ribosylation, 56
Adverse drug reactions (ADRs), 141
AFAP1-AS1, 88
Alfa fetoprotein (AFP), 87
ALK TKI therapy, 6
Androgen deprivation therapy (ADT), 148
Aneuploidy (numerical abnormalities), 113
Angiogenesis, 52, 54
    CSCs, 32
Apoptosis, 31
Array comparative genomic hybridization (aCGH), 119
Artificial intelligence (AI)
    algorithms, 59
    -based tools, 98, 223
    in genetic data interpretation, 151
Ataxia-telangiectasia (A-T), 76

B

Band-specific karyotyping, 114
BCR-ABL fusion gene, 23
Beckwith-Wiedemann syndrome (BWS), 179
Biofluid-based cancer detection
    blood test, 96–97
    cerebrospinal fluid based detection, 96
    liquid biopsy, 94
    optic methods, 94
    radiology, 94
    saliva test, 97
    stool test, 96
    sweat analysis, 97
    tear analysis, 97
    tissue biopsy, 94
    urine test, 95
Biological carcinogens, 58
Biotinylation, 56
Blocker displacement amplification (BDA), 99
Blood test, 96–97
BRAF therapy targeting
    colorectal cancer (CRC)
        EGFR therapy, 35
        FOLFOXIRI plus panitumumab, 35
        vemurafenib monotherapy, 35
        VOLFI trial, 35
    Dabrafenib, 34
    MEK/ERK signaling, 33
    for metastatic melanoma, 34
    V600E mutation, 33
    Vemurafenib, 34
BRCA1 and BRCA2 mutations, 113, 127

Breast cancer
    BRCA1 and BRCA2 hereditary breast and ovarian
        cancer syndrome, 88, 195
        autosomal dominance inheritance pattern,
            70, 71
        basic genetics, 69
        diagnostic approach, 69–70
        diagnostic challenges, 70–71
    genetic counseling in India, *see* India, genetic
        counseling in

C

Camera-based SPECT systems, 93
Cancer aetiology distribution, 67
Cancer biomarkers, 59, 97, 216–217
    analysis, 217
    carbohydrates, 89–90
    epigenetics, 90
    exosomes, 90
    flow cytometry for, 216–217
    genetic biomarkers, 88–89
    immune checkpoint, 90
    in vivo and *in vitro*, 87
    proteins, 87–88
    types and detections, 87–89
Cancer cytogenetics
    aneuploidy (numerical abnormalities), 113
    cancer-linked chromosomal anomalies, 112
    chromosomal instability, 113
    epigenetic dysregulation, 113
    gene mutations, 113
    histone modifications, 113
    monosomy, 113
    Philadelphia chromosome, 112
    polyploidy, 113
    structural alterations, 112–113
    testing methodologies, 112; *see also* Cytogenetics
        diagnostic testing
Cancer detection, molecular diagnostic techniques,
        58
    biofluid-based cancer detection, *see* Biofluid-based
        cancer detection
    biomarkers, *see* Cancer biomarkers
    challenges/limitations, 102–103
    CRISPR-based diagnostics, 101–102
    emerging molecular assays, 58
    FISH, 99, 217
    flow cytometry, 100–101, 216–217
    future aspects, 103
    histopathology-based detection, 97–98
    imaging techniques, *see* Imaging techniques,
        cancer detection
    immunohistochemistry and microarray based
        diagnosis, 217–218
    incidence rate of cancer, 86

liquid biopsy technologies, 58, 217
mortality rates of cancer, 86–87
polymerase chain reaction (PCR), 98–100
Sanger sequencing, 99–100
synthetic biosensors and biomarker analysis, 217
VOC analysis, 217
Cancer diagnosis
    advantages, 215
    early diagnosis, 215
    genetic testing
        challenges and limitations in, 223
        for hereditory cancers, 218–220
        implementation challenges, 223–224
        for somatic variation diagnosis, 219, 221, 222
        as tool for targeted therapy, 221, 223
    imaging techniques, 215, 216
    limitations in existing, 218
    molecular diagnostic advances, 216–218
Cancer genetics
    definition, 46
    DNA, see DNA
    drug resistance, 47
    early detection and prevention, 46
    epigenetic changes, 46
    future directions in cancer research, 61
    personalized medicine, 46
    prognosis and risk stratification, 46
    proto-oncogenes, see Proto-oncogenes
    tumor suppressor genes, see Tumor suppressor
        genes
    understanding cancer biology, 47
Cancer genetic testing; see also individual entries
    accuracy, 150
    advantages, 14–15
    bibliometric analysis, 1
    clinical application-based genetic testing
        pharmacogenomic testing, 10
        predictive testing, 7, 8
        prognostic testing, 7, 9, 10
    comprehension and understanding, 192
    cost of, 150
    coverage of, 150
    decision-making process, 195, 196
    disadvantages, 15
    ethical implications, 197–198
    future roadmap, 15–16
    genetic basis, 2–3
        germline and somatic mutations, 4–6
        mutation spectrum, 3–4
    genetic etiology, 4
    hereditary cancer syndromes, see Hereditary
        cancer syndromes
    hereditary genetic testing, 1
    legal implications, 198–200
    low- and middle-income countries (LMICs), 191
    multifaceted role of, 1, 2
    obstacles and constraints, 204–205
    potential factors contributing to errors, 202–203
    risk communication, 196–197
    social implications, 200–201
    source-based genetic testing, 6–7

technologies in personalized cancer therapy, 11
    comprehensive methods, 10
    FISH, 12–13
    NGS, 2, 13–14
    PCR, 12
    Sanger sequencing, 13
    targeted testing, 10
unintended consequences
    inadequate genetic counseling, 202
    results misinterpreted, 202
    wrong testing ordered, 201–202
Cancer genome landscapes, 4
Cancer immunoediting, 52
Cancer personalized profiling by deep sequencing
    (CAPP-Seq), 117
Cancer stem cells (CSCs), 32
Cancer therapy
    cancer genetic testing technologies in, 11
        comprehensive methods, 10
        FISH, 12–13
        NGS, 2, 13–14
        PCR-based technologies, 12
        Sanger sequencing, 13
        targeted testing, 10
    emerging therapies, 61
    traditional therapies
        chemotherapy, 60
        radiation therapy, 59–60
        surgery, 60
Carbohydrate antigen (CA125), 89–90
Carcinoembryonic antigen (CEA), 96
Caretaker genes, 51
CAR-T cell therapy, 147
Cascade genetic testing, 5
Cell cycle dysregulation, 29
Cell cycle regulators
    CDKs, 27–29
    P53 protein, 28
    pRB pathway, 27–28
    unchecked progression, 29
Cell-free DNA (cf-DNA), 89
Cellular immortality, 31–32
Cerebrospinal fluid (CSF) based detection, 96
Chemical carcinogens, 58
Chemotherapy, 59, 125
CHRDL2 proteins, 88
Chromoanagenesis, 50
Chromoanasynthesis, 50
Chromoplexy, 50
Chromosomal rearrangements, 49
Chromosomal reordering, 23
Chromosomal translocations, 23, 50
Chromothripsis, 50
Circular RNAs (circRNAs), 56
Circulating tumor cells (CTCs), 94, 101
Circulating tumor DNA (ctDNA), 58, 89, 96, 101, 125,
    132
Circulating tumor nucleic acids (ctNAs), 94
CiRS-7 RNA, 89
Clustered regularly interspaced short palindromic
    repeats (CRISPR) based diagnostics, 101

Colorectal cancer (CRC), 194–195
  BRAF therapy targeting, 33–34
Community-based participatory research (CBPR)
    initiatives, 61
Comparative genomic hybridization (CGH), 114–115,
    130
Competitive endogenous RNAs (ceRNAs), 57
Complete blood count (CBC) test, 96
Comprehensive genome profiling (CGP), 124, 125, 128
Computed tomography (CT-Scan), 92–93
Computer-aided detection (CADe) tools, 98
Computer-aided diagnostic (CADx) tools, 98
Conflicts of interest (COI), 185
Conventional cytogenetics, 114
Convolutional neural networks (CNNs), 98
Copy number variations (CNVs), 50, 127, 130
Cowden syndrome (CS), 75–76, 194
CT-colonography (CTC), 92–93
Cultural implications, genetic counseling, 181–182
Cyclin-dependent kinases (CDKs), 27–29
CYP2D6 deficiency, 138
Cytogenetics diagnostic testing (CDT)
  challenges and future directions, 118–119
  clinical implications, 117–118
  conventional cytogenetics, 114
  molecular cytogenetics, 114–116
  sequencing techniques, 116–117

D

DEAD-box RNA helicase protein (DDX21), 36
Direct-to-consumer (DTC) genetic testing, 200–201,
    203, 205
DNA
  functions, 47–48
  genetic mutations and types
    chromoanagenesis, 50
    chromosomal rearrangements, 49
    copy number variations (CNVs), 50
    frame shift mutation, 49
    gene amplifications, 49
    germline mutations, 49
    non-coding indels, 49
    nonstop extension mutations, 50
    point mutations, 48
    somatic mutations, 49
  methylation, 24–25, 54–55, 113
  mismatch repair (MMR) genes, 68
  mutations, 126–127
  repair genes, 46
  structure, 47, 48
DNA methyltransferases (DNMTs), 24, 90
Drug-metabolizing enzyme and transporters,
    140–141

E

Economic implications, 202–203
Empiric risk, 163
Endoscopy-based cancer detection, 94
Endothelial cells, 52

Environmental factors, in cancer development
  biological carcinogens, 58
  chemical factors, 58
  modifiable and non-modifiable factors, 57
  physical factors, 57, 58
Epidermal growth factor receptor (EGFR) functions,
    101
Epigenetic dysregulation, cancer cytogenetics, 113
Epigenetic modifications/alterations, 46, 90
  of chromatin structure, 24, 25
  definition, 24
  DNA methylation, 24–25, 54–55
  histone modification, 25–26, 55–56
  ncRNAs, 26, 56–57
Epigenetics
  as biomarkers, 90
  changes, see Epigenetic modifications/alterations
  definition, 54
Epithelial-mesenchymal transition (EMT), 32, 53–54
Ethical implications
  genetic counseling, 184–185
  genetic testing of children and embryos, 197–198
  psychological and emotional impact, 198
Exosomal CD63, 90
Exosomes, 94
Extracellular matrix (ECM), 52

F

Familial adenomatous polyposis (FAP)
  APC gene, germline mutations in, 75
  attenuated FAP (AFAP), 73
  autosomal recessive inheritance patterns, 72
  basic genetics, 74
  diagnostic approach, 74–75
  diagnostic challenges, 73–74
  hereditary colorectal cancer syndrome, 72
FCGR1A expression, 101
Flow cytometry, 100–101
Fluorescence in situ hybridization (FISH), 12–13, 99,
    115–116, 217
FNIII14. β1-integrin inactivation, 36
Frame shift mutation, 49

G

GALEN algorithm, 98
Gatekeeper genes, 51
Gene amplifications, 23–24, 49, 51
Genetic counseling, 149, 191
  cultural implications, 180–181
  definition, 156
  documentation across phases, 169
  ethical implications, 184–185
  future scope and challenges, 185–186
  hereditary cancer syndromes, 156
  in India, see India, genetic counseling in
  mental health challenges, 182–184
  multifactorial inheritance process, 156
  post-genetic counseling, see Post-genetic
      counseling

post-test counseling, 157
pre-test counseling, *see* Pre-test counseling
responsibilities and roles of counselors, 158
role and importance of, 158
social implications, 180–181
stepwise protocol, 157
test phase
    sample collection and laboratory selection, 164–165
    test selection, 165
Genetic factors in drug metabolism, 142
    1950s–1960s, 138
Genetic profiling
    to guide treatment decisions, 149
    and targeted therapies, 146
Genetic screening, 152–153
Genome sequencing, 10
Genomic instability, 29–30
Genomic profiling
    amalgamation, 125
    as biomarker, 124
    challenges and limitations, 132
    comprehensive, 124, 125, 128
    evolution of cancer treatment, 125
    future perspectives, 133
    general mechanism, 127, 128
    genomics basics and cancer biology, 126–127
    importance and relevance of, 125–126
    techniques, 131
        CGH, 130
        NGS, 128–129
        RNA-seq, 130
        WES, 129–130
        WGS, 129
    treatment outcome benefits and impact, 132
Germline mutations, 4–6, 49, 126
    APC gene, 73
    BRCA1/BRCA2, 69
    lynch syndrome, 68
    PTEN gene, 75
    STK11 (LKB1) gene, 75
    VHL gene, 78
Glucose-6-phosphate dehydrogenase (G6PD) deficiency, 138
Glypican-1 (GPC-1), 90
GREM1 proteins, 88

H

Health Insurance Portability and Accountability Act (HIPAA), 185
Heat shock proteins, 87
Hereditary breast and ovarian cancer (HBOC), 156
Hereditary cancer syndromes
    ataxia-telangiectasia (A-T), 76
    BRCA1 and BRCA2 hereditary breast and ovarian cancer syndrome, 69–71, 195
    challenges to diagnostics, 79
    colorectal cancer, 194–195
    Cowden syndrome (CS), 75–76, 194
    diagnostic criteria limitations, 79–80
    familial adenomatous polyposis (FAP), 72–73

future perspectives, 80
gene involved, mode of inheritance and associated cancer risks, 68
hereditary melanoma, 194
identification, 1, 191
Li-Fraumeni Syndrome (LFS), 71–72, 194
lynch syndrome (HNPCC), 67–69, 194
multiple endocrine neoplasia (MEN), 192–193
MutYH-associated polyposis (MAP), 78–79
Peutz-Jeghers syndrome (PJS), 74–75, 194
tuberous sclerosis complex (TSC), 76–77
von Hippel-Lindau (VHL) syndrome, 77–78, 194
Hereditary melanoma, 194
Hereditary non-polyposis colorectal cancer (HNPCC), 183, 194; *see also* Lynch syndrome
Histone acetylation, 25, 55
Histone demethylation transferases, 26
Histone methylation, 25–26, 56
Histone modification
    acetylation, 25, 55
    ADP ribosylation, 56
    biotinylation, 56
    cancer cytogenetics, 113
    methylation, 25–26, 55
    phosphorylation, 56
    sites and functional implications, 54
    sumoylation, 56
    ubiquitination, 56
Histopathology-based cancer detection, 97
Hormonal therapy, 148
Human chorionic gonadotropin (hCG), 87
Human epidermal growth factor receptor 2 (HER2), 24, 38, 87–88
Hybridization based molecular diagnostic methods, 218

I

Imaging techniques, cancer detection, 58
    CT-Scan, 92–93, 216
    endoscopy-based cancer detection, 94
    FDG-PET, 91
    MRI, 93, 216
    MRS, 216
    PET scan, 91, 93–94, 216
    types, 90–91
    ultrasound, 94
    X-ray, 91–92, 216
Imatinib mesylate (IMAT), 37
Immune cells, 52
Immune checkpoint inhibitors, 147
Immunohistochemistry, 217–218
Immunotherapy, 54, 125, 146, 147
    in melanoma and other cancers, 148–149
India, genetic counseling in
    breast cancer
        anatomy, 171–172
        medullary (brain-like), 172
        peau d'orange, 172
        risk factors and assessment, 172
        scirrhous (woody), 172

subgroups, 172
   terminal duct lobular unit (TDLU), 172
   triple assessment, 173–175
current scenario, 171
future prospects, 171
genetic disorders, 170
leukemia
   acute lymphoid leukemia (ALL), 178
   Beckwith-Wiedemann syndrome (BWS), 178–179
   case scenario, 179–180
   challenge, 180
   childhood leukemia, 178
policy development, 171
small cell lung carcinoma
   anatomy, 176
   case scenario, 176–177
   classification, 176
   discussion, 177
   follow-up, 177
   symptoms, 176
Inherited cancer syndromes, *see* Hereditary cancer syndromes

K

Karyotyping, 114, 119
KRAS gene, 88

L

Lactate dehydrogenase (LDH), 87
Landscape genes, 51
Lapatinib, 37
Legal implications
   genetic discrimination, 198–199
   intellectual property and commercialization, 199–200
Leptomeningeal metastases (LM), 100
Leukemia
   acute lymphoid leukemia (ALL), 178
   Beckwith-Wiedemann syndrome (BWS), 179
   case scenario, 179–180
   challenge, 180
   childhood leukemia, 178
Li-Fraumeni syndrome (LFS), 4–5, 194
   autosomal dominant inheritance pattern, 4
   basic genetics, 71
   diagnostic approach, 71–72
   TP53 gene, 4, 71
LINC00665, 37
Liquid biopsy, 58, 96, 217
Long non-coding RNAs (lncRNAs), 26, 56, 57, 130
Lung cancer, 86
   personalized medicine in, 148
   small cell lung carcinoma, 176–177
   VOC analysis, 217
   X-ray, 91–92
Lynch syndrome
   basic genetics, 68
   diagnostic approach, 69
   DNA-MMR genes mutations, 67
   microsatellite instability (MSI), 68

M

Machine learning, in cancer therapy, 61
Macrophage targeting, cancer therapy, 60
Magnetic resonance imaging (MRI), 93, 216
Magnetic resonance spectroscopy (MRS), 216
Medullary thyroid carcinoma (MTC), 192–193
Metabolic reprogramming, 30
Metastatic non-small cell lung cancer (mNSCLC), 132
Microarray based diagnosis, 217–218
Microfluidic devices, 59
MicroRNA (miRNA), 26, 130
   and regulatory functions, 57
Microsatellite instability (MSI), 26, 68
miR-1224, 37
Mismatch repair (MMR) genes
   lynch syndrome, 68
Mismatch repair (MMR) mechanism, 26
Missense mutations, 49
Mitogen-activated protein kinase (MAPK), 24
Molecular cytogenetics, 114–116
Molecular tumor boards (MTBs), 2
Monoclonal antibodies, 147
Monosomy, 113
Multi-cancer early detection (MCED) tests, 58
Multigene panel testing, 165
Multi-omics approaches, 151–152
Multiple endocrine neoplasia (MEN), 192–193
Mutational signatures, 10
Mutation spectrum, 3–4
MutYH-associated polyposis (MAP), 78–79
MYC proto-oncogene, 23

N

N-acetyltransferase, 138
Neuroblastoma (NB)
   N-myc amplification in, 36–37
Next-generation sequencing (NGS), 2, 10, 13–14, 100, 165
   CDT, 116–117, 119
   genomic profiling, 125–126, 128–129
   pharmacogenomics, 144
N-myc (MYCN) amplification in neuroblastoma, 36–37
Non-coding indels, 49
Non-coding ribonucleic acids (ncRNAs), 26, 56–57
Non sense Mutations, 48
Non-small cell lung cancer (NSCLC), 8, 91, 221, 222
   EGFR mutation, 7, 147, 148
   epigenetic alterations, 90
   HER-2 mutations, 87
Nonstop extension mutations, 50

O

Odds ratio (OR), 163
Oncogene activation, clinical implications
   as biomarkers, 33
   BRAF therapy targeting, *see* BRAF therapy targeting
   miR-1224, 37
   N-myc amplification in neuroblastoma, 36–37

oncogene mutations, 33
proto-oncogenes, 32
targeted therapies, 33
Trastuzumab (Herceptin) development and
efficacy, 37
tyrosine kinase blockers, 37–38
Oncogene mutations, 113
Oncogenes, in cancer development
apoptosis, 31
cancer stem cell invasion, metastasis, and
maintenance, 32
cell cycle dysregulation, 29
cell cycle regulation
overview of, 27
phases, 27
role of regulators, 27–29
uncontrolled cell proliferation, 26
cell proliferation and division, 127
cellular immortality, 31–32
genomic instability, 29–30
metabolic reprogramming, 30
TME modification and immune evasion, 30–31
Oncology genetic testing, *see* Cancer genetic testing
Optical biosensors, 58
Optic methods, cancer detection, 94

P

p53 gene, 27, 51, 88
Personalized medicine in oncology, 145
cancer vaccines, 151
challenges and limitations, 149–150
in drug dosing, 149
EGFR mutations in lung cancer, 148
genetic counseling and risk assessment, 149
genetic profiling, 149
immunotherapy in melanoma and other cancers,
148–149
improved patient outcomes, 148
key components, 146
multi-omics approaches, integration of, 151–152
personalized treatment approaches, 147–148
in preventative oncology, 152–153
targeted therapy in breast cancer, 148
traditional cancer treatment approaches,
limitations of, 146
vs. traditional oncology, 146–147
in treatment decisions, 149
Peutz-Jeghers syndrome (PJS), 74–75, 194
Pharmacodynamics
action mechanism, 142–143
cytotoxicity and apoptosis, 143
definition, 142
resistance mechanisms, 143
Pharmacogenomics
advances in cancer treatments, 144
artificial intelligence in genetic data
interpretation, 151
biomarkers, 140–141
in cancer treatment, 141
challenges and opportunities, 144–145
definition, 139

and drug response, 139, 140
historical context
expansion (1970s–present), 138–139
Fox, Arthur L. (1932), 138
Garrod, Archibald (1909), 138
genetic factors in drug metabolism
(1950s–1960s), 138
Vogel, Friedrich (1959), 138
in modern medicine, 139–140
personalized medicine, 144
pharmacodynamics, 142–143
pharmacokinetics, 142–144
toxicity management, 144
Pharmacogenomic testing, 10
Pharmacokinetics, 142
absorption, 143
blood-brain barrier penetration, 143
definition, 143
and dosing, 144
drug interactions and personalized medicine, 144
excretion, 144
metabolism, 144
Phosphorylation, 56
Physical carcinogens, 57, 59
Piwi-interacting RNAs (piRNAs), 26, 56
Plant-based therapies, 61
Plasma cholinesterase deficiency, 138
Point mutations, 24, 48, 51
Polymerase chain reaction (PCR), 12, 98
Polyploidy, 113
Positron emission tomography (PET) scan, 91, 93–94,
216
Post-genetic counseling
follow-ups and resources, 169
genetic test results, disclosure and explanation
of, 166
legal and social considerations, 169
psychosocial support and coping, 166–167
risk assessment and management, 167
pre-eclampsia, 168
pre-natal screening, 167
Precision oncology, 125, 133
Predictive testing, 7, 8
Pre-metastatic niche formation, 53
Pre-test counseling, 157
cancer history review and risk assessment
comprehensive clinical information, 159, 160
disease risk assessment tools, 159, 161
individuals qualify for cancer screening, 159
presymptomatic testing, 160, 162
susceptibility testing, 162–163
hereditary cancer syndrome risk assessment, 158
informed consent, 158
"non-directive counseling" technique, 159
patient education and informed consent, 163–164
personal and family medical history examination,
158
Prognostic testing, 7, 9, 10
Prostate cancer antigen3 (PCA3), 89
Prostate-specific antigen (PSA), 87, 96
Protein biomarkers, 87–88
Proto-oncogenes, 3, 32, 46

epigenetic changes, *see* Epigenetic modifications
genetic changes
    activated oncogenes, 23
    chromosomal translocations, 23, 50
    gene amplification, 23–24, 51
    point mutations, 24, 50
    microsatellite instability (MSI), 26
PTEN gene, 75

R

Radiation therapy, 59–60, 125
Radiology, cancer detection, 94
RAS proteins, 24
Receptor-targeted nano (RTNs), 36
Relative risk (RR), 162–163
Retinoblastoma protein, 51
RNA sequencing (RNA-seq), 130

S

S-adenosylhomocysteine (SAH), 26
S-adenosylmethionine (SAM), 25–26
Saliva test, 97
Sanger sequencing (SGS), 13, 99–100
Sequencing techniques, cancer cytogenetics, 116–117
Silent mutations, 48
Silicon nanowire biosensors, 59
Single-gene testing, 7, 165
Single-photon emission computed tomography (SPECT), 93
Small cell lung cancer (SCLC), 87, 90, 92, 175–177
Small interfering RNA (siRNA), 26
Small nucleolar RNAs (snoRNAs), 56
Small ubiquitin-like modifier (SUMO) proteins, 56
Social implications
    cultural and religious perspectives, 200
    direct-to-consumer (DTC) genetic testing, 200–201
    genetic counseling, 180–181
    social risks, 200–201
Somatic mutation, 4–5, 49, 126
    genetic profiling, 218
    NRAS and *BRAF*, 10
    testing, 5–6
Somatic variation diagnosis, 219, 221, 222
Sonography, *see* Ultrasound imaging/ ultrasonography
Source-based genetic testing, 6–7
Stool test, 96
Stromal cells, 52
Sumoylation, 55
Susceptibility testing, 162–163
Sweat analysis, 97
Synthetic biosensors, 217

T

Targeted nanocarriers, cancer therapy, 61
Targeted therapies
    in breast cancer, 148

CAR-T cell therapy, 147
    in estrogen receptor (ER) blockade, 148
    genetic profiling and, 146
    hormonal therapy, 148
    Imatinib (Gleevec), 147
    immune checkpoint inhibitors, 147
    immunotherapy, 147
    mechanisms of, 147
    monoclonal antibody for, 221
    oncogene activation, 33
    prostate cancer and androgen deprivation therapy, 148
    small molecule inhibitors for, 221, 223
    Trastuzumab, 147, 148
Tear analysis, 97
Ten-eleven translocation (TET) enzymes, 24
Tissue biopsy, 87, 94
TP53 gene, 71–72, 113, 127, 174, 194
Translocations, 127
Tuberous sclerosis complex (TSC), 76–77
Tumor-derived extracellular vesicles (exosomes), 94
Tumor genomic profiling (TGP), 126
Tumor microenvironment (TME), 46
    cancer cell proliferation, 53
    in cancer therapy, 54
    immune evasion, 54
    modification, 30–31
    and tumor cells interaction, 51–52
    tumor initiation, 52
Tumor mutational burden (TMB), 10
Tumor suppressor gene mutations, 113
Tumor suppressor genes (TSG), 3, 46, 127
    cell proliferation, differentiation, and cancer prevention, 51
    types, 51
Tumor-suppressor proteins, 27
Tyrosine kinase inhibitors (TKIs), 37–38, 147

U

Ubiquitination, 55
Ultrasound imaging/ultrasonography, 94
Urine test, 95–96

V

Variants of unknown significance (VUSs), 70, 132, 186, 204–205
Virtual colonoscopy (VC), *see* CT-colonography
Volatile organic compound (VOC) analysis, 217
von Hippel-Lindau (VHL) syndrome, 77–78, 194

W

Whole-exome sequencing (WES), 10, 129–130
Whole-genome sequencing (WGS), 10, 129

X

X-ray, 91–92
    computed tomography (CT), 216

For Product Safety Concerns and Information please contact our EU
representative GPSR@taylorandfrancis.com
Taylor & Francis Verlag GmbH, Kaufingerstraße 24, 80331 München, Germany

www.ingramcontent.com/pod-product-compliance
Lightning Source LLC
Chambersburg PA
CBHW061407210326
41598CB00035B/6130